T0231176

Asymptomatic Carotid Artery Stenosis

Asymptomatic Carotid Artery Stenosis

Risk Stratification and Management

Edited by

ISSAM D MOUSSA MD
Associate Professor of Clinical Medicine
Co-Director, Endovascular Services
Division of Cardiology
Center for Interventional and Vascular Therapy
Division of Cardiology, Department of Medicine
New York Presbyterian Hospital/Columbia University Medical Center
Columbia University College of Physicians and Surgeons
New York, NY, USA

TATJANA RUNDEK MD PHD
Assistant Professor of Neurology
Director, Non-Invasive Research Neurosonology Laboratory
Department of Neurology
Division of Stroke and Critical Care
Columbia University College of Physicians and Surgeons
New York, NY, USA

JP MOHR MD
Daniel Sciarra Professor of Clinical Neurology
Director, Doris and Stanley Tananbaum Stroke Center
Department of Neurology
Division of Stroke and Critical Care
Columbia University College of Physicians and Surgeons
New York, NY, USA

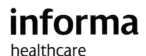

First published in 2007 by Informa Healthcare, Telephone House, 69-77 Paul Street, London EC2A 4LQ, UK.

Simultaneously published in the USA by Informa Healthcare, 52 Vanderbilt Avenue, 7th Floor, New York, NY 10017, USA.

Informa Healthcare is a trading division of Informa UK Ltd. Registered Office: 37–41 Mortimer Street, London W1T 3JH, UK. Registered in England and Wales number 1072954.

A CIP record for this book is available from the British Library.

Library of Congress Cataloging-in-Publication Data available on application

ISBN-13: 9781841846132

Orders may be sent to: Informa Healthcare, Sheepen Place, Colchester, Essex CO3 3LP, UK
Telephone: +44 (0)20 7017 5540
Email: CSDhealthcarebooks@informa.com
Website: http://informahealthcarebooks.com/

For corporate sales please contact: CorporateBooksIHC@informa.com
For foreign rights please contact: RightsIHC@informa.com
For reprint permissions please contact: PermissionsIHC@informa.com

Dedication

To my wife Mireille and little Andreas..for their love and support.

Issam D Moussa

To my mother and father

Tatjana Rundek

Contents

Contributors

Andrei V Alexandrov MD RVT
Director, Stroke Research and Neurosonology
Program
Barrow Neurological Institute
Phoenix, AZ, USA

Lee Birnbaum MD
Stroke Clinical Fellow
Department of Neurology
Division of Stroke and Critical Care
Columbia University College of Physicians and
Surgeons
New York, NY, USA

Kevin Crutchfield MD
Chief Medical Officer
New Health Sciences, Inc
Rockville, MD, USA

E Sander Connoly MD
Associate Professor of Neurological Surgery
Columbia University College of Physicians and
Surgeons
New York, NY, USA

Mitchell SV Elkind MD MS
Associate Professor of Neurology
Department of Neurology
Division of Stroke and Critical Care
Columbia University College of Physicians and
Surgeons
New York, NY, USA

Marie C Eugene DO
New York College of Osteopathic Medicine
Old Westbury, NY, USA

Jennifer A Frontera MD
Stroke Clinical Fellow
Department of Neurology
Division of Stroke and Critical Care
Columbia University College of Physicians and
Surgeons
New York, NY, USA

William A Gray MD
Associate Professor of Clinical Medicine
Director, Endovascular Services
Division of Cardiology
Center for Interventional and Vascular Therapy
New York Presbyterian Hospital/Columbia University
Medical Center
Columbia University, College of Physicians and
Surgeons
New York, NY, USA

Randall T Higashida MD
Clinical Professor of Radiology, Neurological Surgery,
Neurology, and Anesthesiology
University of California
San Francisco Medical Center
Division of Interventional Neurovascular Radiology
San Francisco, CA, USA

Michael R Jaff DO
Director, Vascular Medicine
Massachusetts General Hospital
Boston, MA, USA

Frank Kolodgie MD
Cardiovascular Pathology
Gaithersburg, MD, USA

Bernardo Liberato MD
Director, Neurovascular Service
Hospital Copa D'Or
Rio de Janeiro, Brazil

Randolph Marshall MD
Associate Professor of Clinical Neurology
Co-Director, Cerebral Localization Laboratory
Department of Neurology
Division of Stroke and Critical Care
Columbia University College of Physicians and
Surgeons
New York, NY, USA

Alessandro Mauriello MD
Associate Professor
Department of Pathology
University of Rome Tor Vergata
Rome, Italy

Philip M Meyers MD
Associate Professor, Radiology and Neurological
Surgery
College of Physicians and Surgeons, Columbia
University
Co-Director, Neuroendovascular Service
Neurological Institute and New York Presbyterian
Hospitals
Columbia, NY, USA

JP Mohr MD
Daniel Sciarra Professor of Clinical Neurology
Director, Doris and Stanley Tananbaum Stroke Center
Department of Neurology
Division of Stroke and Critical Care
Columbia University College of Physicians and
Surgeons
New York, NY, USA

Issam D Moussa MD
Associate Professor of Clinical Medicine
Co-Director, Endovascular Services
Division of Cardiology
Center for Interventional and Vascular Therapy
New York Presbyterian Hospital/Columbia University
Medical Center
Columbia University College of Physicians and
Surgeons
New York, NY, USA

Shyam Prabhakaran MD
Stroke Clinical Fellow
Department of Neurology
Division of Stroke and Critical Care
Columbia University College of Physicians and
Surgeons
New York, NY, USA

Tatjana Rundek MD PhD
Assistant Professor of Neurology
Director, Non-Invasive Research Neurosonology
Laboratory
Department of Neurology
Division of Stroke and Critical Care
Columbia University College of Physicians and
Surgeons
New York, NY, USA

Ralph L Sacco MS MD
Professor of Neurology and Epidemiology
Mailman School of Public Health
Gertrude Sergievsky Center
Director, Division of Stroke and Critical Care
Associate Chairman
Department of Neurology
Columbia University College of Physicians and
Surgeons
New York, NY, USA

Giuseppe Sangiorgi MD
Associate Director
Cardiac Catheterization Laboratory
Ospedale San Raffaele
Milan, Italy

H Christian Schumacher MD
Stroke Clinical Fellow
Department of Neurology
Division of Stroke and Critical Care
Columbia University College of Physicians and
Surgeons
New York, NY, USA

Luigi Giusto Spagnoli MD
Director, Department of Pathology
University of Rome Tor Vergata
Rome, Italy

Richard E Temes MD
Stroke Clinical Fellow
Department of Neurology
Division of Stroke and Critical Care
Columbia University College of Physicians and
Surgeons
New York, NY, USA

Santi Trimarchi MD
Associate Director
Department of Vascular Surgery
Policlinico San Donato
San Donato Milanese
Milan, Italy

Renu Virmani MD
Director, Cardiovascular Pathology
CV Path
Gaithersburg, MD, USA

Giuseppe Biondi Zoccai MD
Assistant Professor
Department of Cardiology
University of Turin
Turin, Italy

Foreword

ASYMPTOMATIC CAROTID ARTERY DISEASE: WHY ANOTHER BOOK?

Stroke is the third largest cause of death after heart diseases and cancer and is the leading cause of permanent disability and disability-adjusted loss of independent life-years in Western countries. Approximately 700 000 people in the United States experience a stroke annually, resulting in an estimated $57.9 billion in direct and indirect costs. By the year 2050, an estimated 1 million persons will suffer from stroke every year because of aging in the population and changes in the ethnic distribution. Approximately 25% of the strokes occurring annually are attributable to ischemic events related to occlusive disease of the cervical internal carotid artery (CA).

Asymptomatic carotid stenosis is unique in the surgical literature in that there is statistically significant, level-one evidence from the Asymptomatic Carotid Atherosclerosis Study (ACAS) and Asymptomatic Carotid Surgery Trial (ACST) that patients with asymptomatic CA stenosis derive benefit from carotid endarterectomy (CEA), yet there continue to be prominent physicians who advocate for medical management 'only' of all patients with asymptomatic CA disease. The evidence-based argument is that about 40 patients need to be treated in order to prevent one disabling or fatal stroke at 5 years. However, the number of medically treated patients who need to be treated (e.g. with statins) to prevent a single stroke at 5 years significantly exceeds that of CEA and is about 200, as well delineated in *Asymptomatic Carotid Artery Stenosis, Risk Stratification and Management* edited by Moussa, Rundek, and Mohr. Good patient selection, an institution-specific assessment of the risk of CA intervention, including endarterectomy and stenting, and fastidious periprocedural and postprocedural management of risk factors are all necessary for optimizing patient outcomes.

Risk stratification may help identify subgroups that will benefit from revascularization in asymptomatic CA disease. The editors have devoted five chapters to review all the risk stratification strategies available to the clinician to better select patients for carotid revascularization. One great example of risk stratification is monitoring embolic signals with transcranial Doppler (TCD) imaging. An entire chapter in this book is devoted to this topic (Chapter 9). Although carotid disease is mainly considered an embolic process, there is an additive effect leading to a greater volume of infarction with embolism in the setting of impaired cerebral vascular reserve. At University at Buffalo Neurosurgery, we frequently use acetazolamide-augmented computed tomographic perfusion imaging to aid in the selection of patients with asymptomatic carotid and intracranial stenoses for intervention. The impact of cerebral vascular reserve in the setting of asymptomatic carotid disease needs further study and is well discussed in Chapter 10.

Once candidates have been selected through clinical and physiological imaging criteria, the best approach for intervention needs to be determined for the patient. The role of carotid endarterectomy and carotid artery stenting in the management of patients with asymptomatic CA disease is reviewed in detail in Chapters 13 and 14, respectively. In asymptomatic high-risk patients, the benefit of CA stenting has been shown in the Stenting and Angioplasty with Protection in Patients at High Risk for Endarterectomy (SAPPHIRE) trial. What of low-risk asymptomatic patients? Three prospective, randomized trials in low-risk patients are under way or in the planning phase: the Asymptomatic Carotid Stenosis Stenting versus Endarterectomy Trial (ACT I), the Transatlantic Asymptomatic Carotid Intervention Trial (TACIT), and the Asymptomatic Carotid Surgery Trial – 2. The Carotid Revascularization Endarterectomy versus Stenting Trial (CREST) is ongoing and it compares the efficacy of CA stenting and CEA in preventing stroke, myocardial infarction, or death in both symptomatic and asymptomatic patients with carotid stenosis. The standard of care for carotid intervention will be determined on the basis of evidence obtained from these trials.

In 2007, not every patient with asymptomatic carotid disease needs treatment, but clearly there are subgroups that will benefit from intervention. It is up to us as the treating physicians caring for these patients to identify those patients whose stroke risk is lowered by carotid revascularization. This book provides an excellent foundation on which to build.

Robert D Ecker MD **and L Nelson Hopkins** MD
Department of Neurosurgery and
Toshiba Stroke Research Center
School of Medicine and Biomedical Sciences
University at Buffalo, State University of New York
Buffalo, NY, USA

Preface

Few topics in cardiovascular and cerebrovascular medicine generate as much controversy as the management of patients with asymptomatic carotid artery stenosis (CAS). Despite the publication of several large prospective, randomized clinical trials demonstrating the superiority of carotid endarterectomy (CEA) over medical therapy for the prevention of ischemic stroke in patients with asymptomatic CAS, some physicians remain skeptical about the value of carotid revascularization in these patients. At the crux of this attitude is the argument that the majority of these patients are at low risk for future stroke and that 'too many' patients need to undergo carotid revascularization to prevent one stroke. The pros and cons of this argument have been – and still are – the subject of ongoing discussion.

In the meantime, rather than dismiss the dissenting opinions as illogical or unscientific, we should be seeking a constructive model for interspecialty cooperation to generate the necessary data that would improve our ability to identify asymptomatic patients who would benefit most from carotid revascularization. The literature addressing the various aspects of clinical care of patients with asymptomatic CAS is dispersed among various specialty journals (vascular surgery, neurology, neuroradiology, and cardiology); unfortunately, it is nearly impossible for a busy physician to become acquainted with it all.

This book is the product of a multispecialty effort to provide a 'state of-the-art' review of the epidemiology, natural history, risk stratification strategies, and treatment of patients with asymptomatic CAS. The authors span the specialties of Interventional Cardiology, Neurology, Vascular Medicine, Interventional Neuroradiology and Neurosurgery. A particular emphasis is placed on clinical decision making regarding screening for asymptomatic CAS, management of patients with asymptomatic CAS prior to coronary bypass surgery, and how clinicians can use the various risk stratification strategies to guide decision making regarding the need for carotid revascularization. This effort can help better target carotid revascularization therapies towards high-risk patients and therefore improve its risk-to-benefit ratio.

We hope this book will be of interest to all healthcare professionals who are involved in the management of patients with asymptomatic CAS, including cardiologists, neurologists, vascular surgeons, neurosurgeons, neuroradiologists, and primary care physicians. Ultimately, we hope this book will be a useful resource in the care of patients with asymptomatic CAS and will stimulate further research into the many unresolved questions.

Issam D Moussa MD
Tatjana Rundek MD
JP Mohr MD

Acknowledgments

The concept of this book was transpired from the inter-disciplinary interaction between the faculty at the Center for Vascular & Interventional therapy and those at the Stroke Unit in the Neurological Institute at Columbia University Medical Center. In the process of evaluating patients with asymptomatic carotid artery disease for carotid revascularization questions were constantly raised by my neurology colleagues as to the disconnect between the "scientific evidence" relating to this topic and the varied clinician's attitudes toward the subject. My deepest gratitude goes in particular to my co-editors, JP Mohr and Tatjana Rundek whom I inter-acted with the most and whose invaluable expertise provided the impetus to begin this work. Of course, this book would not have been possible without the contribution of all the expert authors who devoted valuable time and effort to provide state of the art reviews each in their particular area of interest.

On a more personal level, a special gratitude to my mentors: Antonio Colombo, for being my inspiration to get into Interventional Cardiology, and Jeffrey W Moses and Martin B Leon whose vision and leadership created an environment which fosters creativity and nourishes a balance between clinical and academic output. Without this environment I would not have been able to devote the time for this project. Also special thanks to Carol Czarnecki who provided excellent editorial comments and Christina Fernandez who helped obtain permissions for illustrations in this book.

Issam D Moussa

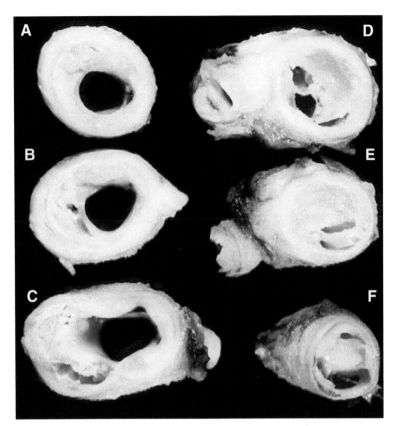

Figure 2.1 Gross bisected specimens of a severe stenotic asymptomatic atherosclerotic lesion at the level of the common carotid (A, B), bifurcation (C, D), and internal carotid artery (E, F).

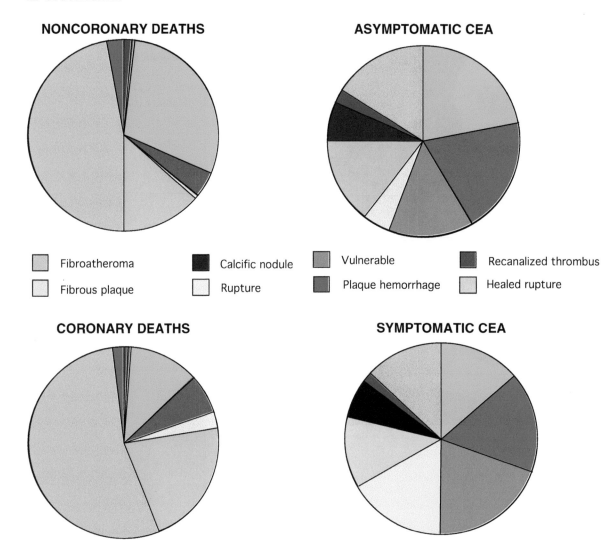

Figure 2.2 Distribution of different plaque types in the coronary and carotid districts based on patient clinical status (non-sudden and sudden coronary death vs symptomatic and asymptomatic carotid patients. CEA, carotid endarterectomy.

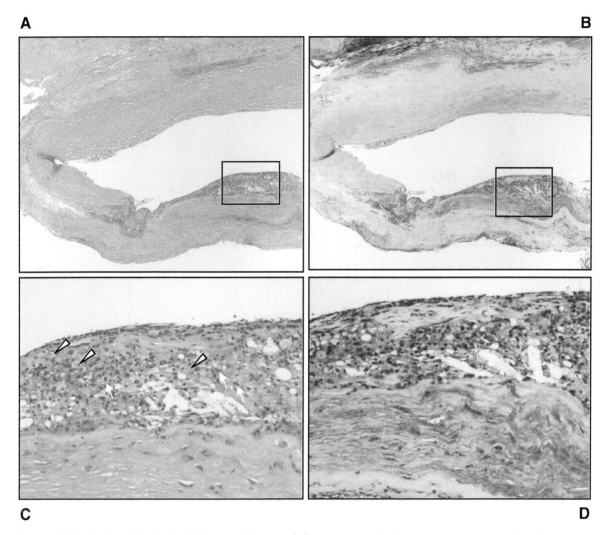

Figure 2.3 Pathological intimal thickening. Micrograph from a surgical endarterectomy specimen. Panel A (hematoxylin eosin staining × 2) and Panel B (Movat pentachrome staining × 2): Low power view of a pathologic intimal thickening characterized by a localized thickening of the intima layer associated to inflammatory cell infiltration (with arrows) and lipid deposition (white triangles) (Panel C and D, high power view of the area within the box in Panel A and Panel B). Necrosis is not evident at this stage.

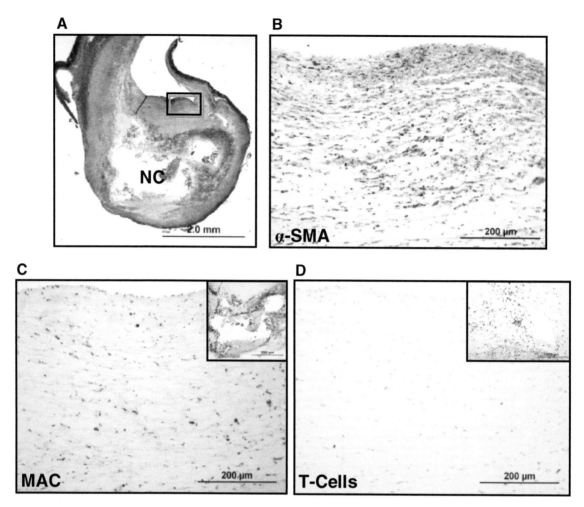

Figure 2.4 Fibrous cap atheroma. (A) Section of human carotid plaque (endarterectomy specimen) shows a fibroatheromatous lesion characterized by a 'true' necrotic core (NC) encapsulated by a relatively thick fibrous cap. (B) The area represented by the black box in A shows abundant immunostaining against smooth muscle actin (α-SMA) within the fibrous cap. (C) A paucity of CD68+ macrophages (MAC) are found within the fibrous cap, with strong reactivity, however, in the periphery of the NC (inset). (D) Similarly, CD45Ro+ T lymphocytes are few within the fibrous cap although T cells are relatively abundant in the shoulder region in areas of vasa vasorum (inset).

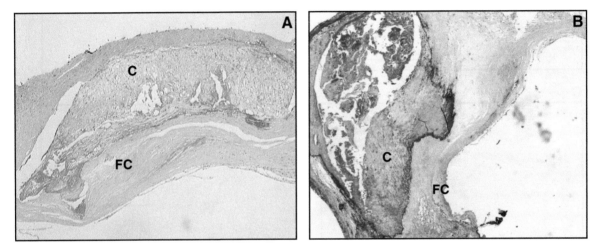

Figure 2.5 Fibrocalcific lesion. (A) Hematoxylin-eosin stain, ×2, and (B) Movat pentachrome stain, ×2, show two plaques with a thick fibrous cap surrounded by extensive calcium deposition characteristic of calcified plate. FC, Fibrous cap; C, calcification.

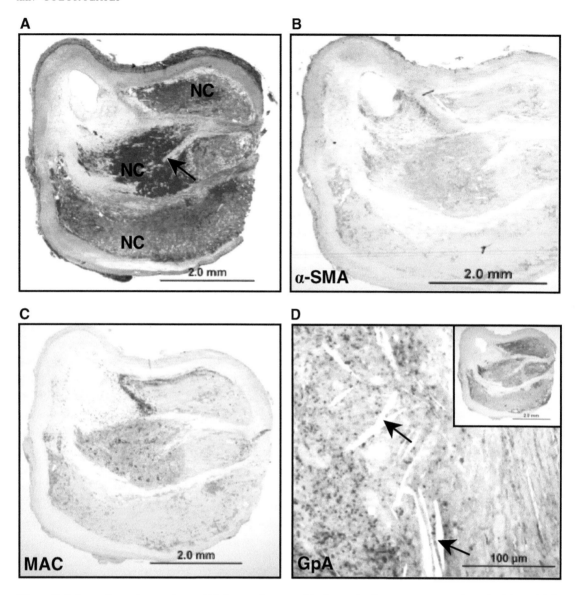

Figure 2.6 Intraplaque hemorrhage. (A) A complex carotid plaque (endarterectomy specimen) with multiple fibrous caps and necrotic cores (NC) and severe intraplaque hemorrhage. The discontinuous fibrous cap (arrow) easily identifies a previous site of plaque rupture. (B) Immunostaining against smooth muscle actin (α-SMA) highlights a healing luminal thrombus from a recent plaque rupture. (C) Macrophages (MAC) are primarily localized to the periphery of the necrotic core near the luminal surface. (D) Antibody against glycophorin A (GpA, a protein specific to erythrocytes) shows intense staining of erythrocyte membranes mostly within the necrotic core intermixed with cholesterol clefts (arrows).

Figure 2.8 Nodular calcification. (A) Low-power view (Movat pentachrome stain) of a human carotid plaque (endarterectomy specimen) with severe calcification. Numerous fragmented calcified plates (arrows) and nodules (arrowheads) are present. (B) Higher-power view (Movat pentachrome stain) within the area of the black box in A showing a region near the luminal surface with extensive nodular calcification underneath a thin fibrous cap (arrow). Eruptive calcified nodules could be a potential cause of luminal thrombi and distal embolization. (C) Several osteoclast-like cells associated with nodules (hematoxylin and eosin stain). (D) Higher-power view (hematoxylin and eosin stain) of the area of the black box in C showing several multinucleated osteoclast-like cells near calcified nodules (arrows).

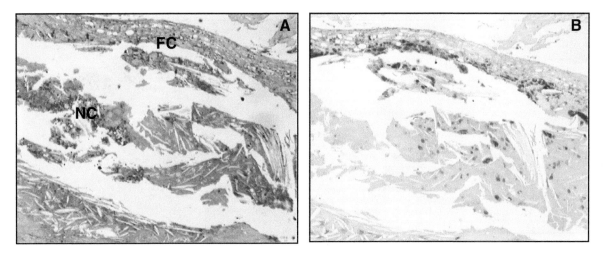

Figure 2.7 Thin fibrous cap atheromata. (A) A vulnerable plaque characterized by a large lipidic-necrotic core (NC) associated to a thin inflamed fibrous cap (FC, Movat pentachrome stain, ×4). (B) High number of macrophagic foam cells, CD68+ are present in the thin fibrous cap of the plaque (CD68 stain, ×4).

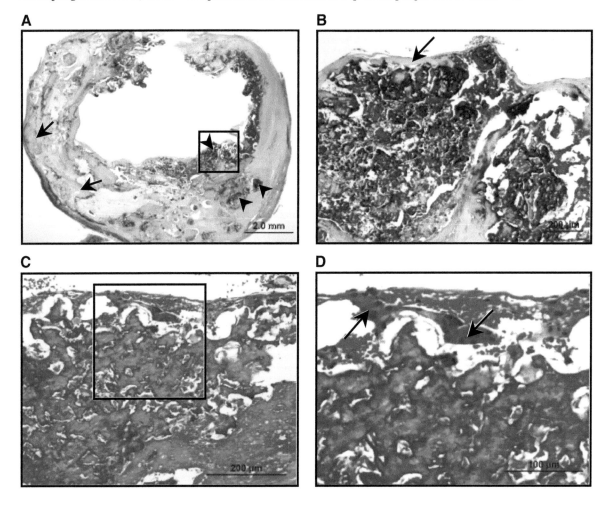

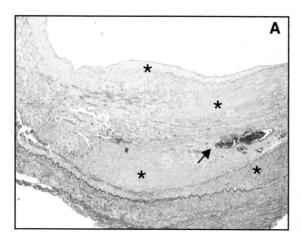
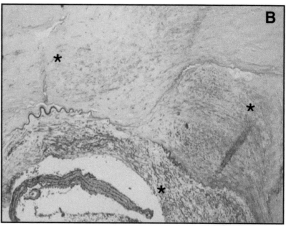

Figure 2.9 Healed plaque with stratified thrombus. (A) and (B) show an organized thrombus characterized by stratified fibrous tissue. Lesions with healed ruptures may exhibit multilayering of lipid and necrotic core (asterisks), suggestive of previous episodes of thrombosis. Old occlusions often show the lumen almost totally occluded by dense collagen and proteoglycan with interspersed capillaries (arrow), arterioles, smooth muscle cells, and inflammatory cells. (Movat pentachrome stain, ×2).

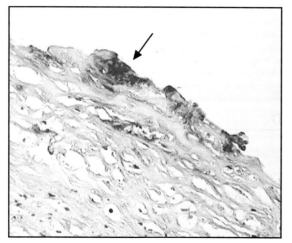

Figure 2.10 Plaque erosion. Acute thrombosis associated with superficial erosion (black arrow), without rupture of the fibrous cap. The endothelium is absent at the erosion site. The exposed intima consists predominantly of smooth muscle and proteoglycans (Movat pentachrome stain, ×4).

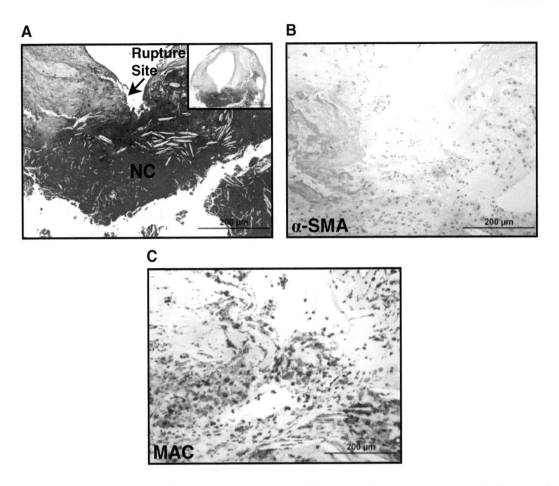

Figure 2.11 Plaque rupture. (A) Section of human carotid plaque (endarterectomy specimen) showing a lesion with a relatively larger necrotic core (NC) and rupture site (arrow). The rupture site is ulcerated with little exposed luminal thrombus. The inset is a lower-power view of the same section (Movat pentachrome staining). (B) Immunostaining against smooth muscle actin (α-SMA) shows a lack of smooth muscle within the fibrous cap at the rupture site. (C) Immunostaining against CD68 shows numerous inflammatory macrophages (MAC) within the fibrous cap.

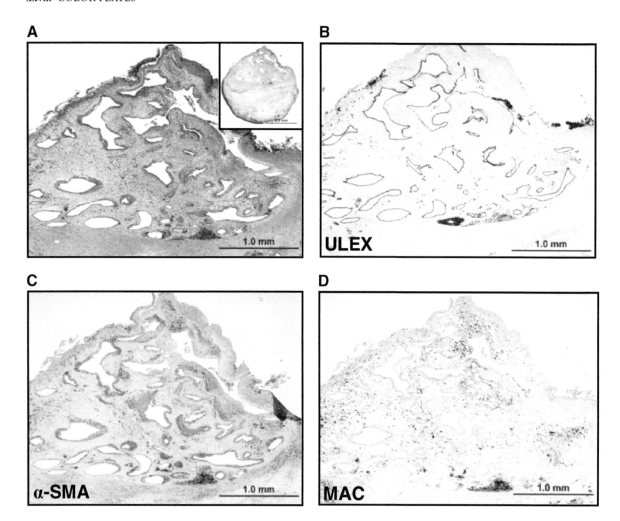

Figure 2.12 Recanalized thrombus. (A) Section of human carotid plaque (endarterectomy specimen) with a recanalized thrombus (Movat pentachrome stain). The inset is a lower-power view of the same section. (B) Indirect immunostaining with anti-*Ulex europaeus* lectin demonstrating numerous vascular channels lined by endothelium. (C) Many recanalized channels are also surrounded by actin-positive smooth muscle cells (α-SMA). (D) Immunostaining against CD68 shows inflammatory macrophages (MAC) within the thrombus and surrounding vascular channels.

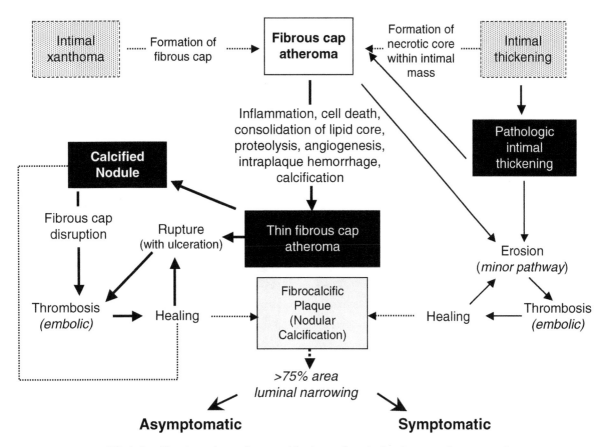

Figure 2.13 Simplified classification scheme for carotid atherosclerosis development from an early, uncomplicated lesion to a more complex, vulnerable atherosclerotic plaque.

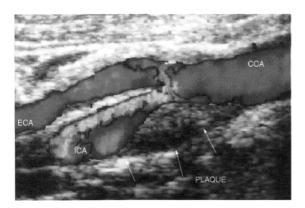

Figure 3.11 Left hemispheric watershed ischemic stroke (arrows) due to high-grade left internal carotid artery stenosis.

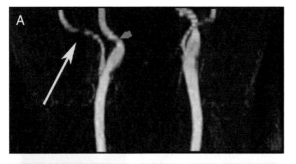

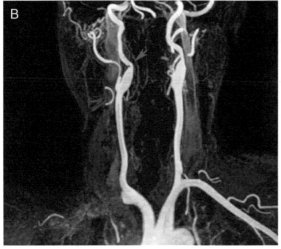

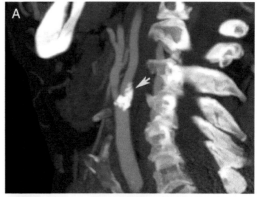

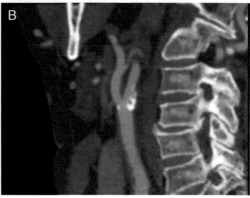

Figure 5.1 (A) Non-contrast carotid MRA (same projection and orientation as the contrast-enhanced MRA in Figure 5.1B). Note that the right ICA lesion (red arrow) is poorly defined because of partial volume averaging and lower spatial resolution. Also note the 'Stair-step' artifact that may simulate a stenosis (yellow arrow). (B) Contrast-enhanced MRA. The stenosis (red arrow) is much more clearly seen on this study because of the higher spatial resolution and absence of artifact.

Figure 5.2 (A) Carotid CTA (same projection and orientation as Figure 5.2B). Note that the thick MIP image makes it look like the carotid artery is completely occluded by a bright calcified plaque (yellow arrow). (B) Carotid CTA. Note that the thin MIP image shows a razor thin plane through the lumen of the vessel and, subsequently, shows the stenosis to be much more mild.

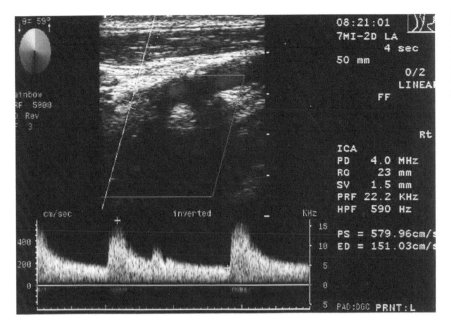

Figure 8.1 High-grade stenosis of the internal carotid artery. Color Doppler shows 80-99% stenosis of the internal carotid artery.

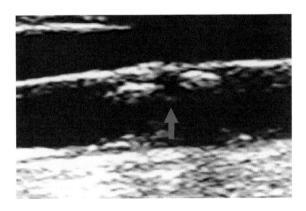

Figure 8.6 An ulcerated plaque (red arrow) with well-defined arterial wall at its base and a recess over 2 mm in the length and depth.

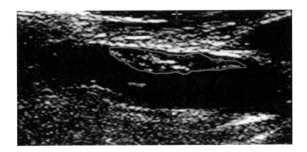

Figure 8.7 Echolucent heterogeneous plaque (outlined in red).

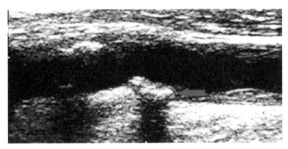

Figure 8.8 Echodense (calcified, bright) homogeneous plaque with acoustic shadowing (red arrow).

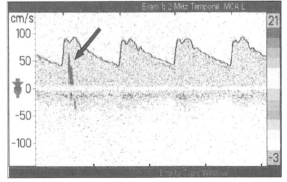

Figure 9.1 Cerebral microembolic signals (MES) or high-intensity transient signals (HITS) detected in the middle cerebral artery (red arrow) in the Doppler spectrum obtained by TCD monitoring.

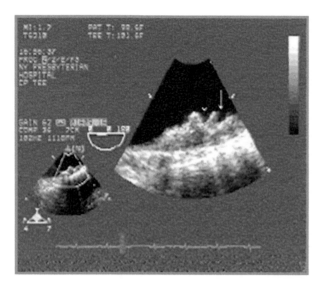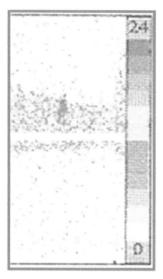

Figure 9.3 Cerebral microembolic signals (MES) detected by TCD in a stroke patient with aortic arch atheroma visualized by transesophageal echocardiography (TEE). TEE courtesy of Marco R Di Tullio MD.

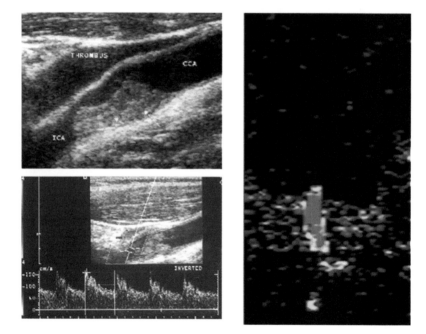

Figure 9.4 Cerebral microembolic signals (MES) detected in the middle cerebral artery (MCA) in an asymptomatic patient with a large irregular atherosclerotic plaque in the carotid artery (60–80% stenosis of the internal carotid artery at the carotid bifurcation) on duplex ultrasound.

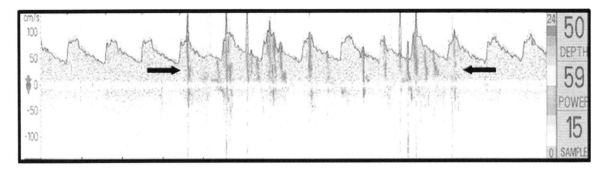

Figure 9.6 Transcranial Doppler (TCD) detection of right-to-left cardiac shunt (PFO; patent foramen ovale). Single-gate spectral TCD waveform display of the middle cerebral artery (MCA) at a depth of 50 mm. Over 15 microemboli of high signal intensity appeared after the intravenous injection of agitated saline (9 ml normal saline mixed with 1 ml air) and rapidly disappeared (between the two arrows). Monitoring started 10 seconds prior to agitated saline injection and continued for 2 minutes after the bolus.

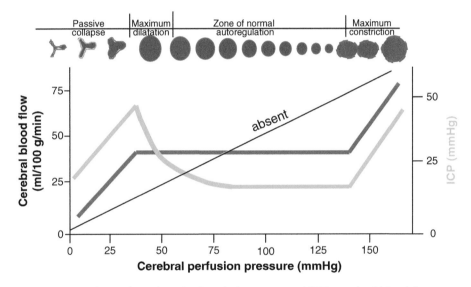

Figure 10.1 Relationship of cerebral perfusion pressure (CPP), cerebral blood flow (CBF), and intracranial pressure (ICP). (Courtesy of Stephan A Mayer MD.)

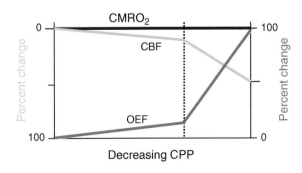

Figure 10.2 Relationship of cerebral blood flow (CBF) and metabolism (oxygen extraction fraction – OEF, cerebral metabolic rate of oxygen – $CMRO_2$) to decreasing cerebral perfusion pressure (CPP).

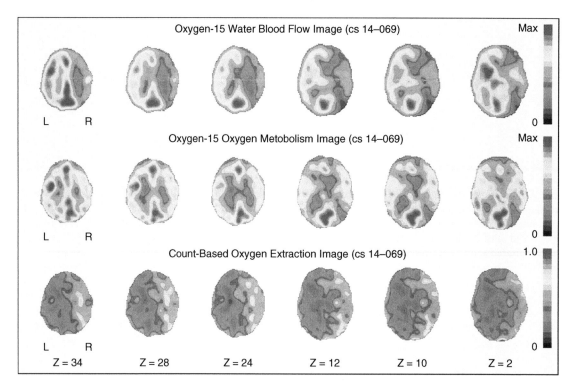

Figure 10.6 Brain PET images for the patient in Figure 10.5 (symptomatic RICA occlusion). Note the reduced blood flow and increased oxygen extraction in the right hemisphere. (Study acquired for the Carotid Occlusion Surgery Study (COSS); Courtesy of William J Powers, Principal Investigator of COSS.)

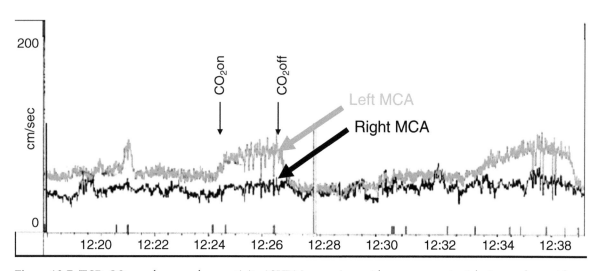

Figure 10.7 TCD-CO_2 cerebrovascular reactivity (CVR) in a patient with asymptomatic right internal carotid artery stenosis. Bilateral recording of mean blood flow velocities (MBFV) in both middle cerebral arteries (MCA) during breath-hold, after CO_2 inhalation, and at rest. Note that MBFV were increased in the left MCA (normal CVR, green arrow) and diminished in the right MCA (black arrow), indicating impaired CVR on the right.

1

Epidemiology and natural history of asymptomatic carotid artery stenosis

Issam D Moussa and JP Mohr

Take-Home Messages

1. Prevalence of asymptomatic carotid artery stenosis (CAS) (>50% DS) varies widely:

General population	2–8%
Patients with coronary artery disease	11–26%
Patients referred for coronary artery bypass surgery	9–28%
Patients with peripheral arterial disease	25–49%

2. Carotid disease progression occurs in 3–32% of patients annually.
3. Carotid disease progression is more common in patients with diabetes mellitus, smoking, and hypertension, as well as in patients with more severe lesions, heterogeneous plaque, and contralateral disease.
4. The annual risk of ipsilateral stroke in patients with asymptomatic CAS is between 2% and 12%. The variability in risk is due to differences in lesion severity, rate of disease progression, plaque characteristics, cerebrovascular reserve, and other unidentified factors.
5. Eighty percent of patients with asymptomatic CAS who experience ipsilateral large artery stroke do so without antecedent transient ischemic attack (TIA).
6. Patients with asymptomatic CAS are at high risk for cardiac morbidity and mortality.

INTRODUCTION

On a routine office visit, your patient informs you that a friend of his just had a stroke and was told that it was caused by a blockage in his carotid artery. The patient states that he is concerned about his own health. He inquires about whether he also has a blockage in his carotid artery, whether he should undergo a test to screen for it, and about his prognosis if he does have a carotid stenosis.

Of the approximately 700 000 new strokes per year that occur in the United States, 15–20% result from carotid occlusive disease. Of these atheroembolic strokes, 75–80% occur without any warning signs of stroke or transient cerebral ischemia.[1,2] Therefore, asymptomatic carotid artery stenosis (CAS) remains a

significant cause of stroke morbidity and mortality, and its prevalence is on the rise.[3]

Your patient's questions are simple yet critical to his/her actual and perceived well-being. However, the answer to these questions is not at all clear-cut. When asked about the prevalence and natural history of a carotid stenosis in a neurologically asymptomatic population, most physicians would quote a prevalence rate of 2–8% and an annual stroke risk of 2%. The fact that we encounter many patients who may not fit into this 'standard profile' is often not thoroughly considered in the decision-making process.

The natural history of asymptomatic CAS varies according to many factors such as age, gender, cardiovascular risk factors, stenosis characteristics, and cerebrovascular reserve, to name a few. Not all asymptomatic internal carotid stenoses act in a similar manner, clinically or anatomically. Some patients will remain asymptomatic despite having carotid stenoses that undergo progression to a higher level of severity, and other patients will have ipsilateral neurological symptoms with stenoses that do not progress to a higher degree of narrowing. Therefore, the key to proper evaluation and management of these ubiquitous lesions is to accurately determine their natural history. In doing so, one should be able to answer the following questions: What lesions will undergo progression to a higher level of severity? How frequently does it occur and to what severity? Does progression of disease predict the development of future ipsilateral neurological events? And what patients should then undergo revascularization?

In the prevention of stroke, few issues have led to more controversy than the management of asymptomatic patients with a carotid artery stenosis. A thorough understanding of the prevalence and natural history of asymptomatic CAS is instrumental to clinical decision-making.

PREVALENCE OF ASYMPTOMATIC CAROTID ARTERY DISEASE

General population

The prevalence of asymptomatic CAS, as defined by >50% diameter stenosis by duplex ultrasound, in general population studies appears to be between 2%

and 8% (Table 1.1).[4–14] Although these studies cannot be directly compared, three observations emerge with respect to predisposing risk factors (Table 1.2):[5–14]

1. Age is the strongest and most consistent risk factor for incident carotid stenosis.[10,11,13,15,16] For example, in the study by Josse et al,[4] the prevalence of asymptomatic CAS was 2.4% in patients aged 55–64 years and 6.1% in patients aged 75–84 years. Similarly, in the study by Salonen et al,[5] the prevalence of asymptomatic CAS was 2.3% in patients aged 54 years and 4.8% in patients aged 60 years. The strong relation of age to atherosclerosis is probably a combination of indirect expression of the continuous exposure to various risk factors[17] as well as the result of an intrinsic process of aging.[18]

2. Male sex ranks second to age in predicting prevalence of carotid stenosis, with the risk of higher-grade stenosis being twice as frequent in men as in women.[11] This difference persists even after adjustment for potential confounders, although the sex difference appears to attenuate in older age.[15,16] The reason for the gender-based differences is unclear and cannot only be explained on the basis of hormonal variations, because the combination of estrogen/progesterone in the HERS study did not delay progression of carotid disease.[19]

3. While traditional cardiovascular risk factors (dyslipidemia, diabetes mellitus, hypertension, smoking, and lifestyle) are clearly associated with higher prevalence of asymptomatic CAS, the strength and consistency of this association vary among studies.

Table 1.1 Prevalence of asymptomatic CAS (>50% DS) in the general population

Study	Setting	No. of patients	Age (years)	Asymptomatic CAS (%)
Josse[4]	General population screening	526	45–84	2.4–6.1
Salonen[5]	Population-based, Finland	412	42–60	2.3–4.8
Colgan[6]	Health fair	348	24–91	4
Fowl[7]	Veterans Volunteers	153	>50	6.5
Jungquist[8]*	Population-based, Sweden	478	68	5
O'Leary[9]	Framingham Study	1189	66–93	8
O'Leary[10]	Cardiac Health Study (CHS)	5201	>65	6.2
Prati[11]	Population-based, Italy	1348	18–99	2.1
Pujia[12]	Retirement homes	239	65–94	5
Willeit[13]	Population-based, Italy	909	40–79	5.8
Mannami[14]	Free-living Japanese population	1694	50–79	4.4

CAS, carotid artery stenosis; DS, diameter stenosis.
*All elderly men; CAS defined as ≥60% DS.

Table 1.2 Effect of traditional cardiovascular risk factors on prevalence of asymptomatic CAS in the general population

Study	Age	Male sex	HTN	DM	Dyslipidemia	Smoking
Salonen[5]	+	−	−	−	+	+
Colgan[6]	+	−	+	−	−	−
Fowl[7]	−	−	−	−	−	+
Jungquist[8]*	NA	NA	−	−	+	+
O'Leary[9]	−	−	−	−	+	−
O'Leary[10]†	+	+	+	+	+	+
Prati[11]‡	+	−	+	−	+	+
Pujia[12]	+	−	+	−	−	−
Willeit[13]§	+	+	+	+	+	+
Mannami[14]‖	+	+	+	±	+	+

*All same age and males. CAS, carotid artery stenosis; HTN, hypertension; DM, diabetes mellitus; HDL, high-density lipoprotein; LDL, low-density lipoprotein; NA, non-applicable.

†Majority of patients with early carotid atherosclerosis.

‡Only HDL protective; LDL not predictive.

§DM, Apolipoprotein b and a1, smoking contributions are dependent on age and gender.

‖DM is predictive in men but not women.

(a) Diabetes mellitus appears to be the most consistent predictive risk factor. De Angelis and associates[20] reported that patients with diabetes were three times more likely to develop carotid stenosis than non-diabetics. Bonora and associates[21] extended these findings to patients with the metabolic syndrome. These investigators found that the metabolic syndrome is burdened by a more frequent incidence and progression of carotid disease. Moreover, they reported that while diabetes mellitus and dyslipidemia were independent predictors of carotid disease, other components of the syndrome (hypertension, obesity, and microalbuminuria) were not when considered individually.

(b) There is agreement among most investigators that smoking is a potent risk factor for carotid atherosclerosis.[22–24] Willeit and colleagues[25] have shown that the number of pack-years of smoking has the strongest association with early carotid artery disease. Notably, the risk burden did not normalize within 5–10 years after cessation, which may lead to speculation that the true atherogenic culprit may not be smoking itself but rather associated disorders, such as chronic infections that are known to persist for years after quitting. Recent evidence also suggests a potential gene–environment interaction in smokers for the development of early carotid therosclerosis through the promotion of endotoxin receptors.[24]

(c) Systolic hypertension has been found to be closely associated with the severity of carotid atherosclerosis.[10,11,13,26] In the study by Su et al,[26] hypertensive patients had an odds ratio of 4.8 for the development of significant carotid stenosis when compared with normotensives.

(d) The impact of lifestyle on development of carotid disease has also been investigated. Luedemann and associates[27] have shown an increased risk of severe asymptomatic CAS in individuals with an unfavorable lifestyle pattern. The interaction between smoking status and lifestyle was interesting in that any beneficial effects of a favorable lifestyle were outweighed by the smoking status for both current and ex-smokers.

Although the association between these risk factors and the development of arterial atherosclerosis in general is an undisputable fact, the lack of consistency among the various studies in confirming this association in relation to carotid disease implores an explanation. Three observations may provide some clarification:

1. Almost all prevalence studies of asymptomatic CAS relied on a single measurement (i.e. a single cholesterol or blood pressure measurement) to define the contribution of risk factors to incidence of carotid disease. This method of analysis may underestimate the strength of association, because the impact of a given risk factor is more likely to be cumulative in nature. Indeed, this observation has been confirmed by Wilson and colleagues,[28] who reported on the increased risk of moderate carotid stenosis (>25%) according to the presence of certain risk factors such as hypertension, cigarette smoking, and cholesterol in the Framingham study. Specifically, the authors reported that the association between these risk factors and the degree of carotid stenosis was more consistent if the time-integrated approach (measurements of risk factors using mean levels collected from examinations over the previous 34 years) was used rather than a single measurement. This was specifically true with total cholesterol and hypertension; for example, in men, the odds ratio for carotid stenosis associated with an increase of 20 mmHg in systolic blood pressure was 2.11 with the time-integrated analysis, but only 1.12 with the single current measurement approach. Also, the odds ratio for carotid stenosis for an increase of 0.26 mmol in total cholesterol was 1.10, significant for the time-integrated analysis but non-significant if current cholesterol levels only were used.
2. The majority of prevalence studies of asymptomatic CAS do not account for the potential role of inflammation as a modulator for carotid disease development. Willeit and associates[25] have demonstrated that while the traditional cardiovascular risk factors are primary instigators of the early stages of atherosclerosis development, they may lose some of their predictive significance when the carotid stenosis becomes obstructive, whereas biological markers of inflammation and enhanced thrombotic activity gain increasing importance. Several biological markers, such as C-reactive protein, homocysteine, fibrinogen, prothrombin fragments, and adhesion molecules, have been implicated as predictors of the presence and severity of carotid disease.[29-31] Furthermore, Roman and colleagues have demonstrated that systemic lupus erythematosus[32] and rheumatoid arthritis,[33] both conditions characterized by chronic inflammation, are associated with accelerated carotid atherosclerosis

independent from age, gender, and other traditional cardiovascular risk factors.
3. The majority of prevalence studies of asymptomatic CAS did not account for the potential role of genetic polymorphisms among patients, which has recently been implied to have a substantive influence on the formation of carotid artery plaque.[34]

Patients with coronary artery disease

Atherosclerotic vascular disease is a systemic disorder typically involving multiple vascular territories in the same patient. Indeed, several studies have confirmed that asymptomatic CAS is more prevalent in patients with established coronary disease. The prevalence of asymptomatic CAS, as defined by >50% diameter stenosis (DS) by duplex ultrasound, in patients with coronary disease is between 8% and 31% (Table 1.3).[35-40] The extent of coronary artery disease, diabetes mellitus, smoking, hypertension, and renal dysfunction have all been identified as predictors of carotid artery disease in this population. Furthermore, it has been suggested that the association between these risk factors and carotid disease is age- and gender-dependent. Zimarino and associates[37] reported that diabetes and smoking were predictive of asymptomatic CAS among younger patients, whereas hypertension was predictive among older subjects. Lanzer[41] reported that while the association between carotid and coronary disease in males was primarily age-dependent, this association in females depended more heavily on the presence of risk factors, specifically type 2 diabetes. Conversely, Tanimoto and colleagues[40] reported that only age and extent of coronary disease were independent predictors of carotid disease. In this study, the investigators screened 632 Japanese patients with established coronary disease and found a 20% prevalence of asymptomatic CAS. As shown in Table 1.4, the prevalence of carotid disease increases dramatically with the number of coronaries diseased.

The relationship between the severity of coronary disease and the prevalence of asymptomatic CAS is also reflected by the high prevalence of carotid disease (9–28%) in patients referred for coronary artery bypass graft (CABG) surgery (Table 1.5).[42-48] However, it is important to point out that it is difficult to establish the true prevalence of carotid disease in patients undergoing CABG for several reasons: first, the criteria for diagnosis of a 'significant' carotid stenosis vary among studies; secondly many of the published series are retrospective and most of the prospective screening studies excluded patients with urgent cardiac symptoms, thereby potentially leading to underestimation of the prevalence of occult carotid disease.

Table 1.3 Prevalence of asymptomatic CAS in patients with CAD

Study	No. of patients	Setting	Carotid stenosis severity (%)	Prevalence (%)
Chen[35]	153	Coronary angiography for suspected CAD	>50	11
			50–79	5
			80–100	6
Kallikazaros[36]	225	Coronary angiography for suspected CAD	>50	18
			50–79	13
			80–100	5
Zimarino[37]	624	Coronary angiography for suspected CAD	>50	14
			50–69	8
			70–100	6
Ambrosetti[38]	168	Cardiac rehabilitation	>50	8–26
Komorovsky[39]	323	Acute coronary syndrome	>50	31
Tanimoto[40]	632	Coronary angiography for suspected CAD	>50	20

CAS, carotid artery stenosis; CAD, coronary artery disease.

Table 1.4 Prevalence of asymptomatic CAS (>50% DS) according to severity of CAD

Extent of CAD	Kallikazaros[36] (n = 225)	Zimarino[37] (n = 624)	Ambrosetti[38] (n = 168)	Komorovsky[39] (n = 323)	Tanimoto[40] (n = 632)
No CAD	3.6%	4.1%	–	–	7%
CAD					
1 vessel	5.3%	14.4%		19%	14.5%
			8%		
2 vessel	13.5%			43%	21.4%
		17%			
3 vessel	24.5%			45%	36%
			26%		
Left main	40%	NR		–	–

CAS, carotid artery stenosis; CAD, coronary artery disease; DS, diameter stenosis, NR, not reported.

Although traditional cardiovascular risk factors consistently predict presence of vascular pathology in individuals with a relatively low prevalence of vascular disease, it is likely that these factors may be of less value in cohorts of higher-risk individuals who already have established vascular disease. This concept is further supported by the findings of Crouse et al[49] who reported that while traditional risk factors account for 30% of the variability in severity of carotid atherosclerosis in patients with coronary disease, much of this variability remains unexplained. These findings are consistent with the concept that genetic factors and/or undiscovered risk factors common to both arterial beds also contribute to the relation between coronary and carotid atherosclerosis in human beings.

Patients with peripheral arterial disease

Patients with peripheral arterial disease (PAD) are likely to have more widespread systemic atherosclerosis and are at greater risk of coronary and carotid artery disease,[48] as well as acute ischemic vascular events.[50]

Table 1.5 Prevalence of asymptomatic CAS (>50% DS) in patients referred for coronary artery bypass graft surgery

Study	No. of patients	Asymptomatic CAS (%)
Barnes[42]	449	19
Faggioli[43]	539	8.7*
Vigneswaran[44]	60	28
D'Agostino[45]	1279	21
Birincioglu[46]	678	13
Rath[47]	1200	9
Kawarada[48]	380	14

*Severe carotid stenosis >75% DS.

The prevalence of asymptomatic CAS, as defined by >50% DS by duplex ultrasound, in patients with PAD appears to be the highest among any other subgroup, and ranges between 14% and 49% (Table 1.6).[7,51–62] In the largest study to date, Cina and colleagues[60] reported a 33% prevalence of asymptomatic CAS in 660 patients with established PAD and no prior neurological events in the 3 years prior to screening. No patients younger than 50 years of age were found to have carotid stenosis >50%, but those older than 80 years had a 41% prevalence of carotid stenosis more than 50%.

The differing prevalence of asymptomatic CAS among patients with PAD may be a consequence of differences in patient demographics, risk factors, and the method of defining these risk factors (questionnaire vs direct measurement) as well as the definition and severity of PAD. The most consistent predictors of asymptomatic CAS in patients with PAD are age and severity of PAD, while the role of other traditional cardiovascular risk factors is less evident.[51,52,54,56,60] Cina and associates[60] identified age more than 70 years, prior remote stroke, diabetes, and a bilateral ankle brachial index (ABI) <0.8 as independent predictors of asymptomatic CAS. A patient who has only one of these risk factors has a 22% risk of having a carotid stenosis >50%, while a patient who has all four risk factors has a 44% risk of having a carotid stenosis >50%. Furthermore, similar to findings in patients

Table 1.6 Prevalence of asymptomatic CAS (>50% DS) in patients with PAD

Study	PAD definition	No. of patients	Asymptomatic CAS (%)
Lower extremity PAD			
Ahn[51]	Ankle brachial index	78	14
Fowl[7]	Ankle brachial index	116	12.9
Klop[52]	Ankle brachial index	374	26.6
Gentile[53]	Pre fem-pop bypass	252	28
Marek[54]	PAD symptoms	188	24.5
Alexandrova[55]	Ankle brachial index	144	50
De Virgilio[56]	PAD symptoms	89	20
Simons[57]	Ankle brachial index	162	14
Ballotta[58]*	Ankle brachial index	132	49
Pilcher[59]	Ankle brachial index/Imaging	200	25
Cina[60]	Ankle brachial index	620	33
Renal artery stenosis			
Louie[61]	Duplex scanning	60	46
Missouris[62]	Angiography	38	45

CAS, carotid artery stenosis; DS, diameter stenosis; PAD, peripheral arterial disease.
*>60% DS.

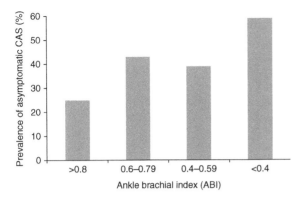

Figure 1.1 Prevalence of asymptomatic CAS according to PAD severity. (Modified from Cina et al.[60])

with coronary disease, they demonstrated that the prevalence of asymptomatic CAS correlates with the severity of PAD (Figure 1.1).

NATURAL HISTORY OF PATIENTS WITH ASYMPTOMATIC CAROTID ARTERY STENOSIS

The purpose of the forthcoming section is to thoroughly examine the natural history of patients with asymptomatic CAS with respect to:

- carotid disease progression
- incidence of cognitive impairment
- incidence of ischemic neurological events
- risk of cardiovascular morbidity and mortality.

A particular emphasis will be placed on the variation of risk estimates among patient populations and the factors that may modulate this risk.

Progression of carotid artery disease

Detection of carotid disease progression in asymptomatic patients is clinically important because rapid progression of disease is associated with a substantially increased risk of ipsilateral neurological events.[63] Furthermore, identifying predictors of disease progression is key to better patient selection for serial duplex surveillance.[64]

Rate of carotid disease progression

The rate at which a carotid stenosis may progress remains the subject of debate despite numerous studies that have directly or indirectly addressed this issue (Table 1.7).[60,65–70] Roederer and colleagues[65] reported one of the earliest studies regarding progression of carotid stenosis in asymptomatic patients. Overall, 31% of patients showed disease progression on one side only

during the follow-up period and 7% on both sides. For lesions with less than 50% stenosis, 1 out of 3 progressed to a more than 50% stenosis after 3 years; when all types of progression were considered, 3 out of 5 patent arteries progressed to a more severe category of disease after 3 years.

The largest natural history study of the progression of asymptomatic carotid stenosis to date was reported by Muluk and associates.[68] These investigators demonstrated that the risk of carotid disease progression is substantial and steadily increases with time. Approximately 9% of the at-risk population had progression each year and this pattern persisted to 7 years of follow-up. This study may even underestimate true progression rates because only 24% of patients had a carotid stenosis >50% at the begining of the study.

Another patient cohort of interest with regard to disease progression comprises patients with unilateral carotid endarterectomy (CEA) who are surveyed for disease progression in the contralateral carotid artery.[71,72] Raman and associates followed 279 patients who underwent unilateral CEA with duplex scanning surveillance for up to 27 months. They found an annual rate of disease progression in the contralateral carotid artery of 8.3% and an annual rate of progression to clinically significant stenosis of 4.4%. Furthermore, nearly three-fourths of patients who had contralateral disease progression started with a stenosis less than 50%, indicating that annual progression may be even more pronounced in those patients with baseline stenoses over 50%.

Progression of carotid stenosis using ultrasound can be defined, measured, and analyzed in more than one way, making direct comparison between studies difficult. Generally, carotid disease progression is defined as an increase in stenosis severity to >50% for carotid arteries, with a baseline <50% stenosis, or as an increase to a higher category of stenosis if the baseline stenosis was >50%. To understand the source of variability in the reported progression rates, several points need to be highlighted:

- Studies of carotid disease progression have used different ultrasound criteria to define stenosis severity.
- The times at which disease progression occurs depends partly on the initial severity of disease. In fact, a moderate lesion is 5 times more likely to progress compared with mild or no lesions. [68,69]
- The differing rate of carotid disease progression is also influenced by differences in the patient's risk profile and intrinsic variability of carotid plaque behavior.[73]

Predictors of carotid disease progression

There is pathological and epidemiological evidence that human carotid atherosclerosis is a product of etiologically

Table 1.7 Rate of carotid disease progression in patients with asymptomatic CAS

Study	No. of patients	Mean FU period (months)	Initial stenosis severity (%)	Progression to a higher category (%)	
				Total	Annual
Roederer[65]	167	36	<50	–	8
			50–79	–	20
			80–99	–	50
Mansour[66]	142	20	50–79	17	8.5
The Asymptomatic Cervical Bruit Study; Lewis[67]	715	38	None	3.25	1.5
			<50	19.5	9.5
			50–79	22.2	11.1
			80–99	9.7	6.5
Muluk[68]	1004	28	None	11.5	3
			<50	38.2	10.9
			50–79	43.5	12.2
			80–99	26.6	7.7
Cina[60]	399	6–9	<50	–	13.5
			50–79	–	3.8
			80–99	–	7.7
Martin-Conejero[69]*	180	26	<30	7	–
			30–70	27	–
Sabeti[70]	1013	8	0–99	9.2	–

CAS, carotid artery stenosis; FU, follow-up.
*Patients with prior contralateral carotid endarterectomy.

distinct processes. Early non-stenotic atherosclerotic lesions grow slowly with concomitant efficient vascular remodeling, which prevents significant lumen obstruction in most patients. This early stage is driven by the classic vascular risk factors[74] supplemented by several less well-established risk conditions, such as iron overload, hypothyroidism, and microalbuminuria.[25] Advanced stenotic lesions, on the other hand, are characterized by occasional marked increases in plaque size, occasionally due to intraplaque hemorrhage[73] and no or inadequate vascular remodeling. At this stage, the predictive significance of the traditional risk factors lessens, while markers of enhanced thrombotic activity (high fibrinogen, low antithrombin, factor V Leiden mutation) and clinical conditions known to interfere with coagulation (high platelet count, diabetes, smoking) gain increasing importance in a synergistic manner.[25]

Furthermore, recent data by Schillinger and colleagues[75] unequivocally confirm a temporal correlation between inflammation and morphological features of rapidly progressive carotid atherosclerosis independent from, but synergistic with, smoking and baseline carotid lesion severity. Specifically, patients with the highest level of high-sensitivity C-reactive protein (hs-CRP) had a 3.65-fold increased risk of carotid disease progression compared with those with the lowest hs-CRP level. The credibility of the importance of these emerging risk factors is supported by the lack of consistent evidence that affirms the role of traditional cardiovascular risk factors in predicting carotid disease progression, as discussed below (Table 1.8).[60,65,68,69,72,75–77]

Age and gender
It has been shown that both carotid stenosis severity and plaque burden increase with age in men and women.[78] However, whether the rapidity of disease progression is different in younger than older patients

Table 1.8 The predictive significance of Framingham risk factors for disease progression in patients with asymptomatic CAS

Study	Age	Male sex	Hypertension	DM	Dyslipidemia	Smoking
Cina[60]	−	−	−	−	−	−
Roederer[65]	+ (younger)	−	−	+	−	+
Muluk[68]	−	−	+ (systolic BP)	−	−	−
Martin-Conejero[69]	+ (younger)	−	−	−	−	−
Raman[72]	−	−	−	−	−	−
Schillinger[75]	+ (older)	−	−	−	−	+
Delcker[76]	−	−	+ (diastolic BP)	+	−	−
Garvey[77]	−	−	+ (pulse pressure)	−	+ (HDL)	−

CAS, carotid artery stenosis; DM, diabetes mellitus; BP, blood pressure; HDL, high-density lipoprotein.

is unclear. Roederer and associates[65] reported that carotid disease progression occurred more often in younger (45%) than older (29%) patients. However, the relationship between age and progression disappeared after accounting for the original disease severity. Similarly, Garvey and associates[77] reported that age was not an independent predictor of carotid disease progression.

It has also been demonstrated that for the same degree of carotid stenosis, men had a higher plaque burden than women.[78] This holds true both for ultrasound-based[78] and angiographic[79] measurements. Epidemiological evidence also supports these biological observations. Garvey and associates[77] reported that carotid disease progression is more pronounced in men than women. However, since only 2% of their patients were female, a population with a greater proportion of women should be assessed to determine the relevance of gender as a predictor of carotid disease progression.

Diabetes mellitus

Although the relationship between diabetes mellitus and the presence of advanced carotid atherosclerosis is indisputable, the literature remains inconsistent with regard to whether diabetes is an independent predictor of carotid disease progression. While Roederer and associates[65] have reported that carotid disease progression is higher in diabetics compared with non-diabetics, others[77] were not able to confirm this relationship. Furthermore, it has been suggested that the injurious effects of diabetes on carotid atherogenesis are independent of glucose control, but rather related to the procoagulant state and attenuated endogenous fibrinolysis in these patients.[25,80]

Blood pressure

In contrast to the unequivocal finding that all components of blood pressure are important predictors of early carotid atherosclerosis[25] and stroke,[81] the strength of association between hypertension and progression of carotid disease varies among studies. While Javid and colleagues[82] have identified hypertension as a significant predictor of the likelihood of carotid atheroma progression, Roederer et al[65] failed to show a significant relationship between any component of blood pressure and progression of carotid disease. Nonetheless, all in all, the preponderance of evidence does support the observation that blood pressure, particularly pulse pressure, is an important predictor of the presence[83] and progression[77] of carotid stenosis.

Cigarette smoking

Cigarette smoking initiates a variety of dose-dependent prothrombotic properties at both the platelet and coagulation levels and is a prominent risk factor of advanced atherogenesis.[84] Smoking has been established as a risk factor for occurrence of severe carotid artery disease[23] and stroke[85] in a dose-dependent manner. Furthermore, the risk burden of advanced atherogenesis normalizes after smoking cessation, consistent with a reversible procoagulant state.[25]

These data are consistent with the findings of Roederer and colleagues[65] who reported that the risk of carotid disease progression was 47% for patients who continued to smoke, 34% for those who quit smoking, and 24% in those who had never smoked. Interestingly, this relationship was not evident in a study of 965 patients reported by Garvey et al.[77] This may be partly due to the fact that 90% of patients in this study admitted to smoking at some point in time.

Lipids

Epidemiological research almost unequivocally suggests a central role for hyperlipidemia in early carotid atherogenesis. However, the reported impact of hyperlipidemia on carotid disease progression has been less consistent. Garvey and associates[77] reported that a low high-density lipoprotein (HDL) level is the only blood lipid level significant for progression of carotid stenosis. They postulated that this may be due to the older age of their patient cohort, since HDL levels remain relatively stable throughout life while low-density lipoprotein (LDL) and total cholesterol levels peak from age 45–60 years and decline thereafter.[74] Furthermore, Willeit and associates[25] found that while hyperlipidemia played a major role in the development of early carotid atherosclerosis, its role in disease progression was less evident. Nonetheless, they found that a lipoprotein (a) (Lp(a)) level >0.32 g/L is one of the strongest risk predictors of advanced carotid atherosclerosis. This finding is substantiated by serial angiography evaluations of coronary arteries that identified elevated Lp(a) as one of the leading indicators of rapid disease progression.[86]

Incidence of cognitive impairment

Cognitive impairment is common in the elderly, with a prevalence of 25% in those ≥65 years old.[87] It is associated with disability, institutionalization, and early death.[88] Cerebral infarction contributes to cognitive impairment in approximately 50% of cases,[88] even in patients without history of stroke or transient ischemic attack.[89] Furthermore, brain hypoperfusion may result in ischemic injury without evidence of infarction.[90] Some studies have suggested that even mild stenosis of the internal carotid artery may be a risk factor for cognitive impairment even in persons without a history of stroke,[91] but other studies have not demonstrated such an association.[92]

Some argue that carotid artery disease is associated with underlying vascular disease and its risk factors that may cause ischemic injury to the brain and cognitive impairment independent of carotid disease.[93–95] However, a recent study by Johnston and colleagues[96] advances intriguing possibilities regarding the relationship between high-grade left internal carotid artery disease and cognitive impairment. This study demonstrates that patients with high-grade left internal carotid artery stenosis did actually suffer from cognitive impairment and decline as assessed by the modified mini-mental state examination. This association was particularly strong and persisted after adjustment for contralateral disease and risk factors for vascular disease. The lack of cognitive impairment in patients with right carotid artery stenosis argues against the hypothesis that high-grade stenosis of the internal carotid artery is simply a marker for vascular disease and its risk factors. Rather, it is consistent with a direct link between stenosis of the internal carotid artery and brain dysfunction that results in cognitive impairment. Of course, it is also possible that a high-grade stenosis of the right internal carotid artery may be associated with impairment in measures of right hemispheric function, but this needs to be studied. Although the exact reasons for the association between left internal carotid stenosis and cognitive impairment are not entirely clear, it is likely that silent cerebral ischemia or hypoperfusion may be a cause.[97] Even though cognitive impairment can be caused by silent brain infarcts secondary to a carotid stentosis,[98,99] the association between cognitive impairment and high-grade left internal carotid artery stenosis was evident in participants without evidence of infarction on magnetic resonance imaging.

Several observational studies have suggested that cognitive function improves in some patients after endarterectomy[100] and recently after carotid stenting[101] but other studies have not demonstrated such an effect.[102] Future studies of therapy for internal carotid artery stenosis should consider performing long-term follow-up to evaluate cognitive impairment in persons with left-sided disease.

Incidence of neurological ischemic events

It is well-established that high-grade internal carotid artery stenosis is a marker for[103,104] as well as a cause of ischemic stroke.[105] In the Cardiovascular Health Study,[103] the presence of carotid stenosis was associated with a 3-fold increase in incidence of stroke irrespective of location and severity of plaque. Similarly, in the Rotterdam study,[104] the presence of carotid plaques increased the risk of anterior circulation cerebral infarction (lacunar and non-lacunar) 1.5-fold, irrespective of plaque location, with no clear difference in risk estimates between ipsilateral and contralateral infarction. However, other clinical studies in patients with more severe internal carotid artery stenosis demonstrated a clear link between asymptomatic CAS and ipsilateral neurological events. Chambers and Norris[106] followed 500 patients with neck bruits and varying degrees of carotid disease. At 1 year, they found that 87% of carotid ischemic events in previously asymptomatic patients occurred either in the carotid distribution ipsilateral to the stenosis in patients with unilateral disease or in either carotid distribution in patients with bilateral disease. Only 13% of events occurred in a carotid distribution without proximal stenosis.

It is clear that the presence of a carotid stenosis in a neurologically asymptomatic patient is both a marker and a cause of ischemic stroke. What remains at the center of debate is the variation in the frequency of ipsilateral ischemic neurological events and whether we can identify patients at high risk for these events prior to their occurrence.

What is the incidence of ipsilateral ischemic neurological events in patients with asymptomatic coronary artery stenosis?

When physicians encounter patients with asymptomatic atherosclerotic vascular disease, they often provide future risk estimates that are derived from population-based studies. Often, the similarities and differences between a particular patient condition and that of the population-based studies that are quoted are not considered. For example, when a patient inquires about the risk of suffering a stroke from an incidentally found, severe yet asymptomatic CAS, most physicians would quote a 2–3% annual risk of stroke. This estimate has been derived from several observational studies[107,108] as well as prospective randomized trials that compared medical therapy with carotid endarterectomy[109–111] in selected patient populations. Although this estimate certainly applies to a great number of patients in clinical practice, it would seem too simplistic to assume that all patients with an asymptomatic CAS have a similar risk of future stroke. The reported annual risk of ischemic stroke associated with asymptomatic CAS varies widely and ranges between 2% and 11.9% (Table 1.9). Three points, however, are worth noting to enable more insightful interpretation of these incidence rates:

1. The rate of ipsilateral ischemic neurological events that are due to asymptomatic CAS can be overestimated because not all ipsilateral strokes are related to the stenosis. In fact, one-third to one-half of these strokes may be related to lacunar infarcts or embolism from the heart.[116]
2. Conversely, the rate of ipsilateral ischemic neurological events can also be underestimated for two reasons: (a) the majority of patients in these studies have moderate carotid stenosis (<80% stenosis); (b) some studies have a very high rate of cardiac mortality that may lead to censoring of patients who may potentially be at high risk for stroke.
3. None of these studies have considered all the potential factors that may modulate stroke risk. Therefore, inter-study variability can simply represent differences in patient/lesion risk profiles.

The discrepancy among these studies is not only limited to the magnitude of future stroke risk but also extends to the factors that modulate this risk. The broad variance in reported stroke risk is worth noting, because this has led to significant discord among different specialties and clinicians with regard to the best management strategy (i.e. observation and medical therapy vs revascularization). This variance should not be dismissed as an act of chance; it is more likely an expression of risk heterogeneity among different patient cohorts.

Can we identify patients at high risk for an ipsilateral ischemic neurological event?

Despite the clear link between the presence of an asymptomatic CAS and ischemic stroke, our ability to predict which individual patient will have an acute ischemic neurological event remains meager at best. Although numerous studies have shown that patients with traditional cardiovascular risk factors are at an increased risk of having cardiovascular and cerebrovascular ischemic events,[118–120] many of these patients may actually remain free of adverse events during long-term follow-up.[121] Conversely, some patients who are at low risk for cardiovascular events, from a traditional risk profile perspective, may suffer an ischemic event. This is best illustrated by Khot and colleagues[17] who demonstrated that 53% of women and 62% of men who underwent coronary revascularization or had an acute coronary syndrome had only one or no traditional cardiovascular risk factors. This gap in predictability is due to the fact that there are still genetic and/or environmental factors that are not precisely measured or remain unknown. This illustrates that clinical decision-making regarding future stroke risk in individual patients cannot only be based on their traditional cardiovascular risk profile.

A complex interaction of factors, patient and lesion related, that are still incompletely understood, determine whether a particular stenosis becomes symptomatic. The most studied of these factors are carotid stenosis severity (see Table 1.9) and carotid stenosis progression (Table 1.10). These factors will be discussed in further detail in the risk stratification section of this book. The biological behavior of the asymptomatic carotid plaque will be discussed in Chapter 2; the hemodynamic factors in Chapter 3; the demographic and clinical variables in Chapter 7; carotid plaque composition, severity, and progression in Chapter 8; impaired cerebrovascular reserve in Chapter 10; plaque predisposition for spontaneous embolization in Chapter 9; and the inflammatory biomarkers in Chapter 11.

Table 1.9 Incidence of ipsilateral ischemic neurological events in patients with asymptomatic CAS according to lesion severity

Study	Study	Measurement method	Stenosis severity (%)	Number of patients	Annual events (%)	
					TIA	Stroke
Roederer[65] (1984)	Natural history study	Doppler US	≤80 >80	262 24	0.13 5.6	0.0 5.6
Chambers and Norris[106] (1986)	Natural history study	Doppler US	30–74 75–100	157 113		1.9 5.3
Hennerici[112] (1987)	Natural history study	Doppler US	50–80 >80	199 36		2.0 8.3
Norris[108] (1991)	Natural history study	Doppler US	50–75 >75	216 177	3.0 7.2	1.3 3.3
Bock[113] (1993)	Natural history study	Duplex US	50–79 80–99 Occluded	61 13 20		2.7 8.8 6.5
Veterans Cooperative Study[109] (1993)	RCT	Angiogram	>50	233		2.3
ACAS[110] (1995)	RCT	Duplex US	60–99	834		2.2
*ECST[114] (1995)	Subanalysis of RCT	Angiogram	30–69 70–99 Occlusion	843 127 55		0.7 1.9 1.2
Mackey et al[115] (1997)	Natural history study	Duplex US	<80 ≥80		2.0 6.3	1.3 3.6
*NASCET[116] (2000)	Retrospective analysis Subanalysis of RCT	Angiogram	60–99	216		3.2
ACST[111] (2004)	RCT	Duplex US	60–99	1560		3.2
ACSRS[117] (2005)	Natural history study	Duplex US	50–69 70–89 90–99	352 344 109	4.0 5.2 4.6	3.4 3.2 11.9

CAS, carotid artery stenosis; TIA, transient ischemic attack; RCT, randomized controlled trial; US, ultrasound.
*Outcome of asymptomatic CAS contralateral to a symptomatic carotid stenosis.

Table 1.10 Impact of carotid disease progression (to >80%) on incidence of ipsilateral TIA/stroke in patients with asymptomatic CAS

Study	Mean follow-up duration (years)	Rate of ipsilateral TIA/stroke	
		Disease progression (%)	No disease progression (%)
Roederer[65]	3.0	46	1.5
Mansour[66]	3.7	37.5	4.2
Mackey[115]	3.6	19.2	2.9
Muluk[68]	2.3	21.0	11.9

CAS, carotid artery stenosis; TIA, transient ischemic attack.

Cardiovascular morbidity and mortality

Numerous pathological[122–124] and epidemiological studies[125–127] have demonstrated a strong association between carotid and coronary disease in terms of prevalence and prognosis. Patients with asymptomatic CAS are at high risk not only for ischemic stroke but also for myocardial infarction and cardiac death.[128] In fact, carotid atherosclerotic disease doubles the risk of death from coronary disease.[121]

The frequency of cardiac vs cerebrovascular events in patients with asymptomatic carotid artery stenosis

Although numerous studies have demonstrated that patients with asymptomatic CAS are at higher risk for cardiac events than for ischemic stroke,[108,129] this observation cannot be generalized to all patients encountered in clinical practice. The risk of future ipsilateral ischemic stroke vs cardiac morbidity and mortality in a particular patient depends on the individual patient's risk profile. While some risk factors, such as hypertension, smoking, and diabetes, are known to increase the risk of both cardiovascular and cerebrovascular events, other factors are prognostically more predictive of one event rather than the other. For example, among patients with asymptomatic CAS, the presence of ischemic heart disease increases the risk of cardiac morbidity and mortality more than that of stroke,[130,131] while a higher grade of carotid stenosis is a more specific predictor for an ischemic stroke rather than a cardiac event.[115]

Illustrating this concept, Chimowitz and colleagues reported that among patients with asymptomatic CAS in the Veterans Affairs (VA) Cooperative study,[129] the 4-year risk of coronary events was significantly higher (40%) among those with a history of CAD than those without a history of CAD (33%). However, they also demonstrated that the rate of myocardial infarction

(MI) or sudden death far exceeds the rate of ipsilateral stroke, regardless of cardiac history. Nonetheless, the high frequency of coronary events in this study should not be generalized to all other patients with asymptomatic CAS, since these patients were all men with very high prevalence of smoking (~90%), peripheral arterial disease (~60%), and diabetes; all known to increase the risk of cardiac events.

Mackey and associates[115] prospectively followed 357 patients with asymptomatic CAS (≥50% stenosis) for ~3 years. Contrary to the findings by Chimowitz et al,[129] the annual rate of ischemic neurological events was higher (6.8%) than the annual rate of MI, unstable angina, and vascular death (4.2%). These differing results are probably due to exclusion of patients with atrial fibrillation, valvular heart disease, and recent MI from the latter study supporting the importance of the individual patient's risk profile in determining the cardiovascular vs cerebrovascular risk.

Cardiac mortality in patients with asymptomatic carotid artery stenosis

There have been numerous natural history studies of patients with asymptomatic CAS. The primary endpoint of many of these studies has been the development of neurological events and particularly stroke or progression of stenosis rather than cardiovascular death, but several of these studies have also reported mortality data. As shown in Table 1.11, the average mortality risk in patients with asymptomatic CAS is 5–6% per year (ranges from 1.5% to 12%). Cardiac death is, by far, the most common cause of mortality in these patients followed by non-vascular and stroke-related mortality (Table 1.11).

These observations have also been confirmed in population-based case–control studies.[135] However, debate continues as to whether the increased risk of cardiac mortality is primarily present in patients with known ischemic heart disease[130] or is independent from

Table 1.11 Long-term mortality in patients with asymptomatic CAS

Mortality	Hennerici[112] (n = 339)	Norris[108] (n = 393)	Mansour[66] (n = 142)	Mackey[115] (n = 15)	Nadareishvili[132] (n = 106)	Dick[133] (n = 525)	Kakkos[134] (n = 1101)
Carotid stenosis >50%	All	All	All	48%	55%	All	All
Follow-up (Mean, years)	2.4	3.3	3.7	3.2	10	3.2	3.2
Total:	24%	15%	14.1%	9.7%	16%	27%	15%
Stroke	12%	7%	30%	–	12%	–	–
Cardiac	50%	64%	40%	–	59%	–	–
Stroke and cardiac	62%	71%	70%	65%	71%	82%	64%
Other	38%	29%	30%	35%	29%	18%	36%

CAS, carotid artery stenosis. Long-term mortality in patients with asymptomatic CAS.

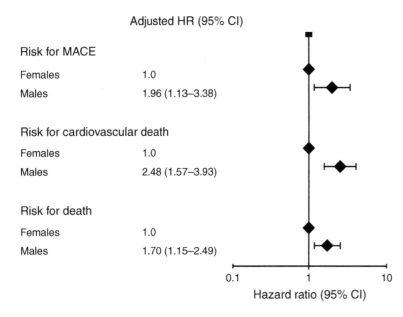

Figure 1.2 Adjusted hazard ratios for major adverse cardiovascular, cerebral, and peripheral vascular events (MACE), vascular mortality, and all-cause mortality in 525 patients with asymptomatic high-grade carotid artery stenosis undergoing conservative medical treatment. (Modified from Dick et al.[133])

the presence of clinically apparent coronary disease.[135] A thorough understanding of the cardiac prognosis of patients with asymptomatic CAS is critical to clinical decision-making with regard to medical management as well as triaging for coronary or carotid revascularization procedures. This topic will be discussed in further detail in Chapters 5 and 7.

Effects of gender on cardiac morbidity and mortality in patients with asymptomatic carotid artery stenosis

Among the various factors (coronary disease, peripheral arterial disease, hypertension) that are associated with increased future risk of fatal cardiovascular events[112,115,132] in patients with asymptomatic CAS, gender seems to play a pivotal role. Dick and associates[133] followed 525 consecutive patients (325 males with a median age of 72 years and 200 females with a median age of 75 years) with asymptomatic >70% carotid stenosis treated conservatively for a median of 38 months. Cumulative major adverse cardiac event-free survival rates in males and females at 1, 3, and 5 years were 83%, 65%, 48% vs 85%, 73%, and 67% (p <0.004), respectively. Males had higher total cardiovascular events, vascular mortality, and all-cause mortality than females, irrespective of age, vascular risk factors, and comorbidities (Figure 1.2).

The role of gender in determining prevalence and prognosis of asymptomatic CAS should be considered in clinical decision-making as well as in future studies.

SUMMARY

Fundamental to the care of patients with asymptomatic carotid artery disease is an appreciation that the prevalence and natural history of this disease vary widely among patients in clinical practice. The differing prevalence and natural history of carotid stenosis in neurologically asymptomatic patients is related to a diverse set of demographic, clinical, anatomical, and physiological variables, as well as genetic predisposition.

Although prevalence of asymptomatic CAS is low in the general population, patients with established atherosclerotic coronary or vascular disease are at a higher risk of having concomitant carotid disease. Patients with asymptomatic CAS are at higher risk for ischemic cerebrovascular and cardiovascular events. Determination of an individual's risk of future event, however, is an imprecise and difficult task. Population-based data cannot be automatically extrapolated to individual patients without consideration of the specific factors that are known to modulate this risk. Risk estimates relating to the prognosis of carotid disease in an asymptomatic individual should be based on the patient's risk profile as well as the results of the specific anatomical and physiological risk stratification modalities (see the Risk Stratification Section).

REFERENCES

1. Foulkes MA, Wolf PA, Price TR, Mohr JP, Hier DB. The Stroke Data Bank: design, methods, and baseline characteristics. Stroke 1998; 19(5): 547–54.
2. Bogousslavsky J, Van Melle G, Regli F. The Lausanne Stroke Registry: analysis of 1,000 consecutive patients with first stroke. Stroke 1988; 19(9): 1083–92.
3. Nagao T, Sadoshima S, Ibayashi S, Takeya Y, Fujishima M. Increase in extracranial atherosclerotic carotid lesions in patients with brain ischemia in Japan. An angiographic study. Stroke 1994; 25(4): 766–70.
4. Josse MO, Touboul PJ, Mas JL, Laplane D, Bousser MG. Prevalence of asymptomatic internal carotid artery stenosis. Neuroepidemiology 1987; 6(3): 150–2.
5. Salonen R, Seppanen K, Rauramaa R, Salonen JT. Prevalence of carotid atherosclerosis and serum cholesterol levels in eastern Finland. Arteriosclerosis 1988; 8: 788–92.
6. Colgan MP, Strode GR, Sommer JD, Gibbs JL, Sumner DS. Prevalence of asymptomatic carotid disease: results of duplex scanning in 348 unselected volunteers. J Vasc Surg 1988; 8(6): 674–8.
7. Fowl RJ, Marsch JG, Love M et al. Prevalence of hemodynamically significant stenosis of the carotid artery in an asymptomatic veteran population. Surg Gynecol Obstet 1991; 172(1): 13–16.
8. Jungquist G, Hanson BS, Isacsson SO et al. Risk factors for carotid artery stenosis: an epidemiological study of men aged 69 years. J Clin Epidemiol 1991; 44(4–5): 347–53.
9. O'Leary DH, Anderson KM, Wolf PA, Evans JC, Poehlman HW. Cholesterol and carotid atherosclerosis in older persons: the Framingham Study. Ann Epidemiol 1992; 2(1–2): 147–53.
10. O'Leary DH, Polak JF, Kronmal RA et al, on behalf of the CHS Collaborative Research Group. Distribution and correlates of sonographically detected carotid artery disease in the Cardiovascular Health Study. Stroke 1992; 23: 1752–60.
11. Prati P, Vanuzzo D, Casaroli M et al. Prevalence and determinants of carotid atherosclerosis in a general population. Stroke 1992; 23: 1705–11.
12. Pujia A, Rubba P, Spencer MP. Prevalence of extracranial carotid artery disease detectable by echo-Doppler in an elderly population. Stroke 1992; 3: 818–22.
13. Willeit J, Kiechl S. Prevalence and risk factors of asymptomatic extracranial carotid artery atherosclerosis: a population-based study. Arterioscler Thromb 1993; 13: 661–8.
14. Mannami T, Konishi M, Baba S, Nishi N, Terao A. Prevalence of asymptomatic carotid atherosclerotic lesions detected by high-resolution ultrasonography and its relation to cardiovascular risk factors in the general population of a Japanese city: the Suita study. Stroke 1997; 28: 518–25.
15. Fabris F, Zanocchi M, Bo M et al. Carotid plaque, aging, and risk factors: a study of 457 subjects. Stroke 1994; 25(6): 1133–40.
16. Joakimsen O, Bonaa KH, Stensland-Bugge E, Jacobsen BK. Age and sex differences in the distribution and ultrasound morphology of carotid atherosclerosis: the Tromso Study. Arterioscler Thromb Vasc Biol 1999; 19(12): 3007–13.
17. Khot UN, Khot MB, Bajzer CT et al. Prevalence of conventional risk factors in patients with coronary heart disease. JAMA 2003; 290(7): 898–904.
18. Grundy SM, Balady GJ, Criqui MH et al. Primary prevention of coronary heart disease: guidance from Framingham. A statement for healthcare professionals from the AHA Task Force on Risk Reduction. American Heart Association. Circulation 1998; 97(18): 1876–87.
19. Byington RP, Furberg CD, Herrington DM et al. Heart and Estrogen/Progestin Replacement Study Research Group. Effect of estrogen plus progestin on progression of carotid atherosclerosis in postmenopausal women with heart disease: HERS B-mode substudy. Arterioscler Thromb Vasc Biol 2002; 22(10): 1692–7.
20. De Angelis M, Scrucca L, Leandri M et al. Prevalence of carotid stenosis in type 2 diabetic patients asymptomatic for cerebrovascular disease. Diabetes Nutr Metab 2003; 16(1): 48–55.
21. Bonora E, Kiechlk S, Willeit J et al. Carotid atherosclerosis and coronary heart disease in the metabolic syndrome. Prospective data from the Bruneck Study. Diabetes Care 2003; 26: 1251–7.
22. Tell GS, Polak JF, Ward BJ et al. Relation of smoking with carotid artery wall thickness and stenosis in older adults. The Cardiovascular Health Study. The Cardiovascular Health Study (CHS) Collaborative Research Group. Circulation 1994; 90(6): 2905–8.
23. Whisnant J, Homer D, Ingall T et al. Duration of cigarette smoking is the strongest predictor of severe extracranial carotid artery atherosclerosis. Stroke 1990; 21: 707–14.
24. Risley P, Jerrard-Dunne P, Sitzer M et al. Carotid Atherosclerosis Progression Study. Promoter polymorphism in the endotoxin receptor (CD14) is associated with increased carotid atherosclerosis only in smokers: the Carotid Atherosclerosis Progression Study (CAPS). Stroke 2003; 34(3): 600–4.
25. Willeit J, Kiechl S, Oberhollenzer F et al. Distinct risk profiles of early and advanced atherosclerosis: prospective results from the Bruneck study. Arterioscler Thromb Vasc Biol 2000; 20: 529–37.

26. Su TC, Jeng JS, Chien KL et al. Hypertension status is the major determinant of carotid atherosclerosis: a community-based study in Taiwan. Stroke 2001; 32: 2265–71.

27. Luedemann J, Schminke U, Berger K et al. Association between behavior-dependent cardiovascular risk factors and asymptomatic carotid atherosclerosis in a general population. Stroke 2002; 33(12): 2929–35.

28. Wilson W, Hoeg J, D'Agostino R et al. Cumulative effects of high cholesterol levels, high blood pressure, and cigarette smoking on carotid stenosis. N Engl J Med 1997; 337: 516–22.

29. van der Meer IM, de Maat MP, Bots ML et al. Inflammatory mediators and cell adhesion molecules as indicators of severity of atherosclerosis: the Rotterdam Study. Arterioscler Thromb Vasc Biol 2002; 22(5): 838–42.

30. Schmidt H, Schmidt R, Niederkorn K et al. Beta-fibrinogen gene polymorphism (C148→T) is associated with carotid atherosclerosis: results of the Austrian Stroke Prevention Study. Arterioscler Thromb Vasc Biol 1998; 18(3): 487–92.

31. Welch GN, Loscalzo J. Homocysteine and atherothrombosis. N Engl J Med 1998; 338(15): 1042–50.

32. Roman MJ, Shanker BA, Davis A et al. Prevalence and correlates of accelerated atherosclerosis in systemic lupus erythematosus. N Engl J Med 2003; 349(25): 2399–406.

33. Roman MJ, Moeller E, Davis A et al. Preclinical carotid atherosclerosis in patients with rheumatoid arthritis. Ann Intern Med 2006; 144(4): 249–56.

34. Hunt KJ, Duggirala R, Goring HH et al. Genetic basis of variation in carotid artery plaque in the San Antonio Family Heart Study. Stroke 2002; 33: 2775–80.

35. Chen WH, Ho DS, Ho SL, Cheung RT, Cheng SW. Prevalence of extracranial carotid and vertebral artery disease in Chinese patients with coronary artery disease. Stroke 1998; 29: 631–4.

36. Kallikazaros I, Tsioufis C, Sideris S, Stefanadis C, Toutouzas P. Carotid artery disease as a marker for the presence of severe coronary artery disease in patients evaluated for chest pain. Stroke 1999; 30: 1002–7.

37. Zimarino M, Cappelletti L, Venarucci V et al. Age-dependence of risk factors for carotid stenosis: an observational study among candidates for coronary arteriography. Atherosclerosis 2001; 159: 165–73.

38. Ambrosetti M, Casorati P, Salerno M et al. Newly diagnosed carotid atherosclerosis in patients with coronary artery disease admitted for cardiac rehabilitation. Ital Heart J 2004; 5(11): 840–3.

39. Komorovsky R, Desideri A, Coscarelli S, Cortigiani L, Celegon L. Impact of carotid arterial narrowing on outcomes of patients with acute coronary syndromes. Am J Cardiol 2004; 93: 1552–5.

40. Tanimoto S, Ikari Y, Tanabe K et al. Prevalence of carotid artery stenosis in patients with coronary artery disease in Japanese population. Stroke 2005; 36: 2094–8.

41. Lanzer P. Vascular multimorbidity in patients with a documented coronary artery disease. Z Kardiol 2003; 92(8): 650–9.

42. Barnes RW, Nix ML, Sansonetti D, Turley DG, Goldman MR. Late outcome of untreated asymptomatic carotid disease following cardiovascular operations. J Vasc Surg 1985; 2(6): 843–9.

43. Faggioli GL, Curl GR, Ricotta JJ. The role of carotid screening before coronary artery bypass. J Vasc Surg 1990; 12(6): 724–9.

44. Vigneswaran WT, Sapsford RN, Stanbridge RD. Disease of the left main coronary artery: early surgical results and their association with carotid artery stenosis. Br Heart J 1993; 70(4): 342–5.

45. D'Agostino RS, Svensson LG, Neumann DJ et al. Screening carotid ultrasonography and risk factors for stroke in coronary artery surgery patients. Ann Thorac Surg 1996; 62: 1714–23.

46. Birincioglu L, Arda K, Bardakci H et al. Carotid disease in patients scheduled for coronary artery bypass: analysis of 678 patients. Angiology 1999; 50(1): 9–19.

47. Rath PC, Agarwala MK, Dhar PK et al. Carotid artery involvement in patients of atherosclerotic coronary artery disease undergoing coronary artery bypass grafting. Indian Heart J 2001; 53(6): 761–5.

48. Kawarada O, Yokoi Y, Morioka N et al. Carotid stenosis and peripheral artery disease in Japanese patients with coronary artery disease undergoing coronary artery bypass grafting. Circ J 2003; 67: 1003–6.

49. Crouse JR, Toole JF, McKinney WM et al. Risk factors for extracranial carotid artery atherosclerosis. Stroke 1987; 18(6): 990–6.

50. Ogren M, Hedblad B, Isacsson SO et al. Ten year cerebrovascular morbidity and mortality in 68 year old men with asymptomatic carotid stenosis. BMJ 1995; 310: 1294–8.

51. Ahn SS, Baker JD, Walden K, Moore WS. Which asymptomatic patients should undergo routine screening carotid duplex scan? Am J Surg 1991; 162: 180–4.

52. Klop RB, Eikelboom BC, Taks AC. Screening of the internal carotid arteries in patients with peripheral vascular disease by colour-flow duplex scanning. Eur J Vasc Surg 1991; 5: 41–5.

53. Gentile AT, Taylor LM, Moneta GL, Porter JM. Prevalence of asymptomatic carotid stenosis in patients undergoing infrainguinal bypass surgery. Arch Surg 1995; 130: 900–4.

54. Marek J, Mills JL, Harvich J, Cui H, Fujitani RM. Utility of routine carotid duplex screening in patients who have claudication. J Vasc Surg 1996; 24: 572–7.

55. Alexandrova NA, Gibson WC, Norris JW, Maggisano R. Carotid artery stenosis in peripheral vascular disease. J Vasc Surg 1996; 23: 645–9.

56. de Virgilio C, Toosie K, Arnell T et al. Asymptomatic carotid artery stenosis screening in patients with lower extremity atherosclerosis: a prospective study. Ann Vasc Surg 1997; 11: 374–7.

57. Simons PCG, Algra A, van der Graaf Y, Eikelboom BC, Grobbee DE, for the SMART Study Group. Carotid artery stenosis in patients with peripheral arterial disease: the SMART study. J Vasc Surg 1999; 30: 519–25.

58. Ballotta E, Da Giau G, Renon L et al. Symptomatic and asymptomatic carotid artery lesions in peripheral vascular disease: a prospective study. Int J Surg Investig 1999; 1(4): 357–63.

59. Pilcher JM, Danaher J, Khaw KT. The prevalence of asymptomatic carotid artery disease in patients with peripheral vascular disease. Clin Radiol 2000; 55: 56–61.

60. Cina CS, Safar HA, Maggisano R, Bailey R, Clase CM. Prevalence and progression of internal carotid artery stenosis in patients with peripheral arterial occlusive disease. J Vasc Surg 2002; 36: 75–82.

61. Louie J, Isaacson JA, Zierler RE, Bergelin RO, Strandness DE Jr. Prevalence of carotid and lower extremity arterial disease in patients with renal artery stenosis. Am J Hypertens 1994; 7(5): 436–9.

62. Missouris CG, Papavassiliou MB, Khaw K et al. High prevalence of carotid artery disease in patients with atheromatous renal artery stenosis. Nephrol Dial Transplant 1998; 13: 945–8.

63. Bertges DJ, Muluk V, Whittle J et al. Relevance of carotid stenosis progression as a predictor of ischemic neurological outcomes. Arch Intern Med 2003; 136: 2285–9.

64. Patel ST, Kuntz KM, Kent KC. Is routine duplex ultrasound surveillance after carotid endarterectomy cost-effective? Surgery 1998; 124: 343–51.

65. Roederer GO, Langlois YE, Jager KA et al. The natural history of carotid arterial disease in asymptomatic patients with cervical bruits. Stroke 1984; 15: 605–13.

66. Mansour MA, Mattos MA, Faught WE et al. The natural history of moderate (50% to 79%) internal carotid artery stenosis in symptomatic, nonhemispheric, and asymptomatic patients. J Vasc Surg 1995; 21: 346–58.

67. Lewis RF, Abrahamowicz M, Cote R, Battista RN. Predictive power of duplex ultrasonography in asymptomatic carotid disease. Ann Intern Med 1997; 127: 13–20.

68. Muluk SC, Muluk VS, Sugimoto H et al. Progression of asymptomatic carotid stenosis: a natural history study in 1004 patients. J Vasc Surg 1999; 29: 208–16.

69. Martin-Conejero A, Reina-Gutierrez T, Serrano-Hernando FJ et al. Disease progression in the contralateral carotid artery after endarterectomy. Ann Vasc Surg 2005; 19(5): 662–8.

70. Sabeti S, Exner M, Mlekusch W et al. Prognostic impact of fibrinogen in carotid atherosclerosis: nonspecific indicator of inflammation or independent predictor of disease progression? Stroke 2005; 36(7): 1400–4.

71. Roth SM, Back RM, Bandyk DF et al. A rational algorithm for duplex scan surveillance after carotid endarterectomy. J Vasc Surg 1999; 30: 453–60.

72. Raman KG, Layne S, Makaroun MS et al. Disease progression in the contralateral carotid artery after endarterectomy. Ann Vasc Surg 2005; 19: 662–8.

73. Takaya N, Yuan C, Chu B et al. Presence of intraplaque hemorrhage stimulates progression of carotid atherosclerotic plaques: a high-resolution magnetic resonance imaging study. Circulation 2005; 111: 2768–75.

74. Wilson P, Anderson K, Harris T, Kannel W, Castelli W. Determinants of change in total cholesterol and HDL-C with age: the Framingham study. J Gerontol 1994; 49: M252–7.

75. Schillinger M, Exner M, Mlekusch W et al. Inflammation and Carotid Artery – Risk for Atherosclerosis Study (ICARAS). Circulation 2005; 111(17): 2203–9.

76. Delcker A, Diener HC, Wilhelm H. Influence of vascular risk factors for atherosclerotic carotid artery plaque progression. Stroke 1995; 26: 2016–22.

77. Garvey L, Makaroun MS, Muluk VS, Webster MW, Muluk SC. Etiologic factors in progression of carotid stenosis: a 10-year study in 905 patients. J Vasc Surg 2000; 31: 31–8.

78. Iemolo F, Martiniuk A, Steinman DA, Spence JD. Sex differences in carotid plaque and stenosis. Stroke 2004; 35: 477–81.

79. Schulz UG, Rothwell PM. Sex differences in carotid bifurcation anatomy and the distribution of atherosclerotic plaque. Stroke 2001; 32: 1525–31.

80. Schneider DJ, Nordt TK, Sobel BE. Attenuated fibrinolysis and accelerated atherogenesis in type II diabetic patients. Diabetes 1993; 42: 1–7.

81. Kannel WB, Dawber TR, Sortie P, Wolf PA. Component of blood pressure and risk of atherothrombotic brain infarction: the Framingham study. Stroke 1976; 7: 327–31.

82. Javid H, Ostermiller WE Jr, Hengesh JW et al. Natural history of carotid bifurcation atheroma. Surgery 1970; 67: 80–6.

83. Franklin S, Sutton-Tyrell K, Belle S, Weber M, Kuller L. The importance of pulsatile components of hypertension in predicting carotid stenosis in older adults. J Hypertens 1997; 15: 1143–50.

84. McGill HC. Smoking and the pathogenesis of atherosclerosis. Adv Exp Med Biol 1990; 273: 9–16.

85. Gorelick P. Stroke prevention. Arch Neurol 1995; 52: 347–55.

86. Terres W, Tatsis E, Pfalzer B et al. Rapid angiographic progression of coronary artery disease in patients with elevated lipoprotein(a). Circulation 1995; 91: 948–50.

87. Graham JE, Rockwood K, Beattie BL et al. Prevalence and severity of cognitive impairment with and without dementia in an elderly population. Lancet 1997; 349: 1793–6.

88. Rockwood K, Wentzel C, Hachinski V et al. Prevalence and outcomes of vascular cognitive impairment. Vascular Cognitive Impairment Investigators of the Canadian Study of Health and Aging. Neurology 2000; 54: 447–51.

89. Price TR, Manolio TA, Kronmal RA et al. Silent brain infarction on magnetic resonance imaging and neurological abnormalities in community-dwelling older adults. The Cardiovascular Health Study. CHS Collaborative Research Group. Stroke 1997; 28: 1158–64.

90. Pullicino PM, Hart J. Cognitive impairment in congestive heart failure? Embolism vs hypoperfusion [Editorial]. Neurology 2001; 57: 1945–6.

91. Mathiesen EB, Waterloo K, Joakimsen O et al. Reduced neuropsychological test performance in asymptomatic carotid stenosis: The Tromsø Study. Neurology 2004; 62: 695–701.

92. Rao R. The role of carotid stenosis in vascular cognitive impairment. Eur Neurol 2001; 46: 63–9.

93. Goldstein LB, Adams R, Becker K et al. Primary prevention of ischemic stroke: a statement for healthcare professionals from the Stroke Council of the American Heart Association. Stroke 2001; 32: 280–99.

94. Rockwood K, Ebly E, Hachinski V, Hogan D. Presence and treatment of vascular risk factors in patients with vascular cognitive impairment. Arch Neurol 1997; 54: 33–9.

95. Knopman D, Boland LL, Mosley T et al. Cardiovascular risk factors and cognitive decline in middle-aged adults. Neurology 2001; 56: 42–8.

96. Johnston SC, O'Meara ES, Manolio TA et al. Cognitive impairment and decline are associated with carotid artery disease in patients without clinically evident cerebrovascular disease. Ann Intern Med 2004; 140: 237–47.

97. de la Torre JC. Critically attained threshold of cerebral hypoperfusion: can it cause Alzheimer's disease? Ann N Y Acad Sci 2000; 903: 424–36.

98. Manolio TA, Burke GL, O'Leary DH et al. Relationships of cerebral MRI findings to ultrasonographic carotid atherosclerosis in older adults: the Cardiovascular Health Study. CHS Collaborative Research Group. Arterioscler Thromb Vasc Biol 1999; 19: 356–65.

99. de Groot JC, de Leeuw FE, Oudkerk M et al. Cerebral white matter lesions and subjective cognitive dysfunction: the Rotterdam Scan Study. Neurology 2001; 56: 1539–45.

100. Greiffenstein MF, Brinkman S, Jacobs L, Braun P. Neuropsychological improvement following endarterectomy as a function of outcome measure and reconstructed vessel. Cortex 1988; 24: 223–30.

101. Grunwald I, Supprian T, Struffert T et al. Cognitive changes after carotid artery stenting. Radiological Society of North America Meeting (RSNA), November 2005: E350.

102. Pettigrew LC, Thomas N, Howard VJ, Veltkamp R, Toole JF. Low mini-mental status predicts mortality in asymptomatic carotid arterial stenosis. Asymptomatic Carotid Atherosclerosis Study investigators. Neurology 2000; 55: 30–4.

103. Manolio TA, Kronmal RA, Burke GL, O'Leary DH, Price TR, for the CHS Collaborative Research Group. Short-term predictors of incident stroke in older adults. The Cardiovascular Health Study Stroke 1996; 27: 1479–86.

104. Hollander M, Bots ML, Iglesias del Sol A et al. Carotid plaques increase the risk of stroke and subtypes of cerebral infarction in asymptomatic elderly. The Rotterdam Study. Circulation 2002; 105: 2872–7.

105. Sacco RL, Benjamin EJ, Broderick JP et al. American Heart Association Prevention Conference. IV. Prevention and Rehabilitation of Stroke. Risk factors. Stroke 1997; 28: 1507–17.

106. Chambers BR, Norris JW. Outcome in patients with asymptomatic neck bruits. N Engl J Med 1986; 315: 860–5.

107. Goldstein LB, Adams R, Becker K et al. Primary prevention of ischemic stroke: a statement for healthcare professionals from the Stroke Council of the American Heart Association. Stroke 2001; 32: 280–99.

108. Norris JW, Zhu CZ, Bornstein NM, Chambers BR. Vascular risks of asymptomatic carotid stenosis. Stroke 1991; 22: 1485–90.

109. Hobson RW, Weiss DG, Fields WS et al. Efficacy of carotid endarterectomy for asymptomatic carotid stenosis. N Engl J Med 1993; 328: 221–7.

110. Executive Committee for the Asymptomatic Carotid Atherosclerosis Study. Endarterectomy for asymptomatic carotid stenosis. JAMA 1995; 273: 1421–8.

111. MRC Asymptomatic Carotid Surgery Trial (ACST) Collaborative Group. Prevention of disabling and fatal strokes by successful carotid endarterectomy in patients without recent neurological symptoms: randomized controlled trial. Lancet 2004; 363: 1491–502.

112. Hennerici M, Hülsbömer HB, Hefter H, Lammerts D, Rautenberg W. Natural history of asymptomatic extracranial arterial disease. Results of a long-term prospective study. Brain 1987; 110(Pt 3): 777–91.

113. Bock RW, Gray-Weale AC, Mock PA et al. The natural history of asymptomatic carotid artery disease. J Vasc Surg 1993; 17(1): 160–9.

114. The European Carotid Surgery Trialists Collaborative Group. Risk of stroke in the distribution of an asymptomatic carotid artery. Lancet 1995; 345: 209–12.

115. Mackey AE, Abrahamowicz M, Langlois Y et al. Outcome of asymptomatic patients with carotid disease. Neurology 1997; 48: 896–903.

116. Inzitari D, Eliasziw M, Gates P et al. The causes and risk of stroke in patients with asymptomatic internal-carotid-artery stenosis. N Engl J Med 2000; 342: 1693–700.

117. Nicolaides AN, Kakkos SK, Griffin M et al, for the Asymptomatic Carotid Stenosis and Risk of Stroke (ACSRS) Study Group. Severity of asymptomatic carotid stenosis and risk of ipsilateral hemispheric ischaemic events: results from the ACSRS study. Eur J Vasc Endovasc Surg 2005; 30: 275–84.

118. Psaty BM, Furberg CD, Kuller LH et al. Traditional risk factors and subclinical disease measures as predictors of first myocardial infarction in older adults: the Cardiovascular Health Study. Arch Intern Med 1999; 159(12): 1339–47.

119. Hsia J, Aragaki A, Bloch M, LaCroix AZ, Wallace R, WHI Investigators. Predictors of angina pectoris versus myocardial infarction from the Women's Health Initiative Observational Study. Am J Cardiol 2004; 93(6): 673–8.

120. Dembroski TM, MacDougall JM, Costa PT Jr, Grandits GA. Components of hostility as predictors of sudden death and myocardial infarction in the Multiple Risk Factor Intervention Trial. Psychosom Med 1989; 51(5): 514–22.

121. Wolf S. Predictors of myocardial infarction over a span of 30 years in Roseto, Pennsylvania. Integr Physiol Behav Sci 1992; 27(3): 246–57.

122. Young W, Gofman JW, Tandy R. The quantification of atherosclerosis III. The extent of correlation of degrees of atherosclerosis within and between the coronary and cerebral vascular beds. Am J Cardiol 1960; 6: 300–8.

123. Mitchell JRA, Schwartz CJ. Relationship between arterial disease in different sites. A study of the aorta and coronary, carotid and iliac arteries. Br Med J 1962: 1293–301.

124. Mathur KS, Kashyap SK, Kumar V. Correlation and the extent and severity of atherosclerosis in the coronary and cerebral arteries. Circulation 1963; 27: 929–34.

125. Howard G, Ryu JE, Evans GW. Extracranial carotid atherosclerosis in patients with and without transient ischemic attacks and coronary artery disease. Arteriosclerosis 1990; 10: 714–19.

126. Tanaka H, Nishino M, Ishida M. Progression of carotid atherosclerosis in Japanese patients with coronary artery disease. Stroke 1992; 23: 946–51.

127. Crouse JR 3rd. Carotid and coronary atherosclerosis. What are the connections? Postgrad Med 1991; 90: 175–9.

128. Belcaro G, Nicolaides AN, Ramaswami G et al. Carotid and femoral ultrasound morphology screening and cardiovascular events in low risk subjects: a 10-year follow-up study (the CAFES-CAVE study). Atherosclerosis 2001; 156: 379–87.

129. Chimowitz MI, Weiss DG, Cohen SL, Starling MR, Hobson RW 2nd. Cardiac prognosis of patients with carotid stenosis and no history of coronary artery disease. Veterans Affairs Cooperative Study Group 167. Stroke 1994; 25(4): 759–65.

130. Hedblad B, Janzon L, Jungquist G, Ogren M. Factors modifying the prognosis in men with asymptomatic carotid artery disease. J Intern Med 1998; 243(1): 57–64.

131. Love BB, Grover-McKay M, Biller J, Rezai K, McKay CR. Coronary artery disease and cardiac events with asymptomatic and symptomatic cerebrovascular disease. Stroke 1992; 23: 939–45.

132. Nadareishvili ZG, Rothwell PM, Beletsky V, Pagniello A, Norris JW. Long-term risk of stroke and other vascular events in patients with asymptomatic carotid artery stenosis. Arch Neurol 2002; 59(7): 1162–6.

133. Dick P, Sherif C, Sabeti S et al. The role of gender is clearly illustrated by gender differences in outcome of conservatively treated patients with asymptomatic high grade carotid stenosis. Stroke 2005; 36: 1178–83.

134. Kakkos SK, Nicolaides AN, Griffin M et al, for the Asymptomatic Carotid Stenosis and Risk of Stroke (ACSRS) Study Group. Factors associated with mortality in patients with asymptomatic carotid stenosis: results from the ACSRS Study. Int Angiol 2002; 59(7): 1162–6.

135. Joakimsen O, Bonaa KH, Mathiesen EB, Stensland-Bugge E, Arnesen E. Prediction of mortality by ultrasound screening of a general population for carotid stenosis: the Tromso Study. Stroke 2000; 31: 1871–6.

2

Pathobiology of the asymptomatic atherosclerotic carotid plaque

Giuseppe Sangiorgi, Alessandro Mauriello, Frank Kolodgie, Santi Trimarchi, Giuseppe Biondi Zoccai, Renu Virmani and Luigi Giusto Spagnoli

---

Take-Home Messages

1. Vascular atherosclerotic lesions can be divided into three groups: (1) non-atherosclerotic intimal lesions; (2) progressive atherosclerotic lesions; and (3) healed atherosclerotic plaque, which is the most prevalent plaque feature in patients with asymptomatic carotid disease.
2. Progression of atherosclerotic disease in the carotid artery occurs primarily through repeated plaque rupture and erosions.
3. Plaques prone to rupture are those with reduced cap thickness, large necrotic-lipid core, and severe inflammatory infiltrate.
4. Recently, intraplaque hemorrhage secondary to rupture of the intraplaque vasa vasorum has been advocated as a mechanism for carotid plaque vulnerability.
5. The timing of transformation of a stable carotid plaque to an unstable one is unpredictable and its triggering mechanisms remain an active area of investigation.
6. Local triggers of plaque instability include shear stress, proteolytic enzymes, and other biological factors. Systemic triggers include inflammatory and non-inflammatory factors such as vascular adhesion molecules, fibrinogen, matrix metalloproteinases (MMPs), and genetic polymorphisms.

INTRODUCTION

The atherosclerotic plaque at the carotid bifurcation is an example of the advanced fibrous plaque found at sites of predilection throughout the arterial system (Figure 2.1). Carotid atherosclerotic plaques are composed of a dense cap of connective tissue embedded with a few smooth muscle cells, overlying a core of lipidic and necrotic debris. Typically, the accumulating plaque burden is initially accommodated by an adaptive positive remodeling with expansion of the vessel external elastic lamina and minimal changes in lumen size.[1] The plaque contains monocyte-derived macrophages, smooth muscle cells, and T lymphocytes. Interaction between these cell types and the connective tissue appears to determine the development and progression of the plaque itself, including important complications, such as thrombosis and rupture.

In this chapter we will review the natural history of atherosclerotic carotid plaque development, the transformation of a stable carotid plaque to a vulnerable one, and the underlying mechanisms that may trigger this transformation.

DEVELOPMENT AND TRANSFORMATION OF THE ATHEROSCLEROTIC CAROTID PLAQUE

A new classification of atherosclerotic plaques has been proposed by Virmani and associates[2,3] modifying the original classification of the American Heart Association (AHA).[4,5] Despite the fact that this modified classification is derived from observations of coronary plaques from patients who died suddenly, it may be applied also to carotid atherosclerotic disease (Figure 2.2).

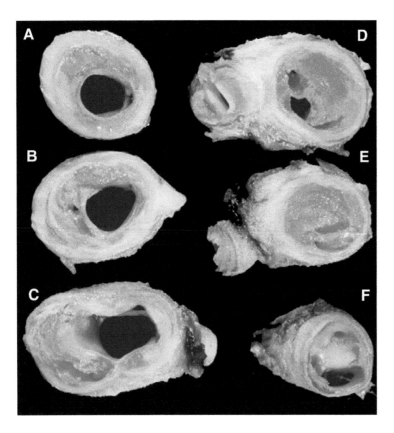

Figure 2.1 Gross bisected specimens of a severe stenotic asymptomatic atherosclerotic lesion at the level of the common carotid (A, B), bifurcation (C, D), and internal carotid artery (E, F). (See color plate section.)

Atherosclerotic lesions have been divided into two groups: non-atherosclerotic intimal lesions and progressive atherosclerotic lesions. A third group of lesions, comprising healed atherosclerotic plaque, is in our experience the most prevalent plaque feature in patients with asymptomatic carotid disease (Table 2.1).

Similarly to what has been found for coronary atherosclerotic plaques, different morphological appearances of carotid lesions largely depend on the status of the fibrous cap, and in particular on its thickness and grade of inflammatory infiltrate, which in turn is largely constituted by macrophages and activated T lymphocytes.

Non-atherosclerotic intimal lesions

Most adult human lesions originate as pre-existing intimal lesions consisting of adaptive intimal thickening that probably remains distinct from intimal xanthomas.

Intimal thickening

While some human lesions may begin as intimal xanthomata, there is an agreement that most adult human lesions originate as pre-existing intimal thickening. Intimal thickening consists mainly of smooth muscle cells in a proteoglycan-rich matrix. It has been demonstrated

that the distribution of these normal, developmental intimal masses in children can be correlated with the distribution of atherosclerotic lesions seen in adult humans.[6] There is very little evidence of cell replication except in early lesions, yet smooth muscle cells of adult lesions are usually clonal.[6] The observations of Tabas et al,[7] who found that the extracellular matrix of intimal thickening may contain enzymes capable of retaining lipids, may justify a role of these lesions in the initial events that contribute to the development of necrotic core. Unfortunately, there are very few investigations on the evolution of early intimal lesions in humans, and none of these clarify their precise pathological mechanisms of development.

Intimal xanthomata

This lesion corresponds to the 'fatty streak' of AHA's scheme and is characterized by an intimal accumulation of fat-laden macrophages. These types of lesions may contain few smooth muscle cells and T lymphocytes. In humans, most of these intimal xanthomata regress,[8,9] since the distribution of lesions in the third decade of life and beyond is very different from the fatty streaks seen in children.

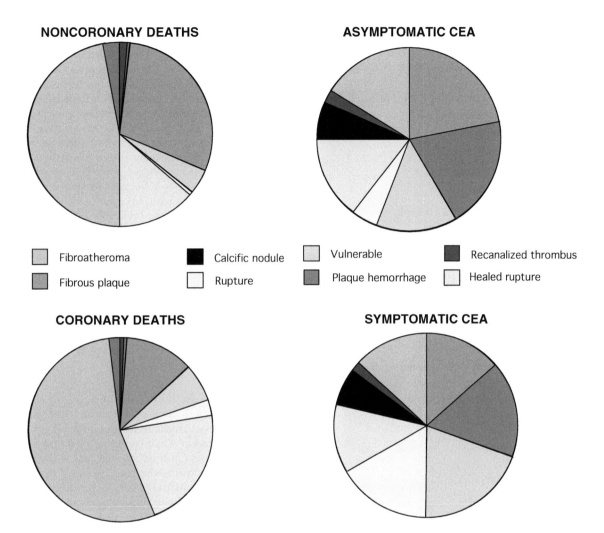

Figure 2.2 Distribution of different plaque types in the coronary and carotid districts based on patient clinical status (non-sudden and sudden coronary death vs symptomatic and asymptomatic carotid patients. CEA, carotid endarterectomy. (See color plate section.)

Progressive atherosclerotic lesions

Stable plaques

Pathological intimal thickening

The pathological intimal thickening (Figure 2.3) is a poorly defined entity sometimes referred to in the literature as 'intermediate lesions'.[4] This type of plaque does not encroach on the lumen and is constituted by an intimal thickening associated with some deep lipid deposition. True necrosis is not evident. The area overlying the lipid core is rich in smooth muscle cells and proteoglycans and may contain a variable number of macrophages

and T lymphocytes.[2] It has been demonstrated that in the coronaries the majority of erosions occur over areas of pathological intimal thickening, giving rise to a clinically significant role for these lesions. Our observations in the carotid artery of asymptomatic patients seem to confirm this (pers comm Sangiorgi G). In 5% of patients with a vulnerable or ruptured plaque in the internal carotid artery, we observed the presence of an underlying pathological intimal thickening lesion.

Fibrous cap atheromata

A fibrous cap atheromata (Figure 2.4) consists of a large lipidic-necrotic core comprising large amounts of

Table 2.1 Various plaques types (modified Virmani classification[2]) obtained from asymptomatic patients and usually observed at the histological examination

Non-atherosclerotic intimal lesions
    Intimal thickening
    Intimal xanthomata

Progressive atherosclerotic lesions
    Stable plaques:

- Pathological intimal thickening
- Fibrous cap atheromata
- Fibrocalcific lesions
- Plaque hemorrhage

    Vulnerable plaques:

- Thin fibrous cap atheromata
- Calcified nodule

    Lesions with acute thrombi:

- Plaque rupture with luminal thrombus
- Plaque rupture with ulceration
- Plaque rupture with organizing thrombus
- Plaque erosion
- Calcified nodule

Healed lesions

    Healed erosion
    Healed rupture
    Total occlusion

extracellular lipid, cholesterol crystals, and necrotic debris, surrounded by a thick fibrous cap consisting principally of smooth muscle cells in a collagenous-proteoglycan matrix, with varying degrees of infiltration of macrophages and T lymphocytes.[2] A variable number of inflammatory cells surround the lipidic-necrotic core. This lesion, according to the AHA classification which distinguishes between lesion types IV and V on the basis of the development of complicating features, may progress and become highly calcified or develop complications such as mural hemorrhage.[5]

Fibrocalcific lesions
Some plaques have thick, fibrous caps overlying extensive accumulations of calcium in the intima close to the media (Figure 2.5). Because the lipid-laden necrotic core, if present, is usually small, this category of lesions has been classified as fibrocalcific rather than atheroma.[2] Tensile strain within an atherosclerotic plaque has been

shown to occur at the interface between tissues of different stiffness and may result in plaque fissuring.[10,11] Lee et al[12] have investigated the mechanical properties of aortic plaque caps and revealed that calcified caps were 4–5 times stiffer than cellular caps. Biomechanical studies have shown that intimal tears often occur at the interface between calcified and adjacent non-calcified arterial tissue.[10] This has led to the observation that changes in the mechanical properties of atherosclerotic plaques, induced by calcification, play a role in the active rupture of the plaque. Indeed, pathological studies reported that calcium is a frequent feature of plaque rupture and a study with electron beam computed tomography (EBCT) revealed that the vast majority of patients with acute myocardial infarction (AMI) or unstable angina have levels of calcium measurable by EBCT.[13] Conversely, Hunt and associates[14] demonstrated that patients with calcification of carotid plaques had fewer symptoms of stroke and transient ischemic attack (TIA) than those without calcification. Also, calcification in carotid plaques is more likely to begin at the surface, resulting in eruption of calcified nodules which are more common in asymptomatic patients.

Plaque hemorrhage
The origin of plaque hemorrhage (Figure 2.6) is still uncertain. It has been suggested that hemorrhage into a plaque occurs from cracks or fissures originating from the luminal surface.[15] The fissuring of the fibrous cap occurs at its thinnest portion, typically at the shoulder region, thereby allowing the entry of blood into the necrotic core. Alternatively, intraplaque hemorrhage has been considered as secondary to rupture of vasa vasorum,[16] a common feature of advanced lesions with plaque rupture and luminal thrombi. Recently, Moreno and associates[17] demonstrated in 269 aortic human plaques the presence of microvessels and inflammatory infiltrate in ruptured plaques when compared with non-ruptured plaques. Microvessel density was increased in lesions with severe macrophage infiltration at the fibrous cap and at the shoulders of the plaque. In addition, microvessel density was also increased in lesions with intraplaque hemorrhage and in thin-cap fibroatheromas, suggesting a contributory role for neovascularization in the process of plaque rupture.

Vulnerable plaques

Thin fibrous cap atheromata
A thin fibrous cap atheromata (Figure 2.7) is characterized by a large necrotic core containing numerous cholesterol clefts. The overlying cap is thin and rich in inflammatory cells, macrophages, and T lymphocytes with few smooth muscle cells.[2,3,18]

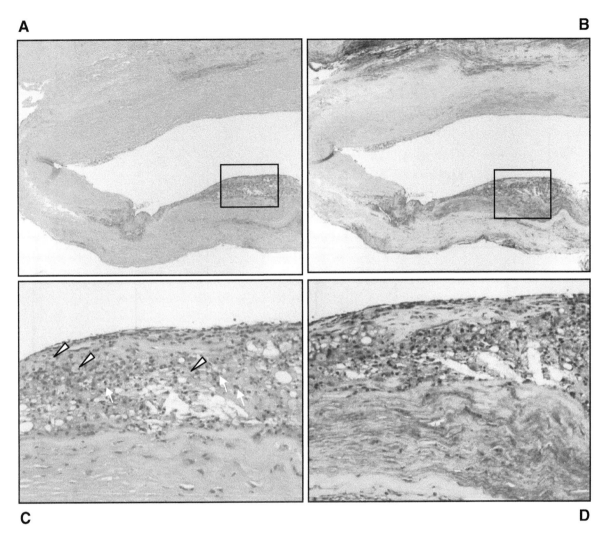

A

B

C

D

Figure 2.3 Pathological intimal thickening. Micrograph from a surgical endarterectomy specimen. Panel A (hematoxylin eosin staining × 2) and Panel B (Movat pentachrome staining × 2): Low power view of a pathologic intimal thickening characterized by a localized thickening of the intima layer associated to inflammatory cell infiltration (with arrows) and lipid deposition (white triangles) (Panel C and D, high power view of the area within the box in Panel A and Panel B). Necrosis is not evident at this stage. (See color plate section.)

A plaque prone to rupture has reduced cap thickness, a large necrotic-lipid core, and a severe inflammatory infiltrate.[19] Burke et al[20] have identified a cut-off value for cap thickness of 65 μm to define a vulnerable coronary plaque. With regard to carotid plaque vulnerability, our own observations identified a thickness of 100 μm for differentiating stable from unstable carotid lesions (pers comm Mauriello A). Different studies have compared carotid plaques removed from symptomatic and asymptomatic patients in an attempt to understand the mechanism underlying plaque activation.[21–28] Studies comparing plaque histology in asymptomatic and symptomatic patients with similar degree of stenosis

are summarized in Table 2.2. Summation analysis demonstrates that plaque rupture or ulceration is much more common in symptomatic patients (48 vs 31%, $p < 0.001$), but lumen thrombus (40 vs 35%) and intra-plaque hemorrhage (48 vs 50%) are equally common in symptomatic and asymptomatic patients. Although there are differences in method of plaque removal and histological analysis, most studies demonstrated that the fibrous cap of symptomatic patients is thinner[26,29–32] and inflammation is more common, with greater number of macrophage and T-cell infiltration in the cap of symptomatic plaques.[25,27,33] The size of the necrotic core appears to be similar in symptomatic and

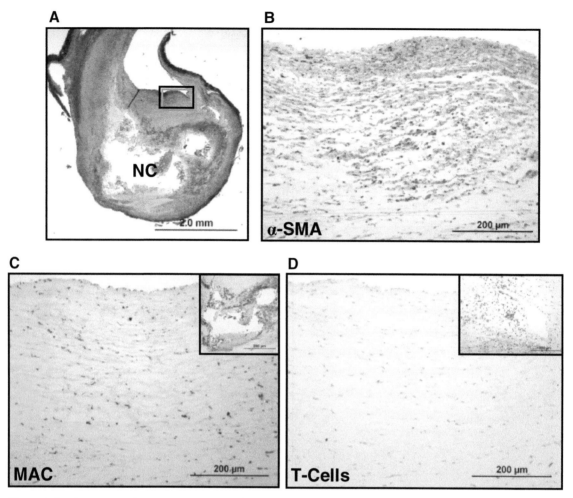

Figure 2.4 Fibrous cap atheroma. (A) Section of human carotid plaque (endarterectomy specimen) shows a fibroatheromatous lesion characterized by a 'true' necrotic core (NC) encapsulated by a relatively thick fibrous cap. (B) The area represented by the black box in A shows abundant immunostaining against smooth muscle actin (α-SMA) within the fibrous cap. (C) A paucity of CD68+ macrophages (MAC) are found within the fibrous cap, with strong reactivity, however, in the periphery of the NC (inset). (D) Similarly, CD45Ro+ T lymphocytes are few within the fibrous cap although T cells are relatively abundant in the shoulder region in areas of vasa vasorum (inset). (See color plate section.)

asymptomatic patients, with no significant difference in the frequency or size of the core in different studies in which similar stenoses have been compared.[21,26,29–34] The quantity of extractable lipid seems to be greater in symptomatic plaques,[30] and this finding is comparable to ultrasound investigations which have demonstrated that echolucent, lipid-rich plaques are often associated with symptoms.[28] Other differences between symptomatic and asymptomatic plaques seem to be related to necrotic core position within the plaque, i.e. in symptomatic patients the necrotic core is nearer to the fibrous cap and the cap thickness is less.

Lesions with thrombi

As reported in Table 2.1, lesions with thrombi are principally due to one of three distinct processes: rupture, erosion, and, less frequently, a calcified nodule. These processes can occur in the setting of a fibrous cap atheroma or, in the case of erosion, pathological intimal thickening. Several studies have established a clear correlation between carotid plaque ulceration, thrombosis and subsequent embolization, and development of ischemic cortical symptoms in the carotid circulation.[21,25,35]

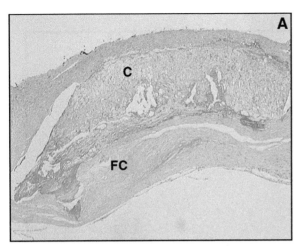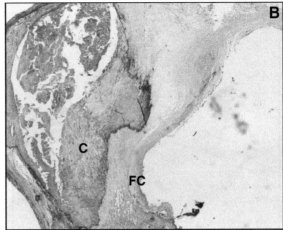

Figure 2.5 Fibrocalcific lesion. (A) Hematoxylin-eosin stain, ×2, and (B) Movat pentachrome stain, ×2, show two plaques with a thick fibrous cap surrounded by extensive calcium deposition characteristic of calcified plate. FC, Fibrous cap; C, calcification. (See color plate section.)

Plaque erosion (Figure 2.10)

Despite the central role of plaque rupture in instigating plaque instability, some have suggested that this event is not always a biological prerequisite for thrombus formation and embolization. In fact, in some series the percentage of specimens derived from symptomatic patients without evidence of plaque surface disruption ranged from 29% to 52%.[19,21,36,37] In contrast, 18–50% of asymptomatic patients revealed plaque rupture. Furthermore, some authors reported the occurrence of intraluminal thrombus formation on a microscopically intact plaque surface.[26] In the coronaries, Farb et al[38] described thrombus formation on unruptured athero-sclerotic plaques as a frequent histological substrate for acute coronary syndromes and defined these plaques as 'eroded.' Plaque erosion has been identified when serial sectioning of a thrombosed arterial segment fails to reveal fibrous cap rupture.[2,26] Typically, the endothelium is absent at the erosion site. The exposed intima consists predominantly of smooth muscle and proteoglycans, and surprisingly, the eroded site contains minimal inflammation.[38] Nevertheless, the cellular and molecular mechanisms for this prothrombotic change of the visually intact intralesional endothelium remains unknown.

Plaque rupture

Most investigators agree that plaque rupture (Figure 2.11) and ulceration is the dominant mechanism that leads to thrombus formation and subsequent embolization and cerebral ischemic events.[21,39] Plaque rupture has been defined by an area of fibrous cap disruption whereby the overlying thrombus is in continuity with the underlying necrotic core.[2,26] Ruptured lesions typically have a large necrotic core and a disrupted fibrous cap infiltrated by macrophages and lymphocytes. The smooth muscle cell content within the fibrous cap at the rupture site may be quite sparse.

Our group has recently demonstrated[40] in 269 carotid atherosclerotic plaques that despite no difference in the degree of stenosis, a thrombotically active carotid plaque associated with high inflammatory infiltrate was observed in 71 (74.0%) of 96 patients with ipsilateral major stroke (and in all 32 plaques from patients operated within 2 months of symptom onset) compared with 32 (35.2%) of 91 patients with TIA or 12 (14.6%) of 82 patients who were asymptomatic (Table 2.3). In addition, a fresh thrombus was observed in 53.8% of patients with stroke operated 13–24 months after the cerebrovascular event. An acute thrombus was associated with cap rupture in 64 (90.1%) of 71 thrombosed plaques from patients with stroke and with cap erosion in the remaining seven cases (9.9%). Ruptured plaques of patients affected by stroke were characterized by the presence of a more severe inflammatory infiltrate, constituted by monocytes, macrophages, and T-lymphocyte cells compared with that observed in the TIA and asymptomatic groups.

Furthermore, pathological investigations comparing endarterectomy tissue samples obtained from patients with or without neurological symptoms has clarified the instability determinants of the carotid plaque, which are indeed similar to those characterizing coronary plaques.[41] The vulnerability of a plaque to rupture is mainly characterized by decreased fibrous cap thickness, large

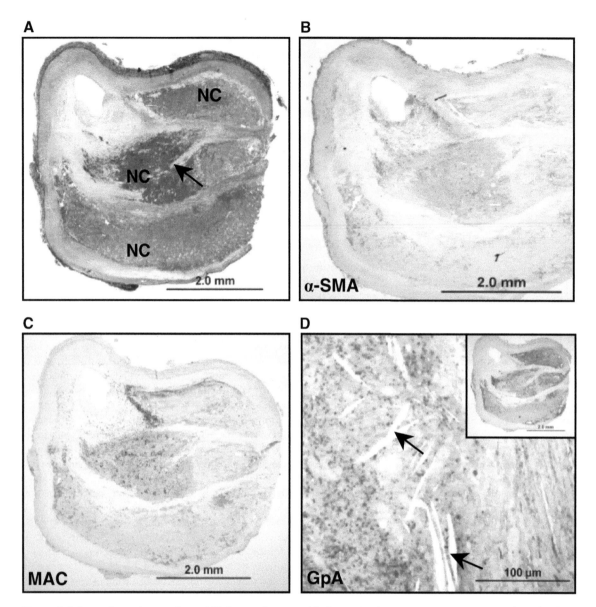

Figure 2.6 Intraplaque hemorrhage. (A) A complex carotid plaque (endarterectomy specimen) with multiple fibrous caps and necrotic cores (NC) and severe intraplaque hemorrhage. The discontinuous fibrous cap (arrow) easily identifies a previous site of plaque rupture. (B) Immunostaining against smooth muscle actin (α-SMA) highlights a healing luminal thrombus from a recent plaque rupture. (C) Macrophages (MAC) are primarily localized to the periphery of the necrotic core near the luminal surface. (D) Antibody against glycophorin A (GpA, a protein specific to erythrocytes) shows intense staining of erythrocyte membranes mostly within the necrotic core intermixed with cholesterol clefts (arrows). (See color plate section.)

lipidic-necrotic core, and increased inflammatory infiltrate (macrophages and T lymphocytes).[19] In addition, the likelihood of plaque rupture is due not only to the intrinsic plaque characteristics (vulnerability) but also to the tensile strength of the plaque and the stress exerted on it.

Calcific nodule

Another rare cause of thrombotic lesion is referred to as a 'calcified nodule' (Figure 2.8). This term identifies a lesion with fibrous cap disruption and thrombi associated with eruptive, dense, calcific nodules.[2] It is unclear whether the fibrous cap wears down from physical

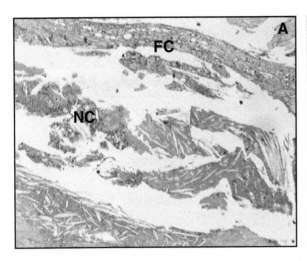
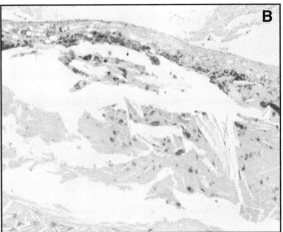

Figure 2.7 Thin fibrous cap atheromata. (A) A vulnerable plaque characterized by a large lipidic-necrotic core (NC) associated to a thin inflamed fibrous cap (FC, Movat pentachrome stain, ×4). (B) High number of macrophagic foam cells, CD68+ are present in the thin fibrous cap of the plaque (CD68 stain, ×4). (See color plate section.)

forces exerted by the nodules themselves, proteases from the surrounding cellular infiltrate, or both.

Healed lesions

Healed ruptures are characterized by a disrupted fibrous cap filled in by smooth muscle cells, proteoglycans, and collagen. Healed ruptures are best identified by picrosirius red staining,[42] whereby newly synthesized type III collagen is seen overlying a ruptured fibrous cap consisting primarily of type I collagen. The matrix within the healed fibrous cap defect may consist of a proteoglycan-rich mass or a collagen-rich scar, depending on the phase of healing. Lesions with healed ruptures may exhibit multilayering of lipid and necrotic core (Figure 2.9), suggestive of previous episodes of thrombosis. Other healed lesions show no evidence of a pre-existing rupture of the fibrous cap, and there is usually no necrotic core. Instead, distinct layers of dense collagen interspersed with smooth muscle cells and proteoglycans often containing fibrin and/or platelets are present; we assume these types of lesions are the result of healed erosions. Old occlusions often show the lumen totally occluded by dense collagen and/or proteoglycan with interspersed capillaries, arterioles, smooth muscle cells, and inflammatory cells. These lesions may also demonstrate earlier phases of organizing thrombi containing fibrin, red blood cells, and granulation tissue. In addition, it is common to find in this type of lesion several recanalization vascular channels covered by endothelium and smooth muscle cells within the organized thrombotic region (Figure 2.12).

Morphological studies of coronary arteries suggest that plaque progression beyond 50% cross-sectional luminal narrowing occurs secondary to repeated ruptures, which may be clinically silent.[43,44] The sites of healed plaque ruptures can be recognized by demonstrating a necrotic core with a discontinuous fibrous cap, which is rich in type I collagen and an overlying intima formed by smooth muscle cells in a matrix rich in proteoglycan and type III collagen.[43] Few angiographic studies have demonstrated plaque progression, and short-term studies have suggested that thrombosis is the likely cause. Mann and Davies showed that the frequency of healed plaque ruptures increases along with lumen narrowing.[44] Burke et al found healed plaque rupture in 61% of hearts from sudden coronary death victims. At least 40–50% of coronary rupture sites show <50% diameter stenosis,[11,38] and the same may be true in carotid disease.

Multiple healed plaque ruptures with layering are also common in carotid segments, and the percent cross-sectional luminal narrowing is dependent on the number of healed repair sites. Therefore, it seems that the progression of atherosclerotic disease to severe stenosis is the result of repeated ruptures.[40]

WHAT TRIGGERS PLAQUE TRANSFORMATION FROM A STABLE TO AN UNSTABLE STATE?

Carotid atherosclerosis is a chronic process that is caused, or at least accelerated, in part by hypertension, cigarette smoking, diabetes, and hyperlipidemia. We and others

Table 2.2 Histological comparison of plaques from symptomatic and asymptomatic patients: summary analysis

Plaque feature	Reference	Symptomatic	Asymptomatic	Significance
Ulceration/plaque rupture	Bassiouny et al[33]	18/31	6/14	NS
	Seeger et al[30]	10/21	11/22	NS
	Sitzer et al[21]	15/27	2/12	0.02
	Carr et al[26]	14/19	8/25	0.004
	Bassiouny et al[31]	19/59	8/40	NS
	Total (%)	76/157 (48)	35/113 (31)	<0.001
Lumen thrombus	Bassiouny et al[33]	17/31	5/14	NS
	Sitzer et al[21]	20/27	5/12	0.05
	Carr et al[26]	12/19	20/25	NS
	Bassiouny et al[31]	5/59	2/40	NS
	Total (%)	54/136 (40)	32/91 (35)	NS
Intraplaque hemorrhage	Bassiouny et al[33]	12/31	12/14	NS
	Von Maravic et al[34]	14/15	21/23	NS
	Feeley et al[29]	25/44	4/8	NS
	Seeger et al[30]	10/21	12/22	NS
	Sitzer et al[21]	6/27	2/12	NS
	Carr et al[26]	16/19	14/25	0.06
	Bassiouny et al[31]	11/59	7/40	NS
	Total (%)	103/216 (48)	72/144 (50)	NS
Fibrous cap				
Fibrous tissue (plaque %)	Feeley et al[29]	66 ± 8	88 ± 14	0.05
Collagen (mg)	Seeger et al[30]	0.17 ± 0.01	0.20 ± 0.01	NS
Cap thinning	Carr et al[26]	18/19	12/25	0.003
Minimum cap thickness (mm)	Bassiouny et al[31]	0.2 ± 0.2	0.4 ± 0.4	<0.006
Median cap volume (mm^3)	Hatsukami et al[32]	170	230	NS
Cap inflammation				
Foam cells	Carr et al[26]	16/19	11/25	0.006
Macrophages (mean ± SD)	Bassiouny et al[31]	1144 ± 1104	385 ± 622	<0.01
Macrophage-rich area (mean ± SD)	Jander et al[25]	18 ± 10	11 ± 4	0.005
T cells (number/mm^2)	Jander et al[25]	71 ± 34	41 ± 31	0.005
ICAM-1 (mean area ± SD)	DeGraba et al[71]	29.5 ± 2.4	15.7 ± 2.7	0.002
Plaque core				
Extractable lipid (mg)	Seeger et al[30]	0.37 ± 0.14	0.29 ± 0.01	<0.001
Cholesterol (mg)	Seeger et al[30]	0.09 ± 0.01	0.06 ± 0.01	<0.005
Necrotic core	Carr et al[26]	18/25	16/19	NS
Mean % necrotic core	Bassiouny et al[31]	22 ± 16	26 ± 18	NS
Median lipid core (mm^3)	Hatsukami et al[32]	60	10	NS
Median necrotic core (mm^3)	Hatsukami et al[32]	60	60	NS

*Different statistical test utilized. Modified from reference 19.

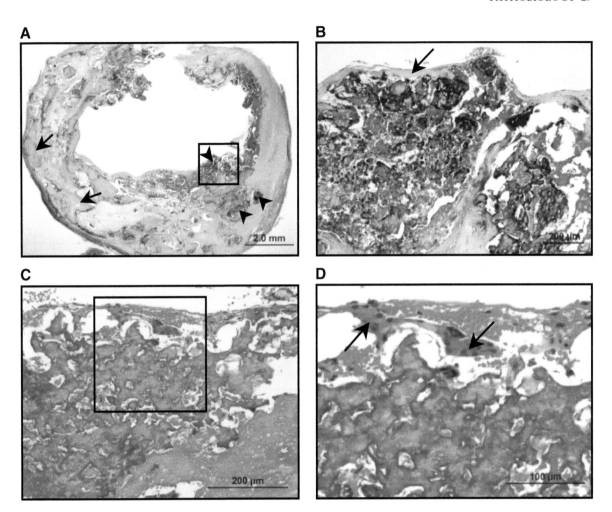

Figure 2.8 Nodular calcification. (A) Low-power view (Movat pentachrome stain) of a human carotid plaque (endarterectomy specimen) with severe calcification. Numerous fragmented calcified plates (arrows) and nodules (arrowheads) are present. (B) Higher-power view (Movat pentachrome stain) within the area of the black box in A showing a region near the luminal surface with extensive nodular calcification underneath a thin fibrous cap (arrow). Eruptive calcified nodules could be a potential cause of luminal thrombi and distal embolization. (C) Several osteoclast-like cells associated with nodules (hematoxylin and eosin stain). (D) Higher-power view (hematoxylin and eosin stain) of the area of the black box in C showing several multinucleated osteoclast-like cells near calcified nodules (arrows). (See color plate section.)

have demonstrated that histological plaque composition strongly correlates with specific cardiovascular risk factors. Fibrous plaques were associated with diabetes, granulomatous plaques infiltrated by giant cells with hypertension, foam cell-rich plaques with hypercholesterolemia, and thrombotic plaques with smoking.[45] However, the risk of plaque transformation from a stable to a vulnerable one is related to the particular 'microenvironment' of the plaque – specifically, the balance between cellular migration/proliferation, extracellular matrix production/degradation, and presence of inflammatory infiltrate (Figure 2.13). Although this

transformation is unpredictable and its triggering mechanisms remain an active area of investigation, local and systemic triggering mechanisms as well as predisposing genetic profiles have been identified (Table 2.4).

Local triggers

Shear stress

Chronic exposure of endothelial cells to high levels of shear stress causes them to exhibit an atheroprotective phenotype.[46] Conversely, low wall shear stress can

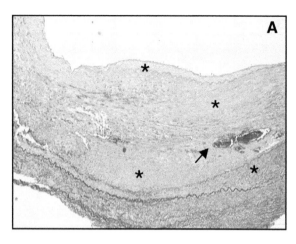 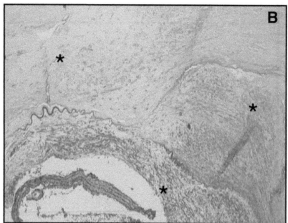

Figure 2.9 Healed plaque with stratified thrombus. (A) and (B) show an organized thrombus characterized by stratified fibrous tissue. Lesions with healed ruptures may exhibit multilayering of lipid and necrotic core (asterisks), suggestive of previous episodes of thrombosis. Old occlusions often show the lumen almost totally occluded by dense collagen and proteoglycan with interspersed capillaries (arrow), arterioles, smooth muscle cells, and inflammatory cells. (Movat pentachrome stain, ×2). (See color plate section.)

Table 2.3 Angiographic stenosis, presence of thrombus, plaque erosion, and plaque rupture by study group

	No. of plaques			p value		
	Patients with major ipsilateral stroke ($n = 96$)	Patients with TIA ($n = 91$)	Asymptomatic ($n = 82$)	Stroke vs TIA	Stroke vs asymptomatic	TIA vs asymptomatic
Angiographic stenosis (%)						
Ipsilateral carotid	86.1	79.5	84.6	0.06	0.32	0.13
Contralateral carotid	60.69	64.2	57.5	0.66	0.44	0.32
Thrombotically active plaque	71 (74)	32 (35.2)	12 (14.6)	<0.001	<0.001	0.002
Cap rupture	64 (66.7)	21 (23.1)	11 (13.4)	<0.001	<0.001	0.004
Cap erosion	7 (7.3)	11 (12.1)	1 (1.2)	0.51	0.09	0.03

TIA, transient ischemic attack.
Modified from Spagnoli et al.[40]

cause arterial damage and subsequent plaque instability through several mechanisms: increased fluid residence time; increased platelet and macrophage adhesion to the arterial wall; and modulation of platelet-derived growth factor and transforming growth factor-β_1.[47] Also, hemodynamic factors seem to influence the cellular composition of the plaque. Indeed, Dirksen et al[48] demonstrated that different plaque areas have different cellular composition. In particular, plaque areas distal to flow are richer in smooth muscle cells, whereas proximal plaque areas are exposed to a greater shear stress and are therefore richer in macrophages. It is now evident from different pathological studies of coronary arteries that plaque rupture occurs at low degrees of narrowing and the degree of narrowing poorly predicts events.[49,50] This can be explained by

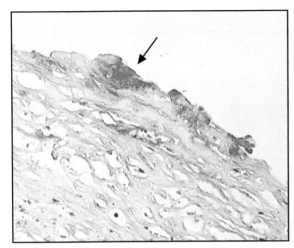

Figure 2.10 Plaque erosion. Acute thrombosis associated with superficial erosion (black arrow), without rupture of the fibrous cap. The endothelium is absent at the erosion site. The exposed intima consists predominantly of smooth muscle and proteoglycans (Movat pentachrome stain, ×4). (See color plate section.)

the greater tension created in the caps of plaques of moderate stenosis compared with that in caps of more severely stenotic plaques with the same cap thickness and at the same blood pressure based on Laplace's law.[11]

Biological factors

Differences in the frequency of thrombosis, cap rupture, cap erosion, and inflammatory infiltrate have been explored in patients with symptomatic and asymptomatic carotid stenosis to elucidate the potential triggering mechanisms for this transformation.

Matrix metalloproteinases

Matrix metalloproteinases (MMPs) are proteolytic enzymes that have several functions, such as digesting extracellular components, processing cell surface proteins, and regulating other cell functions.[51] It is well known that collagen breakdown is dependent on the balance between MMPs and their inhibitors, tissue inhibitors of metalloproteinase (TIMPs). High levels of MMPs have been demonstrated at the site of the inflammatory infiltrate in the fibrous cap.[52] T cells can induce macrophages to secrete MMPs via stimulation of CD40, and, in addition, through production of interleukin-1 (IL-1), which promotes smooth muscle cell (SMC) apoptosis.[53,54]

Growing evidence suggests a central role for these enzymes in determining carotid plaque instability.[55] In this study, MMP-1 transcript levels were nearly 8-fold higher in thin-cap carotid plaques than in thick-cap plaques, and MMP-12 transcript levels were significantly increased in ruptured plaques compared with plaques without cap disruption. Recently, Turu and colleagues[56] confirmed previous findings that unstable carotid plaques (estimated by clinical and morphological methods) had higher metalloproteinase activity. Interestingly, patients with asymptomatic carotid disease, but with plaque progression within the last year prior to endarterectomy, had higher intraplaque MMP-8 activity than patients without progression. Patients with hypertension had higher intraplaque MMP-8 activity, further linking this MMP with the most frequent risk factor in patients with symptomatic carotid disease. Higher expression of MMP-8 in patients with advanced unstable plaques is in agreement with the reported expression of MMP-8 in plaque macrophages in a murine model of atherosclerosis.[57,58] Indeed, various atheroma-associated cells express MMP-8, confirming its potential role in atherogenesis and active plaque remodeling.[59,60] Higher MMP-8 activity may be involved in atherosclerotic plaque progression, but it may be independent from possible plaque rupture. The latter may involve other proteolytic enzymes.[61] It remains unclear whether raised MMP levels cause rupture of the atherosclerotic plaque or are a result of it. Proof of a causative role might come from the demonstration of the efficacy of pharmacotherapy that targets these collagenases.

Pregnancy-associated protein A

Pregnancy-associated protein A (PAPP-A) is a high-molecular-weight, zinc-binding metalloproteinase that is abundantly expressed in advanced atherosclerotic lesions and constitutes a specific activator of insulin-like growth factor (IGF), a mediator of atherosclerosis.[62] In particular, this protease cleaves the bond between IGF-1 and its natural inhibitor, IGFBP-4 (insulin like growth factor binding protein-4), increasing the levels of free IGF-1.[63] It is hypothesized that IGF-1 is one of the most important mediators of transformation from a stable to an unstable plaque. In addition, macrophage stimulation by IGF-1 induces tumor necrosis factor (TNF) synthesis.[64] This cytokine amplifies the plaque destabilization mechanisms both directly and indirectly by other interleukins (IL-1 and IL-6) and interferon-γ (INF-γ) production. The latter induce apoptosis of the SMCs and stimulate macrophages to produce metalloproteinases with a consequent digestion of the collagen and extracellular matrix of the fibrous cap.[65] Recently, Bayes-Genis et al found that PAPP-A was highly expressed in both ruptured and eroded coronary unstable plaques of eight patients who died suddenly from cardiac causes, but was absent or minimally expressed in stable plaques.[66] Beaudeux and associates[67] found

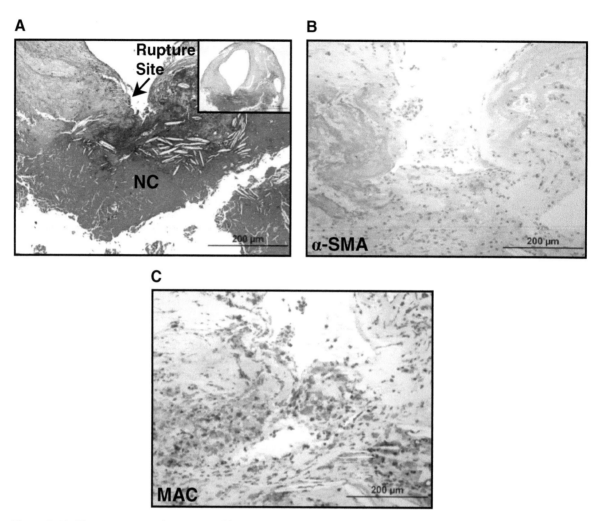

Figure 2.11 Plaque rupture. (A) Section of human carotid plaque (endarterectomy specimen) showing a lesion with a relatively larger necrotic core (NC) and rupture site (arrow). The rupture site is ulcerated with little exposed luminal thrombus. The inset is a lower-power view of the same section (Movat pentachrome staining). (B) Immunostaining against smooth muscle actin (α-SMA) shows a lack of smooth muscle within the fibrous cap at the rupture site. (C) Immunostaining against CD68 shows numerous inflammatory macrophages (MAC) within the fibrous cap. (See color plate section.)

that elevated serum PAPP-A levels are associated not only with the echogenicity of atherosclerotic carotid lesions but also with an enhanced inflammatory state in asymptomatic hyperlipidemic subjects.

Our group has recently demonstrated that there is also an increased expression of PAPP-A in the carotid distribution related either to the presence of complex vulnerable plaques or ruptured plaques with thrombus.[68] Conversely, stable plaques or plaques with organized thrombus did not show PAPP-A expression. In addition, at the confocal microscopic examination, PAPP-A expression was increased in macrophages compared with SMCs and T lymphocytes. This suggests that this marker may serve as a useful method to detect high-risk subgroups of patients bearing vulnerable atherosclerotic carotid plaques before the onset of cerebrovascular events. A multicenter Italian registry (the SUBMARINE study, Serum and Urinary Plaque Vulnerability Biomarkers Detection before and after Carotid Stent Implantation), currently in progress, will assess if in patients affected by recurrent transient ischemic attacks or minor stroke carotid stenting may stabilize the plaque with concomitant reduction in the expression of different biomarkers of vulnerability.

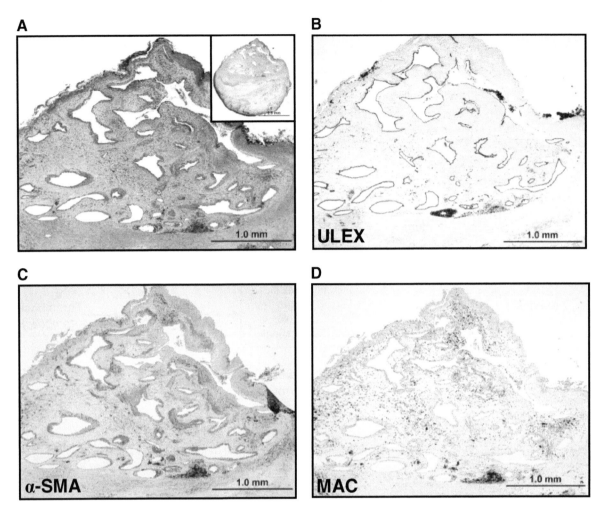

Figure 2.12 Recanalized thrombus. (A) Section of human carotid plaque (endarterectomy specimen) with a recanalized thrombus (Movat pentachrome stain). The inset is a lower-power view of the same section. (B) Indirect immunostaining with anti-*Ulex europaeus* lectin demonstrating numerous vascular channels lined by endothelium. (C) Many recanalized channels are also surrounded by actin-positive smooth muscle cells (α-SMA). (D) Immunostaining against CD68 shows inflammatory macrophages (MAC) within the thrombus and surrounding vascular channels. (See color plate section.)

Circulating transforming growth factor-β_1 levels

Transforming growth factor-β_1, generated locally within the atherosclerotic plaque, is involved in the process of plaque stabilization. Cipollone et al[69] have demonstrated that transforming growth factor-β_1 mRNA levels are increased up to 3-fold in asymptomatic compared with symptomatic plaques. In plaque rupture, exposure of the necrotic core to the circulation promotes thrombosis and subsequent plaque progression. Tissue factor (TF) is mainly present in lipid-rich human atherosclerotic plaques, which are the most thrombogenic substrates, and a significant association of TF expression with plaque infiltration by macrophages and T cells was observed, and TF expression was more important in symptomatic plaques.[70]

Intercellular adhesion molecule-1

The role of intracellular adhesion molecule-1 (ICAM-1) in triggering a symptomatic transformation of a previously stable carotid plaque remains controversial. While some studies[71] have shown that the level of ICAM-1 expression is indeed increased in symptomatic vs asymptomatic carotid plaques, other studies have failed to confirm these findings.[72]

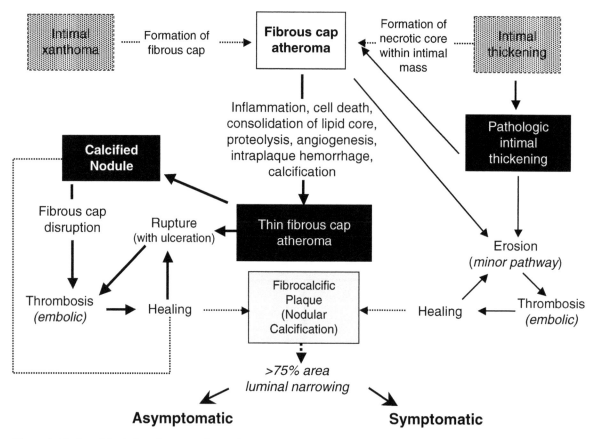

Figure 2.13 Simplified classification scheme for carotid atherosclerosis development from an early, uncomplicated lesion to a more complex, vulnerable atherosclerotic plaque. (See color plate section.)

Systemic triggers

Inflammation plays a key role in triggering plaque instability.[65,73–75] Several systemic proteins have been proposed as markers of a chronic inflammatory state in the arterial wall, such as leukocytes, vascular adhesion molecules, fibrinogen, high-sensitivity C-reactive protein (hsCRP), and serum amyloid A protein. We will only discuss these factors briefly, because they will be discussed in more detail in Chapter 11. We will focus on non-inflammatory systemic triggers of plaque instability such as vascular adhesion molecules, fibrinogen, and MMPs.

Vascular adhesion molecules

Vascular adhesion molecules may be considered potential candidates, since these markers are activated by inflammatory cytokines and then released at the endothelium level.[76–78] The Physicians' Health Study evaluated more than 14 000 healthy subjects, demonstrating that ICAM-1 correlated with cardiovascular risk and that subjects in

the highest quartile had a relative risk of developing an acute event 1.8 greater than subjects in the lowest quartile.[77,79] Furthermore, cytokine IL-18 is another candidate molecule that may influence plaque instability. This inflammatory cytokine is mainly produced by macrophages and monocyte cells and stimulates IFN-γ production, which in turn inhibits collagen production. Mallat and associates[80] demonstrated an elevated expression of IL-18 in unstable carotid plaques compared with stable plaques and that the presence of this marker correlated with clinically symptomatic carotid plaques.

Fibrinogen

The relationship between fibrinogen and the risk of ischemic stroke has been studied in patients with recent TIA or minor ischemic stroke.[81] Fibrinogen predicted subsequent ischemic stroke, with a pooled hazard ratio for value above the median value of 1.34 (95% CI 1.13–1.6; $p < 0.001$). In addition, we demonstrated that patients affected by hyperfibrinogenemia (fibrinogen level

<table>
<tr><td>

Table 2.4 Local and systemic triggering factors for carotid plaque instability

Local triggers

Hemodynamic:
- Shear stress

Biological:
- Matrix metalloproteinases (MMPs)
- Pregnancy-associated protein A (PAPP-A)
- Circulating transforming growth factor-β_1 levels
- Plaque neovascularization
- Intracellular adhesion molecule-1 (ICAM-1)

Systemic triggers

Inflammatory markers:
- High-sensitivity C-reactive protein (hsCRP)
- Leukocytes and monocyte count
- Fibrinogen
- Vascular adhesion molecules
- Serum amyloid A protein

MMPs

Genetic phenotypes

</td></tr>
</table>

> 400 mg/dl) were characterized by a greater inflammatory infiltrate and thinner atherosclerotic plaque cap, with consequent increased risk of thrombosis and rupture compared with patients with lower fibrinogen levels, independently from other risk factors.[82]

C-reactive protein

In the Physicians' Health Study the basal levels of C-reactive protein (CRP) were retrospectively evaluated in healthy subjects. The risk of developing a stroke was two-times greater in the subjects with CRP in the highest quartile compared with subjects in the lowest quartile. Such a type of risk was not modified by smoking status and it was independent from the other risk factors.[74] Recently, Erren et al[83] evaluated the plasma levels of different inflammatory markers in patients affected by both coronary and peripheral atherosclerosis. In 147 patients submitted to coronary angiography, the levels of CRP, fibrinogen, serum amyloid A, and IL-6 were evaluated. All the inflammatory indices were increased in patients with diffuse atherosclerosis compared to patients with only coronary disease or healthy controls, suggesting a higher degree of inflammatory activation in patients with multidistrict atherosclerotic disease.

Matrix metalloproteinases

It has been demonstrated that patients with symptomatic carotid disease have significantly higher plasma MMP-9 levels than asymptomatic patients.[56] This association remains significant irrespective of antiplatelet and/or statin therapy, which suggest that MMP-9 activity may be increased during acute remodeling of thrombosed plaques. However, at an earlier stage, MMP-8 is overexpressed and may lead to plaque destabilization and vulnerability to the deleterious actions of MMP-9. Following ischemic stroke, both MMP-2 and MMP-9 plasma levels have been found to be increased.[84] MMP-2 plasma levels usually recover more rapidly than MMP-9 in the days following stroke, to levels seen on admission.

An interesting finding is that plasma levels of MMPs are independent of systemic changes in inflammatory markers such as CRP, fibrinogen, D-dimers, or white blood cell counts. This agrees with earlier indications that MMP-8 synthesis and release at sites of chronic inflammation, such as atheroma, was associated with prolonged but not acute exposure to proinflammatory cytokines.[59]

Genetic profiles

It has been clearly demonstrated that spontaneous apoptosis of the SMCs in the atherosclerotic plaque is an ongoing process in plaque evolution.[85,86] This process of ongoing programmed cell death, combined with replicative senescence and inflammation, may contribute to thinning of the fibrous cap. Interestingly, Imanashi et al have recently found that the normal intima expresses *c-FLIP*, another antiapoptotic gene, but that this gene is lost in areas of apoptosis of the fibrous cap.[87] Proinflammatory genetic profiles are significantly more common in subjects with a history of stroke. One study[88] evaluated 237 individuals with a history of ischemic stroke and 223 age-matched and gender-matched controls. The polymorphisms of CRP, IL-6, macrophage migration inhibitory factors, monocyte chemoattractant protein 1, ICAM-1, E-selectin, and MMP-3 genes were studied. The odds of stroke increased with the number of high-risk genotypes: carrying one proinflammatory gene variant conferred a risk of 3.3 (1.6–6.9), whereas individuals who carried two and three gene variants had adjusted odds ratios of 21.0 (7.6–57.5) and 50.3 (10.2–248.1), respectively. The impact of inflammatory gene polymorphisms and gene–smoking interactions on common carotid artery intima–media thickness (IMT) has also been studied.[89] An increasing gene load of inflammatory genotypes was associated with a linear increase in serum IL-6 levels and increased carotid artery IMT. Coagulation factors also play an important role, and their genetic expression also determines which patients are likely to have thrombosis vs those that will remain asymptomatic. Indeed, the combination of genetic predisposition to thrombosis and plaque characteristics may be the most important determinant of stroke and TIA.

REFERENCES

1. Schwartz RS, Topol EJ, Serruys PW, Sangiorgi G, Holmes DR. Artery size, neointima, and remodeling: time for some standards. J Am Coll Cardiol 1998; 32: 2087–94.
2. Virmani R, Kolodgie FD, Burke AP, Farb A, Schwartz SM. Lessons from sudden coronary death: a comprehensive morphological classification scheme for atherosclerotic lesions. Arterioscler Thromb Vasc Biol 2000; 20: 1262–75.
3. Naghavi M, Libby P, Falk E et al. From vulnerable plaque to vulnerable patient: a call for new definitions and risk assessment strategies: Part II. Circulation 2003; 108: 1772–8.
4. Stary HC, Chandler AB, Glagov S et al. A report from the Committee on Vascular Lesions of the Council on Arteriosclerosis, American Heart Association. Circulation 1994; 89: 2462–78.
5. Stary HC, Chandler AB, Dinsmore RE et al. A definition of advanced types of atherosclerotic lesions and a histological classification of atherosclerosis. A report from the Committee on Vascular Lesions of the Council on Arteriosclerosis, American Heart Association. Circulation 1995; 92: 1355–74.
6. Schwartz SM, deBlois D, O'Brien ER. The intima. Soil for atherosclerosis and restenosis. Circ Res 1995; 77: 445–65.
7. Tabas I, Li Y, Brocia RW et al. Lipoprotein lipase and sphingomyelinase synergistically enhance the association of atherogenic lipoproteins with smooth muscle cells and extracellular matrix. A possible mechanism for low density lipoprotein and lipoprotein(a) retention and macrophage foam cell formation. J Biol Chem 1993; 268: 20419–32.
8. Armstrong ML, Heistad DD, Megan MB, Lopez JA, Harrison DG. Reversibility of atherosclerosis. Cardiovasc Clin 1990; 20: 113–26.
9. Strong JP, Malcom GT, McMahan CA et al. Prevalence and extent of atherosclerosis in adolescent and young adults: implications for prevention from pathobiological determinants of atherosclerosis in youth study. JAMA 1999; 281: 727–35.
10. Richardson PD, Davies MJ. Influence of plaque configuration and stress-distribution on fissuring of coronary atherosclerotic plaques. Lancet 1989; 2: 941–4.
11. Falk E, Shah PK, Fuster V. Coronary plaque disruption. Circulation 1995; 92: 657–71.
12. Lee RT, Grodzinsky AJ, Frank EH, Kamm RD, Schoen FJ. Structure-dependent dynamic mechanical behavior of fibrous caps from human atherosclerotic plaques. Circulation 1991; 83: 1764–70.
13. Schmermund A, Erbel R. Unstable coronary plaque and its relation to coronary calcium. Circulation 2001; 104: 1682–7.
14. Hunt JL, Fairman R, Mitchell ME et al. Bone formation in carotid plaques: a clinicopathological study. Stroke 2002; 33: 1214–19.
15. Davies MJ, Thomas AC. Plaque fissuring – the cause of acute myocardial infarction, sudden ischaemic death, and crescendo angina. Br Heart J 1985; 53: 363–73.
16. Virmani R, Kolodgie FD, Burke AP et al. Atherosclerotic plaque progression and vulnerability to rupture: angiogenesis as a source of intraplaque hemorrhage. Arterioscler Thromb Vasc Biol 2005; 25: 2054–61.
17. Moreno PR, Purushothaman KR, Fuster V et al. Plaque neovascularization is increased in ruptured atherosclerotic lesions of human aorta: implications for plaque vulnerability. Circulation 2004; 110: 2032–8.
18. Virmani R, Burke AP, Farb AH, Kolodgie FD. Pathology of the unstable plaque. Prog Cardiovasc Dis 2002; 44: 349–56.
19. Golledge J, Greenhalgh RM, Davies AH. The symptomatic carotid plaque. Stroke 2000; 31: 774–81.
20. Burke AP, Farb A, Malcom GT et al. Coronary risk factors and plaque morphology in men with coronary disease who died suddenly. N Engl J Med 1997; 336: 1276–82.
21. Sitzer M, Muller W, Siebler M et al. Plaque ulceration and lumen thrombus are the main sources of cerebral microemboli in high-grade internal carotid artery stenosis. Stroke 1995; 26: 1231–3.
22. Imparato AM, Riles TS, Gortein F. The carotid bifurcation plaque: pathologic findings associated with cerebral ischaemia. Stroke 1979; 10: 238–45.
23. Lusby RJ, Ferrel LD, Ehrenfeld WK, Stoney RJ, Wyle EJ. Carotid plaque hemorrhage: its role in production of cerebral ischemia. Arch Surg 1982; 1178: 1479–88.
24. Avril G, Batt M, Guidoin R et al. Carotid endarterectomy plaques: correlations of clinical and anatomic findings. Ann Vasc Surg 1991; 5: 50–4.
25. Jander S, Sitzer M, Schumann R et al. Inflammation in high-grade carotid stenosis: a possible role for macrophages and T cells in plaque destabilization. Stroke 1998; 29: 1625–30.
26. Carr S, Farb A, Pearce WH, Virmani R, Yao JS. Atherosclerotic plaque rupture in symptomatic carotid artery stenosis. J Vasc Surg 1996; 23: 755–65, discussion 765–6.
27. Carr SC, Farb A, Pearce WH, Virmani R, Yao JST. Activated inflammatory cells are associated with plaque rupture in carotid artery stenosis. Surgery 1997; 122: 757–64.
28. Gronholdt ML. Ultrasound and lipoproteins as predictors of lipid-rich, rupture-prone plaques in the carotid artery. Arterioscler Thromb Vasc Biol 1999; 19: 2–13.
29. Feeley TM, Leen EJ, Colgan MP, Moore DJ, Hourihane D, Shanik GD. Histologic characteristics of carotid artery plaque. J Vasc Surg 1991; 13: 719–24.
30. Seeger JM, Barratt E, Lawson GA, Klingman N. The relationship between carotid plaque composition, plaque morphology and neurologic symptoms. J Surg Res 1995; 58: 330–6.
31. Bassiouny HS, Sakaguchi Y, Mikucki SA et al. Juxtalumen location of plaques necrosis and neoformation in symptomatic carotid stenosis. J Vasc Surg 1997; 26: 585–94.
32. Hatsukami TS, Ferguson MS, Beach KW, Gordon D, Detmer P, Burns D, Alpers C, Strandness E. Carotid plaque morphology and clinical events. Stroke 1997; 28: 95–100.
33. Bassiouny HS, Davies H, Masawa N et al. Critical carotid stenoses: morphologic and chemical similarity between symptomatic and asymptomatic plaques. J Vasc Surg 1989; 9: 202–12.
34. von Maravic C, Kessler C, von Maravic M, Hohlbach G, Kompf D. Clinical relevance of intraplaque hemorrhage in the internal carotid artery. Eur J Surg 1991; 157: 185–8.
35. De Michele M, Ascione L, Guarini P, Perrotta S, Tuccillo B. [Instability determinants of the carotid plaque: from histology to ultrasound [in Italian]. It Heart J 2001; 2: 606–13.
36. Stork JL, Kimura K, Levi CR et al. Source of microembolic signals in patients with high-grade carotid stenosis. Stroke 2002; 33: 2014–18.
37. Spencer MP. Doppler microembolic signals for diagnosis of ulcerated carotid artery plaques. Echocardiography 1996; 13: 551–4.
38. Farb A, Burke AP, Tang AL et al. Coronary plaque erosion without rupture into a lipid core. A frequent cause of coronary thrombosis in sudden coronary death. Circulation 1996; 93: 1354–63.
39. Lammie GA, Sandercock PA, Dennis MS. Recently occluded intracranial and extracranial carotid arteries. Relevance of the unstable atherosclerotic plaque. Stroke 1999; 30: 1319–25.

40. Spagnoli LG, Mauriello A, Sangiorgi G et al. Extracranial thrombotically active carotid plaque as a risk factor for ischemic stroke. JAMA 2004; 292: 1845–52.

41. Carbone LG, Mauriello A, Christiansen M et al. Unstable carotid plaque biochemical and cellular marker of vulnerability. It Heart J 2003; 5(Suppl): 398–406.

42. Junqueira LC, Bignolas G, Brentani RR. Picrosirius staining plus polarization microscopy, a specific method for collagen detection in tissue sections. Histochem J 1979; 11: 447–55.

43. Burke AP, Kolodgie FD, Farb A et al. Healed plaque ruptures and sudden coronary death: evidence that subclinical rupture has a role in plaque progression. Circulation 2001; 103: 934–40.

44. Mann J, Davies MJ. Mechanisms of progression in native coronary artery disease: role of healed plaque disruption. Heart 1999; 82: 265–8.

45. Spagnoli LG, Mauriello A, Palmieri G et al. Relationship between risk factors and morphological patterns of human carotid atherosclerotic plaques: a multivariate discriminant analysis. Atherosclerosis 1994; 108: 39–60.

46. Traub O, Berk BC. Laminar shear stress: mechanisms by which endothelial cells transduce an atheroprotective force. Arterioscler Thromb Vasc Biol 1998; 18: 677–85.

47. Resnick N, Collins T, Atkinson W et al. Platelet-derived growth factor B chain promoter contains a cis-acting fluid shear-stress-responsive element. Proc Natl Acad Sci USA 1993; 90: 7908.

48. Dirksen MT, van der Wal AC, van den Berg FM, van der Loos CM, Becker AE. Distribution of inflammatory cells in atherosclerotic plaques relates to the direction of flow. Circulation 1998; 98: 200–3.

49. Ambrose JA, Tannenbaum MA, Alexopoulus D et al. Angiographic progression of coronary artery disease and the development of myocardial infarction. J Am Coll Cardiol 1988; 12: 56–62.

50. Little WC, Constantinescu M, Applegate RJ et al. Can coronary angiography predict the site of a subsequent myocardial infarction in patients with mild-to-moderate coronary artery disease? Circulation 1988; 78: 1157–66.

51. Somerville RP, Oblander SA, Apte SS. Matrix metalloproteinases: old dogs with new tricks. Genome Biol 2003; 4: 216.

52. Galis ZS, Sukhova GK, Lark MW, Libby P. Increased expression of matrix metalloproteinases and matrix degrading activity in vulnerable regions of human atherosclerotic plaques. J Clin Invest 1994; 94: 2493–503.

53. Bennett MR, Evan GI, Schwartz SM. Apoptosis of human vascular smooth muscle cells derived from normal vessels and coronary atherosclerotic plaques. J Clin Invest 1995; 95: 2266–74.

54. Geng YJ, Henderson LE, Levesque EB, Muszynski M, Libby P. Fas is expressed in human atherosclerotic intima and promotes apoptosis of cytokine-primed human vascular smooth muscle cells. Arterioscler Thromb Vasc Biol 1997; 17: 2200–8.

55. Morgan AR, Rerkasem K, Gallagher PJ et al. Differences in matrix metalloproteinase-1 and matrix metalloproteinase-12 transcript levels among carotid atherosclerotic plaques with different histopathological characteristics. Stroke 2004; 35: 1310–15.

56. Turu MM, Krupinski J, Catena E et al. Intraplaque MMP-8 levels are increased in asymptomatic patients with carotid plaque progression on ultrasound. Atherosclerosis 2005; 187: 161–9.

57. Daugherty A, Dunn JL, Rateri DL, Heinecke JW. Myeloperoxidase, a catalyst for lipoprotein oxidation, is expressed in human atherosclerotic lesions. J Clin Invest 1994; 94: 437–44.

58. Ivan E, Khatri JJ, Johnson C et al. Expansive arterial remodeling is associated with increased neointimal macrophage foam cell content: the murine model of macrophage-rich carotid artery lesions. Circulation 2002; 105: 2686–91.

59. Herman MP, Sukhova GK, Libby P et al. Expression of neutrophil collagenase (matrix metalloproteinase-8) in human atheroma: a novel collagenolytic pathway suggested by transcriptional profiling. Circulation 2001; 104: 1899–904.

60. Malik N, Greenfield BW, Wahl AF, Kiener PA. Activation of human monocytes through CD40 induces matrix metalloproteinases. J Immunol 1996; 156: 3952–60.

61. Rekhter MD, Zhang K, Narayanan AS et al. Type I collagen gene expression in human atherosclerosis. Localization to specific plaque regions. Am J Pathol 1993; 143: 1634–48.

62. Bayes-Genis A, Conover CA, Schwartz RS. The insulin-like growth factor axis: a review of atherosclerosis and restenosis. Circ Res 2000; 86: 125–30.

63. Laursen LS, Overgaard MT, Soe R et al. Pregnancy-associated plasma protein-A (PAPP-A) cleaves insulin-like growth factor binding protein (IGFBP)-5 independent of IGF: implications for the mechanism of IGFBP-4 proteolysis by PAPP-A. FEBS Lett 2001; 504: 36–40.

64. Renier G, Clement I, Desfaits AC, Lambert A. Direct stimulatory effect of insulin-like growth factor-I on monocyte and macrophage tumor necrosis factor-alpha production. Endocrinology 1996; 137: 4611–18.

65. Libby P. Vascular biology of acute coronary syndromes. In: Deckker M, Topol E, eds. Textbook of Interventional Cardiology. Philadelphia: Lippincott and Williams, 1998.

66. Bayes-Genis A, Conover CA, Overgaard MT et al. Pregnancy-associated plasma protein A as a marker of acute coronary syndromes. N Engl J Med 2201; 345: 1022–9.

67. Beaudeux JL, Burc L, Imbert-Bismut F et al. Serum plasma pregnancy-associated protein A: a potential marker of echogenic carotid atherosclerotic plaques in asymptomatic hyperlipidemic subjects at high cardiovascular risk. Arterioscler Thromb Vasc Biol 2003; 23: e7–10.

68. Sangiorgi G, Mauriello A, Bonanno E et al. Pregnancy associated plasma protein-A is markedly expressed by monocyte-macrophage cells in vulnerable and ruptured carotid atherosclerotic plaques: a link between inflammation and cerebrovascular events. J Am Coll Cardiol 2006; 47: 2201–11.

69. Cipollone F, Fazia M, Mincione G et al. Increased expression of transforming growth factor-beta1 as a stabilizing factor in human atherosclerotic plaques. Stroke 2004; 35: 2253–7.

70. Jander S, Sitzer M, Wendt A et al. Expression of tissue factor in high-grade carotid artery stenosis: association with plaque destabilization. Stroke 2001; 32: 850–4.

71. DeGraba TJ, Siren AL, Penix L et al. Increased endothelial expression of intercellular adhesion molecule-1 in symptomatic versus asymptomatic human carotid atherosclerotic plaque. Stroke 1998; 29: 1405–10.

72. Nuotio K, Lindsberg PJ, Carpen O et al. Adhesion molecule expression in symptomatic and asymptomatic carotid stenosis. Neurology 2003; 60: 1890–9.

73. Ross R. Atherosclerosis: an inflammatory disease. N Engl J Med 1999; 340: 115–26.

74. Ridker PM, Cushman M, Stampfer MJ, Tracy RP, Hennekens CH. Inflammation, aspirin, and the risk of cardiovascular disease in apparently healthy men. N Engl J Med 1997; 336: 973–9.

75. Libby P, Aikawa M. New insight into plaque stabilisation by lipid lowering. Drugs 1998; 56: 9–13, discussion 33.

76. Davies MJ, Gordon JL, Gearing AJ et al. The expression of adhesion molecules ICAM-1, VCAM-1, PECAM, E-selectin in human atherosclerosis. J Pathol 1993; 171: 223–9.

77. Ridker PM, Rifai N, Stampfer MJ, Hennekens CH. Plasma concentration of interleukin-6 and the risk of future myocardial infarction in apparently healthy men. Circulation 2000; 101: 1767–72.

78. Ridker PM, Stampfer MJ, Rifai N. Novel risk factors for systemic atherosclerosis: a comparison of C-reactive protein, fibrinogen, homocysteine, lipoprotein(a), and standard cholesterol screening as predictors of peripheral arterial disease. JAMA 2001; 285: 2481–5.

79. Peter K, Nawroth P, Conradt C et al. Circulating vascular cell adhesion molecule-1 correlates with the extent of human atherosclerosis in contrast to circulating intercellular adhesion molecule-1, E-selectin, P-selectin and thrombomodulin. Arterioscler Thromb Vasc Biol 1997; 17: 505–12.

80. Mallat Z, Corbaz A, Scoazec A et al. Expression of interleukin-18 in human atherosclerotic plaques and relation to plaque instability. Circulation 2001; 104: 1598–603.

81. Rothwell PM, Howard SC, Power DA et al. Fibrinogen concentration and risk of ischemic stroke and acute coronary events in 5113 patients with transient ischemic attack and minor ischemic stroke. Stroke 2004; 35: 2300–5.

82. Mauriello A, Sangiorgi G, Palmieri G et al. Hyperfibrinogenemia is associated with specific histological composition and complications of atherosclerotic carotid plaques in patients affected by transient ischemic attacks. Circulation 2000; 101: 744–50.

83. Erren M, Reinecke H, Junker R et al. Systemic inflammatory parameters in patients with atherosclerosis of the coronary and peripheral arteries. Arterioscler Thromb Vasc Biol 1999; 19: 2355–63.

84. Horstmann S, Kalb P, Koziol J, Gardner H, Wagner S. Profiles of matrix metalloproteinases, their inhibitors, and laminin in stroke patients: influence of different therapies. Stroke 2003; 34: 2165–70.

85. Taylor AJ, Farb AA, Angello DA, Burwell LR, Virmani R. Proliferative activity in coronary atherectomy tissue. Clinical, histopathologic, and immunohistochemical correlates. Chest 1995; 108: 815–20.

86. O'Brien ER, Alpers CE, Stewart DK et al. Proliferation in primary and restenotic coronary atherectomy tissue. Implications for antiproliferative therapy. Circ Res 1993; 73: 223–31.

87. Imanishi T, McBride J, Ho Q et al. Expression of cellular FLICE-inhibitory protein in human coronary arteries and in a rat vascular injury model. Am J Pathol 2000; 156: 125–37.

88. Flex A, Gaetani E, Papaleo P et al. Proinflammatory genetic profiles in subjects with history of ischemic stroke. Stroke 2004; 35: 2270–5.

89. Jerrard-Dunne P, Sitzer M, Risley P et al. Inflammatory gene load is associated with enhanced inflammation and early carotid atherosclerosis in smokers. Stroke 2004; 35: 2438–43.

3

Cerebrovascular anatomy and physiology and mechanisms of first-ever ischemic stroke in patients with carotid artery stenosis

Tatjana Rundek, Philip M Meyers and Kevin Crutchfield

Take-Home Messages

1. Fundamental to caring for patients with carotid occlusive disease is an integrated understanding of cerebrovascular anatomy, cerebrovascular physiology, and the mechanism of carotid disease-related strokes.
2. An understanding of cerebrovascular anatomy involves knowledge of the major cerebral vessels, circle of Willis and other potential collateralization pathways, and the most common anomalies that can be encountered in this circulation.
3. An understanding of cerebrovascular physiology should entail knowledge of the mechanisms of cerebral blood flow regulation, and the factors that can impact these mechanisms in health and disease.
4. The first warning sign of a previously asymptomatic carotid occlusive disease is often a complete stroke. Warning TIAs occur in only 20–30% of patients.
5. The mechanism of cerebral ischemia in patients with carotid occlusive disease is often artery-to-artery embolization. However, cerebral hemodynamic insufficiency may also contribute to the occurrence and severity of ischemic injury.
6. Among patients with asymptomatic carotid artery stenosis (CAS), various metabolic and hemodynamic disease states can cause cerebral ischemia (atrial fibrillation, left ventricular thrombus), or increase brain vulnerability to ischemic injury (sleep apnea, thyroid disorders, and nutritional deficiencies).

INTRODUCTION

Fundamental to caring for patients with carotid artery disease is a basic understanding of cerebrovascular anatomy and physiology as well as knowledge of the mechanisms and patterns of ischemic stroke in these patients. The brain is a highly metabolic organ, utilizing 20% of the body's energy at rest with limited metabolic substrate reserve. This limited anaerobic capacity makes the brain intrinsically dependent upon a continuous supply of blood to meet its energy demands. The unique anatomy of the cerebrovascular system allows for instantaneous, dynamic regulation of flow through collateralization

from multiple inputs and connections. Blood will always flow from an area of high pressure into an area of a lower pressure, so that alterations in the vascular structure may alter which cerebral territories are at greatest risk by altering the pressure gradient. The healthy cerebrovascular system has developed mechanisms to compensate for external stressors that may limit the central nervous system (CNS) energy delivery or utilization. In disease, these mechanisms may be maximally stressed so that the introduction of another stressor may lead to vascular inefficiency and subsequent brain ischemia.

This chapter will review the unique anatomy and physiology of the cerebrovascular system, the mechanisms and patterns of first-ever ischemic stroke in patients with carotid disease, and the common systemic conditions that may impair the system's innate abilities to preserve cerebral perfusion.

CEREBROVASCULAR ANATOMY

It is through familiarity with the normal cerebrovascular anatomy as well as its common variants and anomalies that identification of pathology can be readily accomplished. The focus of this section is to cover basic neurovascular anatomy, the common variants which may be misinterpreted as disease, and the cerebrovascular collateral circulation in patients with carotid occlusive disease.

The aortic arch and great vessels

The three major arterial branches from the aortic arch are the innominate artery, the left common carotid artery, and the left subclavian artery (Figure 3.1). The innominate artery is typically the first branch of the arch

and bifurcates into the right subclavian and right common carotid arteries. An aberrant right subclavian artery is a common arch abnormality and can occur in 0.5–1.0% of cases. The right vertebral artery is the first branch off of the right subclavian artery and is dominant in 25% of cases. The right carotid artery arises from the proximal innominate artery and may occasionally arise directly from the arch. The left common carotid artery is typically the second vessel arising from the arch and has a number of variants, including a common origin with the innominate, hypoplastic, or absent. The left subclavian artery is the last vessel arising from the arch and gives rise to the left vertebral artery, which is dominant in 50–60% of cases.

Anterior cerebrovascular circulation

External carotid artery

The external carotid artery supplies most of the extracranial head and neck and has several branches, including the superior thyroid, ascending pharyngeal,

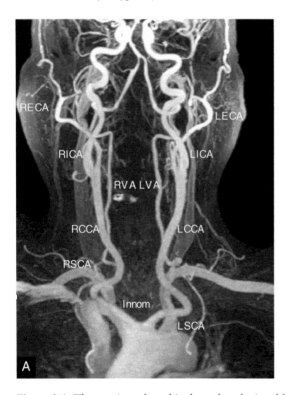 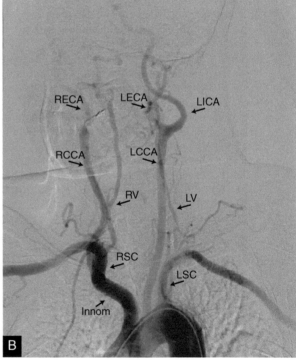

Figure 3.1 The aortic arch and its branches depicted by (A) contrast-enhanced MR angiography (courtesy of Steven Wolf MD) and (B) digital substraction angiography. LSCA, left subclavian artery; RSCA, right subclavian artery; Innom, innominate artery; LVA, left vertebral artery; RVA, right vertebral artery; LCCA, left common carotid artery; RCCA, right common carotid artery; LICA, left internal carotid artery; RICA, right internal carotid artery; LECA, left external carotid artery; RECA, right external carotid artery.

lingual, facial, occipital, posterior auricular, superficial temporal, and internal maxillary arteries.

The external carotid artery provides intracranial, anterior collateral flow through the middle meningeal artery anastomosis with the lacrimal branch of the supratrochlear branch of the ophthalmic artery as well as extracranial, supraorbital branch anastomosis with the superficial temporal artery branch of the external carotid artery. The ophthalmic artery provides blood flow to the orbit, as well as critical, ipsilateral internal to external collateral channels.

Internal carotid artery

The internal carotid artery (ICA) has a number of segments that warrant individual attention, as each can commonly become involved with differing pathological processes. The carotid bulb involves the distal 2–4 cm of the common carotid artery, the dilatation at the ICA bulb, and the proximal 2–4 cm of the ICA. As shown in Figure 3.2, the cervical segment typically has no branches and remains smooth and non-dilated. In about 10% of cases the cervical ICA originates from the common carotid bifurcation medial to rather than lateral to the external carotid. The petrous segment begins when the ICA enters the carotid canal in the temporal bone (Figure 3.2C). Importantly, the intrapetrous segment may give rise to an aberrant ICA by taking a posterolateral instead of an anteromedial course through the temporal bone. This aberrant course can be readily identified by angiography and has important clinical application in its differentiation from glomus tumors and prevention of unwitting biopsy. The cavernous segment begins where the ICA exits from the carotid canal and terminates in the subarachnoid space. Important branches off the cavernous ICA include the ophthalmic artery, the posterior communicating artery (PComm), and the anterior choroidal artery. The ophthalmic artery provides an anastomosis between the internal and external carotid arteries, forming an important collateral pathway in the situation of occlusion of the internal carotid artery. The PComm can be hypoplastic in up to 30% of cases. The PComm may also persist in its embryonic form as the fetal origin of the posterior cerebral artery (PCA) in 20–25% of cases. In rare cases, the anterior choroidal may be hypoplastic and supply vascular territory in the PCA distribution. The ICA terminates at the bifurcation of the anterior and middle cerebral arteries, defining the anterior cerebral flow territory, which represent the final collateral pathway for carotid flow distribution.

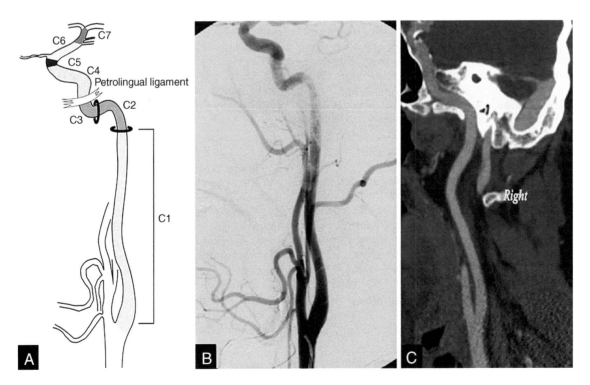

Figure 3.2 Anatomy of the internal carotid artery (ICA). (A) The various segments of the ICA. (B) Digital subtraction angiography of the ICA. (C) CT angiography of the right ICA (courtesy of Steven Wolf MD).

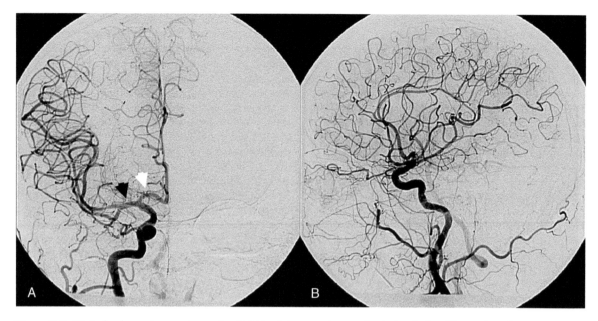

Figure 3.3 Digital subtraction angiography (DSA) of the anterior cerebral circulation illustrating the anterior cerebral artery (ACA, white arrow) and the middle cerebral artery (MCA, black arrow) in the AP view (A) and the lateral view (B).

Anterior cerebral artery (ACA)

The ACA comprises two segments, the A1 and A2. The A1 segment gives rise to the medial lenticulostriates, which supply the caudate head and the anterior limb of the internal capsule. The A2 segment curves around the genu of the corpus callosum and gives rise to the recurrent artery of Heubner in 50% of cases. Common variants of the ACA include a hypoplastic or absent A1 in 5–18% and duplicated AComm arteries in 10% of individuals (Figure 3.3).

Middle cerebral artery (MCA)

The MCA comprises the horizontal (M1) segment, which gives rise to the lateral lenticulostriates, which supply the putamen and globus pallidus, insular (M2) segment within the insula and exiting from the sylvian fissure, and the opercular (M3) segment emerging from the sylvian fissure and supplying the hemispheric surface (see Figure 3.3).

Posterior cerebrovascular circulation

Vertebral arteries

The vertebral arteries (VA) originate from their respective subclavian arteries, with the left VA being dominant in the majority of cases. The VA enter the transverse foramina at C6 and exit at C2, where they turn laterally then cephalad though C1. Each passes through the foramen magnum to join the basilar artery. Extracranially, the VA gives rise to the posterior meningeal artery, which can be enlarged with dural malformations or tumors. Intracranially, the VA gives rise to the posterior inferior cerebellar artery (PICA). A hypoplastic VA can be seen in up to 40% of angiograms. Additionally, 1% of vertebral arteries end in the PICA see Figure 3.5).

Basilar artery

The basilar artery is formed by the union of the right and left vertebral arteries and extends cephalad rostrally to the pons and midbrain to terminate at the origins of the right and left PCAs. The basilar artery is approximately 3 cm in length and can vary from 1.5 to 4 mm in diameter. Diameters greater than this are abnormal and indicate the presence of dolichoectasia. The main branches of the basilar artery are the anterior inferior cerebellar artery (AICA), pontine perforating branches, and the superior cerebellar arteries (SCAs). Important variants include SCAs arising from the PCAs and basilar hypoplasia in the setting of a fetal PCA.

Posterior cerebral artery

In the majority of cases, the posterior cerebral arteries (PCAs) originate from the basilar artery. They comprise a P1 or peduncular segment, a P2 or ambient segment, and a P3 or quadrigeminal segment. The P1 segment typically gives rise to the posterior thalamoperforating arteries, which supply the thalamus and midbrain, and the medial posterior choroidal artery, which supplies the tectum, midbrain, posterior thalamus, pineal gland, and the choroid of the third ventricle. The P2 segment gives rise to the lateral posterior choroidal artery, which supplies the posterior thalamus and the choroid plexus of the lateral ventricles, and the thalamogeniculate arteries, which supply the medial geniculate body, pulvinar, crus cerebri, and occasionally the lateral geniculate body. The posterior cerebral artery becomes supratentorial just before combining with the posterior communicating arteries providing for anterior–posterior collateral flow.

The posterior vessels provide for all the infratentorial structures as well as the supratentorial occipital lobes. Extracranial collateral flow may occur via an anastomosis of the occipital artery off the external carotid artery and the posterior meningeal artery off the vertebral arteries. There is also a minimal, more proximal collateral channel from the thyrocervical trunk to the vertebral artery. With the exception of a slightly redundant input and the collateral channels mentioned, there is limited ability of the posterior circulation to dynamically regulate cerebral blood flow.

Cerebral collateral circulation

A basic understanding of the anatomy of the cerebral collateral circulation is required to make informed decisions regarding prognosis of patients with carotid occlusive disease as well as outcome of carotid revascularization therapies. The cerebral collateral circulation refers to the network of vascular channels that preserve cerebral blood flow when major conduits fail. The course and anatomic characteristics of collaterals vary extensively. The collateral vessels are formed during the prenatal period, although pathophysiological conditions may cause secondary changes. The collateral ability of a vessel is ultimately determined by luminal caliber.[1] The arterial anatomy of the collateral circulation includes extracranial sources of cerebral blood flow (Figure 3.4) and intracranial routes of ancillary perfusion (Figure 3.5) that are commonly divided into primary or secondary collateral pathways.[2]

Primary collaterals

These collaterals include the arterial segments of the circle of Willis. The circle of Willis, first described by the English physician Thomas Willis in 1664, serves to link the anterior circulation, comprising the ICA, ACA, and anterior communicating artery (AComm), with the

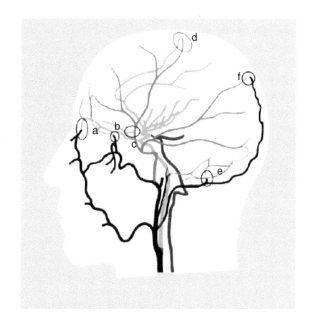

Figure 3.4 Extracranial arterial collateral circulation. Shown are anastomoses from the facial (a), maxillary (b), and middle meningeal (c) arteries to the ophthalmic artery and dural arteriolar anastomoses from the middle meningeal artery (d) and occipital artery through the mastoid foramen (e) and parietal foramen (f). (Adapted from Liebeskind et al.[2])

posterior circulation, comprising the PComm, the horizontal P1 segments of the PCA, and the basilar artery. Only 20–25% of individuals have a complete circle of Willis. Anatomic studies note the absence of the anterior communicating artery in 1% of subjects, absence or hypoplasia of the proximal anterior cerebral artery in 10%, and absence or hypoplasia of either posterior communicating artery in 30%.[3] The majority of the circle of Willis is superior to the tentorium cerebelli, but the proximal posterior cerebral arteries are infratentorial. Space-occupying or pressure-mediated pathologies in either space may alter the collateral flow efficacy of the circle of Willis.

Interhemispheric blood flow across the anterior communicating artery and reversal of flow in the proximal anterior cerebral artery provide collateral support in the anterior portion of the circle of Willis (Figure 3.6). Published data have demonstrated improved outcomes in treatment of ICA stenosis when this channel is open.[4] The posterior communicating arteries may supply collateral blood flow in either direction between the anterior and posterior circulations. Additional inter-hemispheric collaterals include the proximal posterior cerebral arteries at the posterior aspect of the circle of Willis.

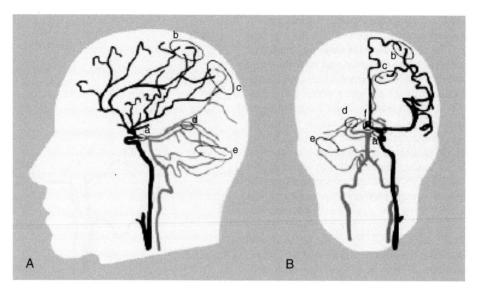

Figure 3.5 Intracranial arterial collateral circulation in lateral (A) and frontal (B) views. Shown are posterior communicating artery (a); leptomeningeal anastomoses between anterior and middle cerebral arteries (b) and between posterior and middle cerebral arteries (c); tectal plexus between posterior cerebral and superior cerebellar arteries (d); anastomoses of distal cerebellar arteries (e); and anterior communicating artery (f). (Adapted from Liebeskind DS et al.[2])

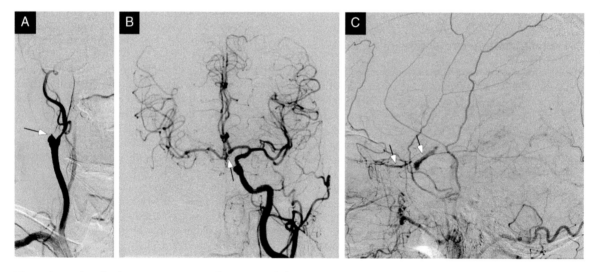

Figure 3.6 Digital subtraction angiography (DSA) of the anterior portion of the circle of Willis: (A) occlusion of the RICA (arrow); (B) intracranial DSA, illustrating the left anterior cerebral artery (ACA) and middle cerebral artery (MCA) and left to right hemisphere collaterals through the anterior communicating artery (ACA) (arrow); (C) notice filling of the distal RICA through the right ophthalmic artery (arrows).

Secondary collaterals

This circulation is divided into:[5]

1. The ophthalmic artery (Figure 3.6C).
2. The leptomeningeal (also known as superficial or pial) arteries, which consist of the terminal branches

of the anterior, middle, and posterior cerebral arteries forming an anastomotic network on the surface of the hemispheres and yielding branches that penetrate the cortex and subjacent white matter; the deepest ones form the medullary (or superficial perforating) arteries (Figure 3.7).

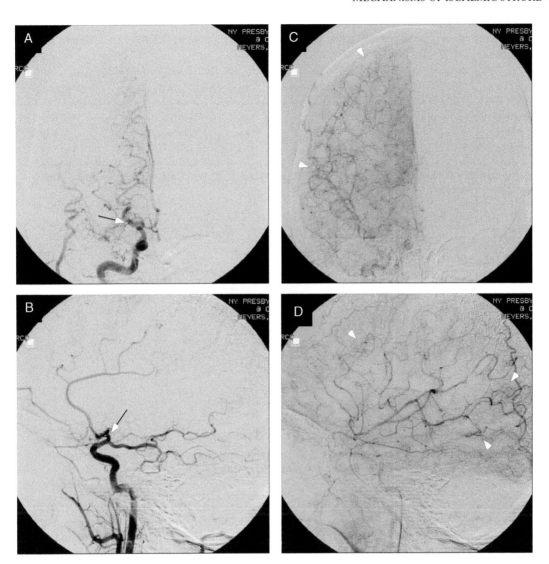

Figure 3.7 Occluded right middle cerebral artery (MCA) in anteroposterior view (A) and lateral view (B). Note the leptomeningeal collaterals in the anteroposterior view (C) and lateral view (D).

3. The perforating (or deep perforating) arteries, arising from the circle of Willis or from its immediate branches, perforating the brain parenchyma as direct penetrators, and supplying the diencephalon and the basal ganglia.

Patterns of collateral blood flow in patients with asymptomatic carotid artery stenosis

In patients with CAS, the cause of stroke is primarily thromboembolic; however, it is recognized that the presence of low regional cerebral blood flow is also a risk factor.[6] As a consequence, the occurrence of ischemic stroke in these patients may be due not only to the embolic process but also to the influence of differences in collateral pathways distal to the stenosis.

A magnetic resonance angiography (MRA) study by Hendrikse and colleagues described the primary cerebral collateral pathways in patients with asymptomatic CAS vs those with symptomatic CAS or normal subjects (Table 3.1).[7] Patients with asymptomatic CAS had a higher prevalence of collateral flow via the anterior communicating artery compared with other groups (Figure 3.8). The contribution of the posterior communicating artery to collateral flow was small in all patients studied. Although this report documents the

Table 3.1 Prevalence of collateral flow patterns via ipsilateral circle of Willis in patients with and without carotid artery stenosis

	Asymptomatic CAS (n = 19)	Symptomatic CAS (n = 21)	Controls (n = 53)
AComm only	7 (37%)	2 (10%)	0
PComm only	1 (5%)	3 (14%)	5 (9%)
AComm or PComm	8 (42%)	5 (24%)	5 (9%)

CAS, carotid artery stenosis; AComm, anterior communicating artery; PComm, posterior communicating artery. Adapted from Hendrikse et al.[7]

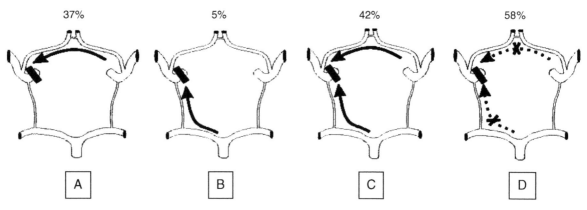

Figure 3.8 Patterns of collateral flow in patients with severe asymptomatic carotid stenosis via the circle of Willis, categorized as (A) via the A1 segment of the ACA only, (B) via the posterior communicating artery (PComm) only, (C) via both the A1 segment and the PComm and (D) no collateral flow via the circle of Willis. (Adapted from Hendrikse et al.[7])

importance of circle of Willis collaterals to symptomatology in patients with carotid occlusive disease, the relationship of collaterals to risk of future stroke in patients with asymptomatic CAS remains unknown.

CEREBROVASCULAR PHYSIOLOGY

Given the physical and rheologic properties of blood, a non-Newtonian fluid,[8] maintenance of laminar flow in the cerebrovascular tree is critical to maximize peripheral delivery of metabolic substrate. The ability of the cerebral vessels to autoregulate and display vasomotor reactivity is dependent upon anatomic and physiological properties of the cerebral blood vessels. Cerebral vessels are divided into three discreet functional groups (Figure 3.9).[9]

1. The conductance vessels, which are the large, muscular arteries that extend from the aortic root to the level of the arterioles.

2. The resistance vessels, which are represented by the small arteries and the arterioles that control volumetric flow by narrowing and increasing resistance to flow.

3. The capacitance vessels, which are represented by the cerebrovenous system.

Conductance vessels physiology

The conductance vessels are divided into the more proximal, elastic arteries, with their ability to dampen the great pressures generated during cardiac systole, and the more distal muscular arteries that form the circle of Willis. Differences in the composition and relative proportions of fibrin, collagen, and smooth muscles differentiate the type and function of the conductance vessels. The main role of these vessels is to move blood forward by the maintenance of a pressure gradient. Physiologically, the circle of Willis and all its branches, down to the level of the arterioles, constitute the conductance or conduit vessels of the brain.

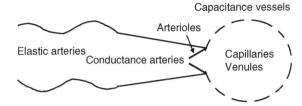

Figure 3.9 Schematic representation of the functional groups of the cerebrovascular system.

Vessels have intrinsic energy demands, especially the large, elastic muscular arteries or 'Windkessel' vessels that provide a dampening of the high-pressure wave generated by the forceful contraction of the heart in systole as well as accessory pumping function for the vascular system.[9] The further away from the heart the vessel is located, this action dissipates, with no visible distention of the cerebral vessels. A virtual stretch and constriction of the vascular smooth muscles (myogenic reflex) of the muscular arteries of the circle of Willis will increase tension in the vascular smooth muscle; the extent of this input into the kinetics of the system needs to be fully determined, but clearly helps to maintain the pressure gradient as well as efficient laminar flow. The stretch and contraction of the large elastic vessels creates an accessory pressure boost to the vascular system, and this harmonic activity – known in physics as a transverse propagation wave – has been reported to have a significant effect on the maintenance of efficient laminar flow through reduction of turbulence.[8]

Alterations in metabolism may have an effect on the relative tensions generated by the muscular and elastic arteries, by increasing smooth muscle tone. With the diminution of available adenosine triphosphate (ATP), smooth muscles will increase contracture or tension. This action causes an increase in proximal pressure wave propagation as well as an increase in conductance vessel resistance, with the final result of an early reflected pressure wave. This leads to increased intravascular pressure, with vessel distention and hypertrophy.[8]

Dynamic regulation, autoregulation, and vasomotor reactivity

The cerebrovascular system has developed at least three mechanisms for the preservation of the perfusion pressure gradient:

- dynamic regulation, which is predominantly a function of structural anatomy and occurs in the larger conductance vessels of the brain
- autoregulation, which is a physiological phenomenon of segmental and capacitance vessel regulators

to offset disturbances in perfusion pressure to maintain constant regional flow
- vasomotor reactivity, which refers to the ability of the resistance vessels to meet changing metabolic demands.

The terms autoregulation and vasomotor reactivity describe different phenomena with distinct prognostic implications,[10] and should not be used interchangeably. Autoregulation is a muscular, conductance artery phenomenon where cerebral blood flow rate is constant regardless of changes in the cerebral perfusion pressure gradient.[11] This may be secondary to myogenic mechanisms, but other factors, including potassium channels,[12] and adenosine levels[13] are involved as well. Chronically increased intravascular pressure diminishes the ability of this mechanism to compensate, whereas vasomotor reactivity is an arteriole response to neurogenic or chemical stimuli associated with healthy cerebral vessels and its alterations are associated with pathological states and an increased risk of cerebrovascular events.

Neuronal and chemical control of autoregulation and vasomotor reactivity

Autoregulation and vasomotor reactivity are modulated by neuronal input, stretch forces (myogenic), and the local chemical environment. Regional expansion of the capacitance vessel volume will diminish overall local vascular resistance by opening more parallel channels, creating a greater pressure gradient, and thereby increasing flow into that region. All these mechanisms are in dynamic equilibrium: a change in capacitance (or impedance) in one region will dynamically affect the entire system, given a constant intravascular volume.

Central neurogenic control is mediated by cholinergic and noradrenergic nerve terminals at the resistance vessels, the arterioles. When stimulated, the resistance vessels open and allow for an increase in volumetric flow into the territory involved. With an increase in the number of parallel resistance vessels now open, the perfusion pressure into the region drops unless a compensatory increase in proximal perfusion pressure were to occur. In pulsatile systems, this is expressed as a pulse pressure gradient to impedance relationship. When imbalanced, a perfusion to impedance mismatch is present and leads to low flow or conversely, the hyperemic flow state. Interventions such as carotid endarterectomy (CEA) have been noted to improve vasomotor reactivity over time.

Vasomotor reserve control is a chemical response of the capacitance vessels that opens the resistance vessels in much the same way as the neurogenic mechanisms described above. The most classic example of this resistance and capacitance vessel response is to hypercapnia, with a resultant increase in flow through the conductance vessels to meet the new pressure demand. This constitutes the basis for the present vasomotor reserve testing (see Chapter 10) that is performed to measure the ability of the system to respond to a metabolic stressor. If already compromised by an external stressor, such as diminished flow from a proximal vascular lesion with low-grade ischemia, then the system may be maximally or near maximally dilated or opened already to meet the increased demands of the new stressor, thereby limiting the response of the vascular territory. Low-grade hypoxemia or ischemia may also cause the same. From a hemodynamic perspective, adequate metabolic substrate delivery is dependent upon a balanced interaction between cerebral perfusion pressure and blood flow impedance, relying on both autoregulation and vasomotor reactivity.

MECHANISMS AND PATTERNS OF FIRST-EVER STROKE IN PATIENTS WITH PREVIOUSLY ASYMPTOMATIC CORONARY ARTERY STENOSIS

Mechanisms of ICA-related ischemic stroke

It has been shown that up to 40% of ischemic strokes in patients with previously asymptomatic CAS are lacunar or cardioembolic and about 60% are related to carotid stenosis.[14] The relative importance of hemodynamic, as opposed to thromboembolic mechanisms of CAS-related strokes, has been a subject of debate.[15] There is mounting evidence, however, that the mechanism of ischemic stroke in the majority of these patients is artery-to-artery embolization.[16] Nonetheless, it is well known that many of these patients may actually have asymptomatic embolization without sustaining clinical or subclinical ischemic injury.[17] Although one may argue that this may be due to the size of the embolized particle as well as the site of embolism, there is evidence that there are hemodynamic and metabolic factors that may render the brain susceptible to ischemic injury in some patients more than others.

Clinical presentation of ICA-related cerebral ischemia

Patients with previously asymptomatic CAS often present with a completed stroke as opposed to a transient ischemic attack (TIA) as the first manifestation of their disease.[18] Other patients, however, may present with a TIA that may or may not be followed by a completed stroke. The reasons for this variability in clinical presentation remain unclear. Some investigators, however, have suggested that the frequency of TIAs in patients with previously asymptomatic CAS is related to lesion severity.[19] These investigators found that the frequency of TIAs increases in parallel with the degree of lesion severity up to a critical degree of 90%; thereafter, the frequency of TIAs decreases.

With respect to the relationship between location and etiology of cerebral ischemia, Anderson and colleagues have shown that retinal symptoms are more typical than hemispheric symptoms for carotid stenosis.[20] Furthermore, the retinal vs hemispheric location of initial symptoms was strongly predictive of the location of subsequent events in patients with carotid stenosis, even when new symptoms are contralateral to the original ones.

Imaging patterns of ICA-related ischemic stroke

Recent studies have clearly illustrated that different stroke patterns on magnetic resonance imaging (MRI) can predict the cause of stroke, as defined by the TOAST classification.[21] In a study by Tsiskaridze and colleagues,[19] 173 patients who experienced their first-ever stroke and who had >50% ipsilateral carotid artery stenosis were evaluated for patterns of cerebral infarcts. Anterior pial infarcts occurred in 31% of patients, posterior pial infarcts in 19%, subcortical infarcts in 20%, large hemispheral infarcts in 12%, and borderzone infarcts in 10%. The topography of large-artery ischemic strokes in patients with carotid disease can be one of two patterns:

1. Territorial distribution without borderzone involvement, which is a typical pattern of ICA-related stroke consistent with an artery-to-artery embolization (Figure 3.10).
2. Borderzone distribution (watershed), with or without territorial involvement (Figure 3.11). Watershed infarcts (WS) involve the junction of the distal fields of two non-anastomosing arterial systems. Classic neuropathological studies describe two distinct WS areas:[22]

   - cortical watershed (CWS) infarcts between the cortical territories of the ACA, MCA, and PCA
   - internal watershed (IWS) infarcts in the white matter along and slightly above the lateral ventricle, between the deep and the superficial arterial systems of the MCA, or between the superficial systems of the MCA and ACA.

In autopsy studies, watershed infarcts represent about 10% of all brain infarcts.[23] However, because WS infarction is seldom fatal, this is probably an underestimate, and imaging studies in severe internal

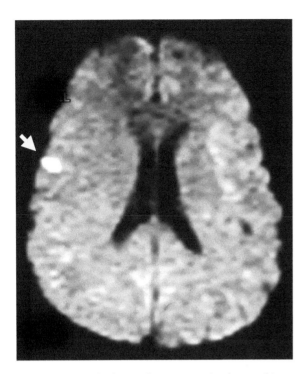

Figure 3.10 Right hemispheric cortical infarct (white arrow) in a patient with carotid occlusive disease.

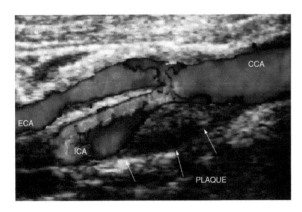

Figure 3.11 Left hemispheric watershed ischemic stroke (arrows) due to high-grade left internal carotid artery stenosis. (See color plate section.)

carotid artery disease report an incidence ranging from 19% to 64%.[24–26] Although the pathological and imaging characteristics of WS infarcts are well-described, their pathogenesis remains a subject of debate. Based on the well-established observation that severe systemic hypotension can cause bilateral WS infarction, hemodynamic failure is classically considered to cause WS infarcts in ICA disease.[27] In contrast, embolism from ICA disease

preferentially affects the stem and large branches of the MCA, producing cortical and/or deep striatocapsular infarcts.[28]

Nonetheless, in sharp contrast with the above view, several pathological reports emphasize the association of WS infarction with microemboli arising from unstable carotid plaques.[29–32]

Therefore, there is considerable controversy regarding the pathophysiology of WS infarcts in critical carotid disease, with both the low-flow and the multiembolic mechanisms being considered, based on substantial evidence for both. However, most likely, a synergetic association of these two mechanisms is involved.[6] Future studies combining imaging of brain perfusion, diffusion-weighted imaging, and ultrasound detection of microembolic signals will help resolve these issues.

EFFECT OF SYSTEMIC DISEASE STATES ON THE CEREBROVASCULAR SYSTEM

Metabolic disorders

Metabolic disturbances diminish the ability of endothelial and smooth muscle cells to efficiently generate ATP, leading to significant alterations in the physiological performance of the cerebrovascular system. These changes include diminished proximal perfusion pressure generation, increased vascular resistance with a diminution of capacitance vessel volume, or expansion of the capacitance vessel volume with resultant drop in the capillary perfusion pressure gradient. The number of metabolic derangements that could lead to this state is numerous, but some of the more common treatable disturbances that are not addressed elsewhere in this book include sleep apnea, thyroid disease, and nutritional deficiencies.

Sleep apnea

Sleep apnea has been shown to lead to a number of cardiovascular and metabolic disturbances that increase the likelihood of stroke.[33,34] More specifically, sleep apnea has been shown to be an independent risk factor for stroke and death.[35] Sleep apnea is associated with decreased cerebral blood flow, paradoxical embolization, and hypercoagulability, all alterations that may increase the risk of stroke. Although the underlying mechanisms for the cerebrovascular hemodynamic alterations remain ill-defined, findings from a study using transcranial Doppler (TCD) and dynamic vascular analysis (DVA) have showed that chronic sleep apnea in subjects with cerebrovascular events may affect cerebrovascular dynamics in a pattern consistent with diminished proximal force of flow.[36] Stiffening of the proximal elastic arteries secondary to hypertension[8] associated with the apnea could account for this kinetic state, as would diminished cardiac output.

Hypercarbia causes increased intracranial pressure (ICP) and increased intracranial vascular resistance during apnea.[37] Apnea also causes an increase of the pressure in the right atrium, which not only increases the right-to-left shunting but also decreases venous return to the heart with overall diminished cardiac output, causing a drop in proximal perfusion pressure consistent with the findings observed in a DVA study. Since successful treatment of apnea has been shown to improve endothelial function,[38] screening for and treating apnea or other causes of diminished metabolic support of the large muscular arteries could improve efficiency of the proximal elastic arteries, improving laminar flow characteristics and cerebral perfusion.

Thyroid disease

Thyroid homeostasis is vital to proper mitochondrial energy production.[39] Disruptions of this homeostasis leads to significant alterations in cardiovascular and, subsequently, cerebrovascular dynamics.[40–42] These cerebrovascular changes improve after thyroid hormone replacement. Using the data from DVA, a diminution of forward perfusion pressure with diminished cerebrovascular dynamics secondary to hypothyroidism was observed (internal data of New Health Sciences, Inc. – available upon request).

Vitamin deficiencies

The B vitamins are utilized by mitochondrial enzymes in the efficient production of ATP as well as the metabolism of amino acids. Diminution of these vitamins may lead to decreased amounts of ATP available for maintenance of efficient myogenic tone and increased levels of homocysteine, which increases vascular resistance.[43] Thiamine deficiency, for example, causes low cardiac output[44] with early hyperdynamic or high output failure, with an initial decreased vascular resistance and increased intravascular volume. This would lead to the drop in proximal perfusion pressure with a concomitant diminution of elasticity secondary to increased intravascular volume. Folate deficiency leads to increased levels of homocysteine, with concomitant increased risk of vascular events.[45] Data from DVA studies (internal data of New Health Sciences, Inc. – available upon request) has shown increased muscular artery resistance that diminishes after just 6 weeks of oral folic acid therapy.

Cardiac diseases

Proximal vascular diseases such as congestive heart failure have been shown to diminish cerebral vasomotor reactivity to inhaled CO_2[46] and have a characteristic low dynamic flow pattern with DVA testing.[47] Other causes of diminished proximal perfusion pressure of the intracranial vessels are dysrhythmia, decreased cardiac output from any cause, and aortic valve disease. A patent foramen ovale (PFO) may also increase the risk of vascular events and, unless screened efficiently, will increase the likelihood of an adverse event in endovascular trials. Concurrent sleep apnea increases right-to-left shunting[48] as well as increased coagulability, making the likelihood of a CNS complication even higher. This combination makes patients with PFOs more likely to suffer embolic events in the setting of sleep apnea. TCD and carotid ultrasonography with intravenous administration of microbubbles have made the non-invasive screening of PFO available in the office setting. The impact of PFO on cerebral flow dynamics and cerebrovascular disease needs further investigation.

SUMMARY

Fundamental to caring for patients with carotid occlusive disease is an integrated understanding of cerebrovascular anatomy, cerebrovascular physiology, mechanisms of carotid disease-related strokes, and the underlying systemic disease states that may predispose patients to a cerebral ischemic event. An understanding of cerebrovascular anatomy should involve knowledge of the major cerebral vessels, circle of Willis, and the potential collateralization pathways in occlusive carotid disease. An understanding of cerebrovascular physiology should entail knowledge of cerebral blood flow regulation in health and disease. Physicians should also be familiar with patterns of clinical presentation as well as topography of brain ischemia on imaging. Lastly, it is important to emphasize that, irrespective of the direct cause of cerebral ischemia, systemic metabolic and hemodynamic alterations can greatly increase the vulnerability of the brain to ischemic injury. These conditions should be identified and treated.

REFERENCES

1. Hoksbergen AW, Fulesdi B, Legemate DA, Csiba L. Collateral configuration of the circle of Willis: transcranial color-coded duplex ultrasonography and comparison with postmortem anatomy. Stroke 2000; 31: 1346–51.
2. Liebeskind DS. Collateral circulation. Stroke 2003; 34: 2279–84.
3. Lippert H, Pabst R. Arterial Variations in Man. Munich, Germany: JF Bergmann Verlag, 1985: 92–3.

4. Kluytmans M, van der Grond J, van Everdingen K et al. Cerebral hemodynamics in relation to patterns of collateral flow. Stroke 1999; 30: 1432–9.

5. Tatu L, Moulin T, Bogousslavsky J, Duvernoy H. Arterial territories of the human brain: cerebral hemispheres. Neurology 1998; 50(6): 1699–708.

6. Caplan LR, Hennerici M. Impaired clearance of emboli (washout) is an important link between hypoperfusion, embolism, and ischemic stroke. Arch Neurol 1999; 55: 1475–82.

7. Hendrikse J, Eikelboom BC, van der Grond J. Magnetic resonance angiography of collateral compensation in asymptomatic and symptomatic internal carotid artery stenosis. J Vasc Surg 2002; 36 (4): 1–7.

8. McDonald's Blood Flow in Arteries, 5th edn. New York: Oxford University Press, 2005.

9. Milnor WR. Cardiovascular Physiology, 1st edn, New York: Oxford University Press, 1990.

10. Poon WS, Ng SC, Chan MT, Lam JM, Lam WW. Cerebral blood flow (CBF)-directed management of ventilated head-injured patients. Acta Neurochir Suppl 2005; 95: 9–11.

11. Lassen NA, Friberg L, Kastrup J, Rizzi D, Jensen JJ. Effects of acetazolamide on cerebral blood flow and brain tissue oxygenation. Postgrad Med J 1987; 63: 185–7.

12. Plane F, Johnson R, Kerr P et al. Heteromutimeric Kv1 channels contribute to myogenic control of arterial diameter. Circ Res 2005; 96(2): 216–24.

13. Phillis JW. Adenosine and adenine nucleotides as regulators of cerebral blood flow: roles of acidosis, cell swelling and KATP channels. Crit Rev Neurobiol 2004; 16(4): 237–70.

14. Inzitari D, Eliasziw M, Gates P et al. The causes and risk of stroke in patients with asymptomatic internal-carotid-artery stenosis. N Engl J Med 2000; 342: 1693–700.

15. Barnett HJ. Hemodynamic cerebral ischemia. An appeal for systematic data gathering prior to a new EC/IC trial. Stroke 1997; 28(10): 1857–60.

16. Kang DW, Chu K, Ko SB et al. Lesion patterns and mechanism of ischemic internal carotid artery disease. Arch Neurol 2002; 59: 1577–82.

17. Markus HS, Droste DW, Brown MM. Detection of asymptomatic cerebral embolic signals with Doppler ultrasound. Lancet 1994; 343(8904): 1011–12.

18. Mackey AE, Abrahamowicz M, Langlois Y et al. Outcome of asymptomatic patients with carotid disease. Neurology 1997; 48: 896–903.

19. Tsiskaridze A, Devuyst G, de Freitas GR, van Melle G, Bogousslavsky J. Stroke with internal carotid artery stenosis. Arch Neurol 2001; 58(4): 605–9.

20. Anderson DC, Kappelle LJ, Eliasziw M et al. Occurrence of hemispheric and retinal ischemia in atrial fibrillation compared with carotid stenosis. Stroke 2002; 33: 1963–8.

21. Kang DW, Chalela JA, Ezzeddine MA, Warach S. Association of ischemic lesion patterns on early diffusion-weighted imaging with TOAST stroke subtypes. Arch Neurol 2003; 60: 1730–4.

22. Zulch KJ. Uber die entstenhung und lokalisation der hirninfarkte. Acta Neurol Chir 1961; 7(Suppl): 1–117.

23. Jorgensen L, Torvik A. Ischaemic cerebrovascular diseases in an autopsy series. 2. Prevalence, location, pathogenesis, and clinical course of cerebral infarcts. J Neurol Sci 1969; 9: 285–320.

24. Bogousslavsky J, Regli F. Unilateral watershed cerebral infarcts. Neurology 1986; 36: 373–7.

25. Ringelstein EB, Zeumer H, Angelou D. The pathogenesis of strokes from internal carotid artery occlusion. Diagnostic and therapeutical implications. Stroke 1983; 14: 867–75.

26. Wodarz R. Watershed infarctions and computed tomography. A topographical study in cases with stenosis or occlusion of the carotid artery. Neuroradiology 1980; 19: 245–8.

27. Bladin CF, Chambers BR. Frequency and pathogenesis of hemodynamic stroke. Stroke 1994; 25: 2179–82.

28. Mull M, Schwarz M, Thron A. Cerebral hemispheric low-flow infarcts in arterial occlusive disease. Lesion patterns and angiomorphological conditions. Stroke 1997; 28: 118–23.

29. Beal MF, Williams RS, Richardson EP Jr, Fisher CM. Cholesterol embolism as a cause of transient ischemic attacks and cerebral infarction. Neurology 1981; 31: 860–5.

30. Pollanen MS, Deck JH. Directed embolization is an alternate cause of cerebral watershed infarction. Arch Pathol Lab Med 1989; 113: 1139–41.

31. Masuda J, Yutani C, Ogata J, Kuriyama Y, Yamaguchi T. Atheromatous embolism in the brain: a clinicopathologic analysis of 15 autopsy cases. Neurology 1994; 44: 1231–7.

32. Pollanen MS, Deck JH. The mechanism of embolic watershed infarction: experimental studies. Can J Neurol Sci 1990; 17: 395–8.

33. Yaggi HK, Mohsenin V. Obstructive sleep apnea and stroke. Lancet Neurol 2004; 3: 333–42.

34. Kasikcioglu H, Karasulu L, Durgan E et al. Aortic elastic properties and left ventricular diastolic dysfunction in patients with obstructive sleep apnea. Heart Vessels 2005; 20(6): 239–44.

35. Yaggi HK, Concato J, Kernan WN et al. Obstructive sleep apnea as a risk factor for stroke and death. N Engl J Med 2005; 353(19): 2034–41.

36. Mozayeni BR, Mohsenin V, Tegeler C, Crutchfield KE. Cerebrovascular dynamics differentiate sleep apnea subtypes. Cerebrovasc Dise 2005; 15: 12.

37. Lee AG, Golnik K, Kardon R et al. Sleep apnea and intracranial hypertension in men. Ophthalmology 2002; 109(3): 482–5.

38. Duchna HW, Orth M, Schultze-Werninghaus G, Guilleminault C, Stoohs RA. Long-term effects of nasal continuous positive airway pressure on vasodilatory endothelial function in obstructive sleep apnea syndrome. Sleep Breath 2005; 9(3): 97–103.

39. Psarra AM, Solakidi S, Sekeris CE. The mitochondrion as a primary site of action of steroid and thyroid hormones: presence and action of steroid and thyroid hormone receptors in mitochondria of animal cells. Mol Cell Endocrinol 2006; 246(1-2): 21–33.

40. Danzi S, Klein I. Thyroid hormone and the cardiovascular system. Minerva Endocrinol 2004; 3: 139–50.

41. Fazio S, Palmieri FA, Lombardi G, Biondi B. Effects of thyroid hormone on the cardiovascular system. Recent Prog Horm Res 2004; 59: 31–50.

42. Giannattasio C, Rivolta MR, Failla M et al. Large and medium sized artery abnormalities in untreated and treated hypothyroidism. Eur Heart J 1997; 18(9): 1492–8.

43. Arcaro G, Fava C, Dagradi R et al. Acute hyperhomocysteinemia induces a reduction in arterial distensibility and compliance. J Hypertens 2004; 22(4): 775–81.

44. Mendoza CE, Rodriguez F, Rosenberg DG. Reversal of refractory congestive heart failure after thiamine supplementation: report of a case and literature review. J Cardiovasc Pharmacol Ther 2003; 8(4): 313–16.

45. Balander-Gouaille C, Bottiglieri T. Homocysteine Related Vitamins and Neuropsychiatric Disorders. Paris: Springer-Verlag, 2003.

46. Xie A, Skatrud JB, Khayat R et al. Cerebrovascular response to carbon dioxide in patients with congestive heart failure. Am J Respir Crit Care Med 2005; 172: 371–8.

47. Crutchfield KE, Razumovsky AY, Tegeler CH, Mozayeni BR. Differentiating vascular pathophysiological states by objective analysis of flow dynamics. J Neuroimaging 2004; 14(2): 97–107.

48. Beelke M, Angeli S, Del Sette M et al. Prevalence of patent foramen ovale in subjects with obstructive sleep apnea: a transcranial Doppler ultrasound study. Sleep Med 2003; 4(3): 219–23.

4

Who should be screened for asymptomatic carotid artery stenosis?

Issam D Moussa and Michael R Jaff

Take-Home Messages

1. The decision to screen a particular patient for asymptomatic carotid artery stenosis (CAS) requires individualized clinical judgment incorporating the current evidence with the particulars of that patient's condition.
2. Screening unselected individuals in the general population for asymptomatic CAS is not justified because of the low prevalence of disease.
3. Carotid duplex screening should be strongly considered in 'high-risk' patients, such as:

    (a) patients with carotid bruits
    (b) elderly patients with coronary artery disease
    (c) elderly patients with peripheral arterial disease
    (d) patients undergoing coronary artery bypass surgery or major vascular surgery.

INTRODUCTION

Interest in screening for extracranial CAS has increased after the publication of studies demonstrating that carotid endarterectomy (CEA) can prevent stroke in asymptomatic patients with extracranial carotid disease.[1–3] The interest in screening has grown further with the addition of carotid artery stenting to the armamentarium of carotid revascularization.[4] The benefit of screening, namely stroke prevention, depends on several factors: the prevalence of asymptomatic CAS in specific populations; the natural history of carotid disease; the

sensitivity and specificity of the screening method (most often, duplex ultrasonography); the need to confirm the diagnosis (magnetic resonance arteriography [MRA], computed tomographic angiography [CTA], contrast arteriography); the costs of screening; and the cost-effectiveness of carotid revascularization (CEA vs carotid stenting). It is essential to recognize that all studies that addressed this topic constructed decision-making models to test the cost-effectiveness of screening individuals for asymptomatic CAS to identify candidates for CEA. It cannot be presumed that these models would apply to individuals with asymptomatic CAS who are candidates for carotid artery stent revascularization.

THE ARGUMENT AGAINST SCREENING FOR ASYMPTOMATIC CAROTID ARTERY STENOSIS IN THE GENERAL POPULATION

Proponents of this position argue that although CEA has been shown to confer benefit in reducing stroke risk over medical therapy, the absolute benefit is small and does not justify screening the general population, predominantly due to the very low prevalence of significant asymptomatic CAS. The prevalence of asymptomatic CAS in the general population is 2–8% for stenosis $\geq 50\%$ and 1–2% for stenosis $\geq 80\%$ (Chapter 1). In a review of the published literature, Hill[5] determined that the annual stroke or death rate from undetected asymptomatic CAS is 0.16% for stenosis $\geq 50\%$. Furthermore, the estimated number of patients that need to be screened to prevent one stroke ranges from 850 to 1700. Supporting this strategy, Lee et al[6] reported on the cost-effectiveness of screening 65-year-old men for asymptomatic CAS to identify candidates for CEA. Screening this patient population was associated with a cost-effectiveness rate of $120 000 per quality-adjusted life-year (QALY), which is less cost-effective than most accepted health interventions. These findings should be interpreted in the context of the assumptions that were made in this analysis:

- an asymptomatic CAS that warrants intervention was defined as a stenosis of $\geq 60\%$
- the clinical outcome measures included any stroke, death, and serious adverse events from angiography and CEA (including myocardial infarction, but excluding transient ischemic attacks [TIAs])
- the presumption that the benefit of CEA would last only up to 10 years.

Although screening the general population for asymptomatic CAS is not cost-effective and may actually cause harm,[7] this conclusion cannot be generalized to all patients encountered in clinical practice. A more selective approach to screening for asymptomatic CAS is warranted.

THE ARGUMENT FOR SCREENING FOR ASYMPTOMATIC CAROTID ARTERY STENOSIS IN HIGH-RISK PATIENTS

Philosophically, most experts agree that waiting for a first neurological event prior to consideration of revascularization for CAS is a flawed strategy. Data supporting the proven benefit of carotid revascularization over medical therapy, although modest, currently exists. Furthermore, using a TIA as the only trigger for revascularization has several drawbacks:

1. Most strokes in patients with asymptomatic CAS occur without a preceding TIA.[8]
2. A TIA cannot often be assessed objectively, is confounded by many other transitory phenomena, and may occur during sleep, when it may not be recognized.[9,10]
3. Even when a patient recognizes a TIA, the patient may not seek immediate medical attention, increasing the risk of stroke to 5–8% during the first week.[11,12]
4. Up to 22% of patients with TIA sustain brain parenchymal damage on computed tomographic (CT) scanning, suggesting that a TIA can result in end-organ damage.[13]

Is screening high-risk patients cost-effective?

In general, the prevalence of a disease has a much greater impact on the predictive value of a test than its diagnostic accuracy. For example, for a test with a sensitivity and specificity of 93%, the ratio of true positives to false positives is 1:7 if the prevalence is 1% and 3:1 if the prevalence is 20% (Figure 4.1).[7] Therefore, a more selective approach to screening by targeting population groups with conditions known to be associated with an increased prevalence of asymptomatic CAS, increased risk of disease progression, and higher rates of future stroke, is likely to be more cost-effective. Obuchowski and associates[14] evaluated a decision model for screening asymptomatic persons for CAS (>60%). They concluded that screening provides benefit if 20% of the population screened has CAS. At lower prevalence rates, they found that screening is not cost-effective. Feussner and Matchar[15] concluded in their study that screening will not provide a benefit unless the prevalence of severe stenosis is $\geq 35\%$. However, in their analysis in 1988, the perioperative stroke rate associated with CEA was 4.1%, which is higher than that reported in the Asymptomatic Carotid Atherosclerosis Study (ACAS) and the Asymptomatic Carotid Surgery Trial (ACST).[2,3] As a result of improving surgical techniques and reduced perioperative stroke rates, new models have evaluated this question. Derdeyn and Powers[16] developed a computer model to evaluate the cost-effectiveness of screening 1000 men over a 20-year period. A one-time screening program in an asymptomatic population with a high prevalence (20%) of $\geq 60\%$ stenosis cost $35 130 per incremental QALY, which is considered cost-effective. The point with the greatest cost-effectiveness in this model was a peak systolic velocity (PSV) of 230 cm/s (Figure 4.2). Neither one-time screening of a low-prevalence (4%) population nor annual screening was considered cost-effective in their analysis (Table 4.1).

Which patients should be screened for the presence of asymptomatic carotid artery stenosis?

Patients with carotid bruits

Should auscultation for carotid bruits be a part of physical examination?
Neck auscultation is an imperfect screening test for CAS. The problem is explained by three factors. First is the considerable inter-observer variation among clinicians in the interpretation of the intensity, pitch,

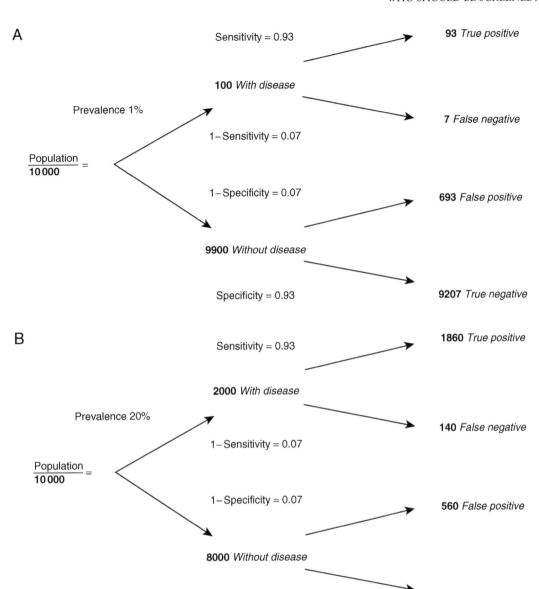

Figure 4.1 Outcomes from screening a population of 10 000 people with a test of 93% sensitivity and specificity: (A) prevalence = 1% (pretest probability = 0.01); (B) prevalence = 20% (pretest probability = 0.20). (Adapted from Whitty et al.[7])

and duration of the bruit heard. Secondly, the auscultable bruit depends on the turbulence created by the stenosis being in the audible range for the human ear, which for most is in the range of 70–80% but not when less or more severe. When less severe, there is not enough turbulence for a bruit to be heard; when more severe, the stenosis impairs anterograde flow and there is

not enough volume of flow to create the bruit. Lastly, similar sounds can be produced by anatomic variation, tortuosity, venous hum, goiter, and transmitted cardiac murmurs.

Various medical organizations have published guidelines for and against neck auscultation for carotid bruits as a screening method for asymptomatic CAS.

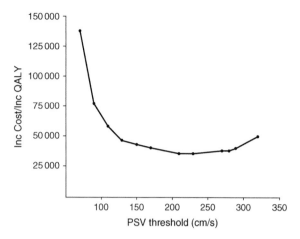

Figure 4.2. Incremental (Inc) cost per incremental quality-adjusted life-year (QALY) as a function of the peak systolic velocity (PSV) threshold of screening Doppler ultrasound. (Adapted from Derdeyn and Powers.[16])

Table 4.1 Base case cost-effectiveness of screening and treatment		
Prevalence of asymptomatic CAS	Incremental QALYs gained	Cost per QALY gained
High prevalence (20%):		
Annual screen	7	$457 773
One-time screen	30	$35 130
Low prevalence (4%):		
Annual screen	−9	NA
One-time screen	7	$52 588

CAS, carotid artery stenosis; QALYs, quality-adjusted life-years.

Modified from Derdeyn and Powers.[16]

All costs and QALYs are discounted annually at 3% present value.

While the American Academy of Family Physicians recommend auscultation for carotid bruits in people aged ≥40 years with risk factors for cerebrovascular or cardiovascular disease, or those with history of cardiovascular disease, The US Preventive Services Task Force offers a 'C' recommendation for screening, stating that there is insufficient evidence to recommend for or against screening for asymptomatic CAS utilizing physical examination.[17]

Nonetheless, it is clinically prudent to identify patients with cervical bruits because they are markers of systemic vascular disease. Therefore, auscultation for cervical bruits must remain part of every general physical examination. The balance of evidence suggests that the presence of an asymptomatic carotid bruit is associated with increased long-term incidence of stroke, myocardial infarction, and death.[18,19] Patients with cervical bruits are three times more likely to have an ischemic stroke than an age- and sex-matched population without a bruit.[20] The risk of ischemic stroke in diabetic patients with bruits is even worse, where these patients have more than 6 times the risk of first stroke in the first 2 years after the bruit was detected than patients without a bruit.[21]

There is poor correlation between the location of the bruit and the location of the stroke. Management of these patients must be individualized.

How prevalent are carotid bruits in neurologically asymptomatic individuals?

The prevalence of carotid bruits in asymptomatic individuals varies according to age and other cardiovascular risk factors. Sandok and colleagues[22] evaluated the prevalence of cervical bruits in 509 asymptomatic individuals in Olmsted County, Minnesota. The prevalence of asymptomatic carotid arterial bruits increased with age: 0.9% at 45–54 years old; 2.1% at 55–64 years old; 3.8% at 65–74 years old; and 5% at ≥75 years old. The risk was higher in females (4.4%) than in males (1.6%). The prevalence of carotid bruits is significantly higher in patients with established atherosclerotic vascular disease. Gutierrez and colleagues[23] reported a prevalence of 24% among 300 neurologically asymptomatic patients prior to peripheral vascular surgery.

How prevalent is carotid artery stenosis in asymptomatic patients with a carotid bruit?

The prevalence of carotid artery stenosis in patients with carotid bruits is significantly higher than that in patients without carotid bruits.[24,25] It is estimated that about 30–40% of asymptomatic patients with a carotid bruit will have an internal CAS >50%.[8,26,27] However, these studies also demonstrate that many patients with asymptomatic bruits do not have significant carotid disease. Moreover, hemodynamically significant carotid stenotic lesions may exist in the absence of an audible bruit. Severe carotid stenoses (90–99%) that are associated with slow flow are often not associated with an audible bruit.[28,29] Using 70–99% stenosis on carotid angiogram as a reference standard, auscultation of a carotid bruit has been found to have a sensitivity of only 63–76% and a specificity of only 61–76% for clinically significant stenosis.[17] Therefore, it is critical to remember that the absence of a carotid bruit does not rule

Table 4.2 Prevalence of asymptomatic CAS in patients with CAD

Study	No. of patients	Setting	Carotid stenosis severity (%)	Prevalence (%)
Chen et al[30]	153	Coronary angiography for suspected CAD	>50	11
			50–79	5
			80–100	6
Kallikazaros et al[31]	225	Coronary angiography for suspected CAD	>50	18
			50–79	13
			80–100	5
Zimarino et al[32]	624	Coronary angiography for suspected CAD	>50	14
			50–69	8
			70–100	6
Ambrosetti et al[33]	168	Cardiac rehabilitation	>50	8–26
Komorovsky et al[34]	323	Acute coronary syndrome	>50	31
Tanimoto et al[35]	632	Coronary angiography for suspected CAD	>50	20

CAS, carotid artery stenosis; CAD, coronary artery disease.

Table 4.3 Prevalence of asymptomatic CAS (>50% DS) according to severity of CAD

Extent of CAD	Kallikazaros et al[31] (n = 225)	Zimarino et al[32] (n = 624)	Ambrosetti et al[33] (n = 168)	Komorovsky et al[34] (n = 323)	Tanimoto et al[35] (n = 632)
No CAD	3.6%	4.1%	–	–	7%
1 vessel	5.3%	14.4%	8%	19%	14.5%
2 vessel	13.5%	17%	–	43%	21.4%
3 vessel	24.5%	NR	–	45%	36%
Left main	40%		26%	–	–

CAS, carotid artery stenosis; CAD, coronary artery disease; DS, diameter stenosis; NR, not reported.

out high-grade significant carotid stenosis and should not be used as a reason to deny screening, especially if other risk factors exist.

Elderly patients with severe coronary or peripheral arterial disease

Patients with systemic atherosclerotic vascular disease (coronary artery or peripheral vascular disease) are high-risk groups for the presence of asymptomatic CAS. The prevalence of significant asymptomatic CAS (≥60%) in these patients ranges between 5 and 19% (Tables 4.2–4.4).[30–48] Age, severity of atherosclerotic disease, diabetes, tobacco use, and hypertension have all been identified as additional risk factors associated with increased prevalence of asymptomatic CAS in this population. Furthermore, it has also been clearly established that these patients are also at high risk for future

Table 4.4 Prevalence of asymptomatic CAS (>50% DS) in patients with PAD

Study	PAD definition	No. of patients	Asymptomatic CAS (%)
Lower extremity PAD			
Ahn et al[37]	Ankle brachial index	78	14
Klop et al[38]	Ankle brachial index	374	26.6
Gentile et al[39]	Pre fem-pop bypass	252	28
Marek et al[40]	PAD symptoms	188	24.5
Alexandrova et al[41]	Ankle brachial index	144	50
De Virgilio et al[42]	PAD symptoms	89	20
Simons et al[43]	Ankle brachial index	162	14
Ballotta et al[44]*	Ankle brachial index	132	49
Pilcher et al[45]	Ankle brachial index/imaging	200	25
Cina et al[46]	Ankle brachial index	620	33
Renal artery stenosis			
Louie et al[47]	Duplex scanning	60	46
Missouris et al[48]	Angiography	38	45

CAS, carotid artery stenosis; DS, diameter stenosis; PAD, peripheral arterial disease.
*>60% DS.

Table 4.5 Multivariate determinants of asymptomatic CAS

Variable	Odds ratio (95% CI)	Risk score
Age	4.1 (2.6–6.7)	4
Sex (male)	1.4 (0.9–2.0)	NS
Current smoker	2.0 (1.2–3.5)	1
Coronary artery disease	2.4 (1.5–3.9)	2
Hypercholesterolemia	1.9 (1.2–2.9)	1

CAS, carotid artery stenosis; CI, confidence interval.
Adapted from Qureshi et al.[50]

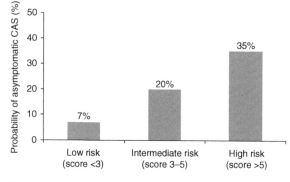

Figure 4.3 Post-test probability for detection of significant asymptomatic carotid artery stenosis (CAS) based on total risk score. (Adapted from Qureshi et al.[50])

ischemic cardiovascular and cerebrovascular events. In one series of 149 patients with atherosclerotic renal artery stenosis, the likelihood of finding severe CAS was 19%, and increased as the renal artery stenosis severity increased (7% in mild renal artery stenosis; 28% in severe renal artery stenosis).[49]

Although there is agreement that the above risk factors increase the likelihood of asymptomatic CAS, most physicians are still uncertain about specific patient populations who should be targeted in screening efforts. Qureshi and colleagues[50] developed a carotid screening stratification scheme in an attempt to further define these populations. These investigators used data collected from 1443 persons enrolled in the Western New York Stroke Screening Program. A scoring system based on factors that were found to be independently predictive of asymptomatic CAS, including age, history of coronary artery disease, smoking status, male gender, and hypercholesterolemia, was developed from 887 participants (Table 4.5). This scoring system was then validated in 444 participants prospectively. This scoring system defines three risk groups with different probabilities for having significant asymptomatic CAS (Figure 4.3). Individuals who have multiple risk factors (risk score >5) have a 35% probability of significant asymptomatic CAS; those in the intermediate-risk group had a probability of about 20%; and the low-risk group (risk score <3) represented a group with a low probability (7%) of having asymptomatic CAS.

In a similar community-based screening program, Rockman and colleagues screened 610 patients who were older than 60 years of age and had a history of either hypertension, heart disease, or cigarette smoking, or a family history of stroke.[51] Screening included blood pressure determination, an electrocardiogram, and a carotid duplex. Asymptomatic CAS was more prevalent (10.8%) than new hypertension (2.6%) or new atrial fibrillation (0.5%). The presence of cardiac disease increased the odds of identifying asymptomatic carotid stenosis by 2.5-fold, similar to the effect of current smoking, and higher than the effect of hypertension (1.9-fold). More than one of every five patients with known hypertension and heart disease had asymptomatic CAS.

Therefore, screening for asymptomatic CAS should be strongly considered in elderly patients with coronary artery disease, particularly in the presence of hypertension or smoking. It should be clear, however, that medical societies have yet to endorse any specific recommendations for screening for asymptomatic CAS.

Patients undergoing coronary artery bypass surgery

Asymptomatic CAS is prevalent among patients undergoing coronary artery bypass graft (CABG) surgery (Table 4.6).[52-57] Screening patients prior to CABG for presence of asymptomatic CAS is attractive because carotid stenosis is a risk factor for stroke after CABG. Knowledge of significant CAS prior to CABG seems appropriate and responsible. Although only approximately 1.5–2% of CABG patients suffer significant stroke, this rate can reach 5% in patients with severe bilateral asymptomatic CAS.[58] If the majority of these strokes occur in patients with severe asymptomatic CAS, then the potential to prevent stroke in this population would be significant. This has significant implications considering the morbidity and mortality from stroke and the annual number of cardiac surgery operations performed. It is clear, however, that not all patients with asymptomatic CAS at the time of CABG suffer a neurological event, and not all patients with stroke following CABG have an associated carotid stenosis of any degree. Stroke following CABG is multifactorial in etiology and the actual proportion of risk that can be attributed to carotid stenosis needs to be determined before considering such intervention.[59]

Is asymptomatic CAS a risk factor for post-coronary artery bypass graft neurological events?

The reported perioperative risk of stroke related to asymptomatic CAS in patients having CABG surgery varies widely. Some studies have shown no increased risk of ipsilateral stroke,[52,60,61] whereas other studies have shown a higher risk.[62-64] Methodologically sound natural history studies regarding the impact of asymptomatic CAS on incidence of stroke after CABG are not available. A critical analysis of the published cohort studies on the relationship between asymptomatic CAS and stroke after CABG reveals very few studies which meet criteria to qualify for consideration in clinical decision-making.[60,61,63,65-67] In a case–control study,[65] Hill and colleagues demonstrated that while a carotid stenosis of 50–90% increases the risk of ipsilateral stroke 5.2-fold, a carotid stenosis of 80–90% increases the risk of ipsilateral stroke by 24.3-fold. In this study, other variables that were found to be predictive of stroke were age >65 years, comorbid peripheral vascular disease, hypertension, and the female gender. Furthermore, the association between asymptomatic CAS and stroke remains significant after multivariate adjustment of other variables. In a recent review article by Naylor and colleagues,[58] the risk of perioperative

Table 4.6 Prevalence of asymptomatic CAS (>50% DS) in patients referred for coronary artery bypass graft surgery[69]

Study	No. of patients	Asymptomatic CAS (%)
Barnes et al[52]	449	19
Faggioli et al[53]	539	8.7*
D'Agostino et al[54]	1279	21
Birincioglu et al[55]	678	13
Rath et al[56]	1200	9
Kawarada et al[57]	380	14

CAS, carotid artery stenosis; DS, diameter stenosis.
*Refers to severe carotid stenosis (>75% DS).

stroke was <2% in patients without significant carotid disease, increasing to 3% in predominantly asymptomatic patients with a unilateral 50–99% stenosis; to 5% in those with bilateral 50–99% stenoses, and 7–11% in patients with carotid occlusion.

Although a properly conducted prospective natural history study is still needed for confirmation, the available evidence certainly supports a casual relationship between asymptomatic CAS and post-CABG ipsilateral neurological events.

Should all patients undergoing coronary artery bypass graft surgery be screened for asymptomatic carotid artery?

Routine screening of patients before CABG has demonstrated a prevalence of 9–28% for patients with asymptomatic CAS of ≥50% (see Table 4.6) and approximately 8% for those with a stenosis of ≥80%.[68] This prevalence is expected to increase with an aging population of patients requiring cardiac surgery who suffer from increasingly diffuse and complex disease.

Whether all patients undergoing CABG should be screened is debatable; prevalence of asymptomatic CAS in patients undergoing CABG increases with age, left main coronary artery involvement,[69] concomitant peripheral arterial disease,[68] diabetes, tobacco use, and the presence of carotid bruits. In a study by Durand and colleagues[70] designed to evaluate the merits of selective vs systematic screening in CABG patients, the authors found that selectively screening patients with either an age ≥65 years old or the presence of a carotid bruit would significantly reduce the screening load with negligible impact on neurological outcomes.

SUMMARY

The decision to screen a particular patient for asymptomatic CAS requires individualized clinical judgment incorporating the current evidence with the particulars of that patient's condition. Although it is true that the incidence of stroke and death resulting from asymptomatic CAS is proportional to the prevalence and prognosis of untreated disease, the prevalence of asymptomatic CAS in the general population and the risk of subsequent ipsilateral stroke or death suggest that the yearly risk to any given individual is low. The high number of patients who would require screening to prevent stroke or death in one patient makes general screening for asymptomatic CAS unjustified. However, limiting screening to patients at high risk for asymptomatic CAS such as those with carotid bruits and/or

peripheral or coronary arterial disease improves the diagnostic yield and may improve clinical outcome with an appropriate management strategy.

REFERENCES

1. Hobson RW, Weiss DG, Fields WS et al, for Veterans Affairs Cooperative Study Group. Efficacy of carotid endarterectomy for asymptomatic carotid stenosis. N Engl J Med 1993; 328(4): 221–7.
2. Executive Committee for the Asymptomatic Carotid Atherosclerosis Study. Endarterectomy for asymptomatic carotid stenosis. JAMA 1995; 273: 1421–8.
3. MRC Asymptomatic Carotid Surgery Trial (ACST) Collaborative Group. Prevention of disabling and fatal strokes by successful carotid endarterectomy in patients without recent neurological symptoms: randomized controlled trial. Lancet 2004; 363: 1491–502.
4. Yadav JS, Wholey MH, Kuntz RE et al; Stenting and Angioplasty with Protection in Patients at High Risk for Endarterectomy Investigators. Protected carotid-artery stenting versus endarterectomy in high-risk patients. N Engl J Med 2004; 351(15): 1493–501.
5. Hill AB. Should patients be screened for asymptomatic carotid artery stenosis? Can J Surg 1998; 41: 208–13.
6. Lee TT, Solomon NA, Heidenreich PA, Oehlert J, Garber AM. Cost-effectiveness of screening for carotid stenosis in asymptomatic persons. Ann Int Med 1997; 126(5): 337–46.
7. Whitty CJ, Sudlow CL, Warlow CP. Investigating individual subjects and screening populations for asymptomatic carotid stenosis can be harmful. J Neurol Neurosurg Psychiatry 1998; 64: 619–23.
8. Mackey AE, Abrahamowicz M, Langlois Y et al. Outcome of asymptomatic patients with carotid disease. Neurology 1997; 48: 896–903.
9. Fisher CM. Transient ischemic attacks. Perspective. N Engl J Med 2002; 347: 1642–3.
10. Toole JF. The Willis Lecture: transient ischemic attacks, scientific method, and new realities. Stroke 1991; 22: 99–104.
11. Johnston SC, Gress DR, Browner WS, Sidney S. Short-term prognosis after emergency department diagnosis of TIA. JAMA 2000; 284(22): 2901–6.
12. Eliasziw M, Kennedy J, Hill MD, Buchan AM, Barnett HJ; North American Symptomatic Carotid Endarterectomy Trial Group. Early risk of stroke after a transient ischemic attack in patients with internal carotid artery disease. CMAJ 2004; 170(7): 1105–9.
13. Taghavy A, Hamer H. Parenchymal "damage" in transient ischemic attacks (TIAs) and prolonged reversible ischemic neurologic deficits (PRINDs): the role of cranial CT and EEG. Int J Neurosci 1992; 66(3-4): 251–61.
14. Obuchowski NA, Modic MT, Magdinec M, Masaryk TJ. Assessment of the efficacy of noninvasive screening for patients with asymptomatic neck bruits. Stroke 1997; 28: 1330–9.
15. Feussner JR, Matchar DB. When and how to study the carotid arteries. Ann Intern Med 1988; 109: 805–18.
16. Derdeyn CP, Powers WJ. Cost-effectiveness of screening for asymptomatic carotid atherosclerotic disease. Stroke 1996; 27: 1944–50.
17. US Preventive Services Task Force. Screening for asymptomatic carotid artery stenosis. In: DiGuiseppi C, Atkins D, Woolf SH, eds. Guide to Clinical Preventive Services, 2nd edn. Alexandria, VA: International Medical Publishing, 1996: 53–61.
18. Heyman A, Wilkinson WE, Heyden S et al. Risk of stroke in asymptomatic persons with cervical arterial bruits: a population study in Evans County, Georgia. N Engl J Med 1980; 302: 838–41.
19. Wolf PA, Kannel WB, Sorlie P, McNamara P. Asymptomatic carotid bruit and risk of stroke. The Framingham Study. JAMA 1981; 245: 1442–5.
20. Wiebers DO, Whisnant JP, Sandok BA, O'Fallon WM. Prospective comparison of a cohort with asymptomatic carotid

bruit and a population-based cohort without carotid bruit. Stroke 1990; 21: 984–8.

21. Gillett M, Davis WA, Jackson D, Bruce DG, Davis TME. Prospective evaluation of carotid bruit as a predictor of first stroke in type 2 diabetes: the Fremantle Diabetes Study. Stroke 2003; 34: 2145–51.

22. Sandok BA, Whisnant JP, Furlan AJ, Mickell JL. Carotid artery bruits: prevalence survey and differential diagnosis. Mayo Clin Proc 1982; 57(4): 227–30.

23. Gutierrez IZ, Barone DL, Makula PA, Currier C. The risk of perioperative stroke in patients with asymptomatic carotid bruits undergoing peripheral vascular surgery. Am Surg 1987; 53(9): 487–9.

24. Gauthier JC, Rosa A, Lhermitte F. Auscultation carotidienne. Rev Neurol (Paris) 1975; 131: 175–84.

25. Davies KN, Humphrey PR. Do carotid bruits predict disease of the internal carotid arteries? Postgrad Med J 1994; 70(824): 433–5.

26. Fell G, Breslau P, Knox RA et al. Importance of noninvasive ultrasonic Doppler testing in the evaluation of patients with asymptomatic carotid bruits. Am Heart J 1981; 102: 221–6.

27. Roederer GO, Langlois YE, Jager KA et al. The natural history of carotid arterial disease in asymptomatic patients with cervical bruits. Stroke 1984; 15: 605–13.

28. Pessin MS, Panis W, Prager RJ, Millan VG, Scott RM. Auscultation of cervical and ocular bruits in extracranial carotid occlusive disease: a clinical and angiographic study. Stroke 1983; 14(2): 246–9.

29. Sauve JS, Thorpe KE, Sackett DL et al. Can bruits distinguish high-grade from moderate symptomatic carotid stenosis? The North American Symptomatic Carotid Endarterectomy Trial. Ann Int Med 1994; 20(8): 633–7.

30. Chen WH, Ho DS, Ho SL, Cheung RT, Cheng SW. Prevalence of extracranial carotid and vertebral artery disease in Chinese patients with coronary artery disease. Stroke 1998; 29: 631–4.

31. Kallikazaros I, Tsioufis C, Sideris S, Stefanadis C, Toutouzas P. Carotid artery disease as a marker for the presence of severe coronary artery disease in patients evaluated for chest pain. Stroke 1999; 30: 1002–7.

32. Zimarino M, Cappelletti L, Venarucci V et al. Age-dependence of risk factors for carotid stenosis: an observational study among candidates for coronary arteriography. Atherosclerosis 2001; 159: 165–73.

33. Ambrosetti M, Casorati P, Salerno M et al. Newly diagnosed carotid atherosclerosis in patients with coronary artery disease admitted for cardiac rehabilitation. Ital Heart J 2004; 5(11): 840–3.

34. Komorovsky R, Desideri A, Coscarelli S, Cortigiani L, Celegon L. Impact of carotid arterial narrowing on outcomes of patients with acute coronary syndromes. Am J Cardiol 2004; 93: 1552–5.

35. Tanimoto S, Ikari Y, Tanabe K et al. Prevalence of carotid artery stenosis in patients with coronary artery disease in Japanese population. Stroke 2005; 36: 2094–8.

36. Lanzer P. Vascular multimorbidity in patients with a documented coronary artery disease. Z Kardiol 2003; 92(8): 650–9.

37. Ahn SS, Baker JD, Walden K, Moore WS. Which asymptomatic patients should undergo routine screening carotid duplex scan? Am J Surg 1991; 162: 180–4.

38. Klop RB, Eikelboom BC, Taks AC. Screening of the internal carotid arteries in patients with peripheral vascular disease by colour-flow duplex scanning. Eur J Vasc Surg 1991; 5: 41–5.

39. Gentile AT, Taylor LM, Moneta GL, Porter JM. Prevalence of asymptomatic carotid stenosis in patients undergoing infra-inguinal bypass surgery. Arch Surg 1995; 130: 900–4.

40. Marek J, Mills JL, Harvich J, Cui H, Fujitani RM. Utility of routine carotid duplex screening in patients who have claudication. J Vasc Surg 1996; 24: 572–7.

41. Alexandrova NA, Gibson WC, Norris JW, Maggisano R. Carotid artery stenosis in peripheral vascular disease. J Vasc Surg 1996; 23: 645–9.

42. de Virgilio C, Toosie K, Arnell T et al. Asymptomatic carotid artery stenosis screening in patients with lower extremity athero-sclerosis: a prospective study. Ann Vasc Surg 1997; 11: 374–7.

43. Simons PCG, Algra A, van der Graaf Y, Eikelboom BC, Grobbee DE, for the SMART Study Group. Carotid artery stenosis in patients with peripheral arterial disease: the SMART study. J Vasc Surg 1999; 30: 519–25.

44. Ballotta E, Da Giau G, Renon L et al. Symptomatic and asymptomatic carotid artery lesions in peripheral vascular disease: a prospective study. Int J Surg Investig 1999; 1(4): 357–63.

45. Pilcher JM, Danaher J, Khaw KT. The prevalence of asymptomatic carotid artery disease in patients with peripheral vascular disease. Clin Radiol 2000; 55: 56–61.

46. Cina CS, Safar HA, Maggisano R, Bailey R, Clase CM. Prevalence and progression of internal carotid artery stenosis in patients with peripheral arterial occlusive disease. J Vasc Surg 2002; 36: 75–82.

47. Louie J, Isaacson JA, Zierler RE, Bergelin RO, Strandness DE Jr. Prevalence of carotid and lower extremity arterial disease in patients with renal artery stenosis. Am J Hypertens 1994; 7(5): 436–9.

48. Missouris CG, Papavassiliou MB, Khaw K et al. High prevalence of carotid artery disease in patients with atheromatous renal artery stenosis. Nephrol Dial Transplant 1998; 13: 945–8.

49. Zierler RE, Bergelin RO, Polissar NL et al. Carotid and lower extremity arterial disease in patients with renal artery athero-sclerosis. Arch Intern Med 1998; 158: 761–7.

50. Qureshi AI, Janardhan V, Bennett SE et al. Who should be screened for asymptomatic carotid artery stenosis? Experience from the Western New York Stroke Screening Program. J Neuroimaging 2001; 11: 105–11.

51. Rockman CB, Jacobowitz GR, Gagne PJ et al. Focused screening for occult carotid artery disease: patients with known heart disease are at high risk. J Vasc Surg 2004; 39: 44–51.

52. Barnes RW, Nix ML, Sansonetti D, Turley DG, Goldman MR. Late outcome of untreated asymptomatic carotid disease following cardiovascular operations. J Vasc Surg 1985; 2(6): 843–9.

53. Faggioli GL, Curl GR, Ricotta JJ. The role of carotid screening before coronary artery bypass. J Vasc Surg 1990; 12(6): 724–9.

54. D'Agostino RS, Svensson LG, Neumann DJ et al. Screening carotid ultrasonography and risk factors for stroke in coronary artery surgery patients. Ann Thorac Surg 1996; 62: 1714–23.

55. Birincioglu L, Arda K, Bardakci H et al. Carotid disease in patients scheduled for coronary artery bypass: analysis of 678 patients. Angiology 1999; 50(1): 9–19.

56. Rath PC, Agarwala MK, Dhar PK et al. Carotid artery involvement in patients of atherosclerotic coronary artery disease undergoing coronary artery bypass grafting. Indian Heart J 2001; 53(6): 761–5.

57. Kawarada O, Yokoi Y, Morioka N et al. Carotid stenosis and peripheral artery disease in Japanese patients with coronary artery disease undergoing coronary artery bypass grafting. Circ J 2003; 67: 1003–6.

58. Naylor AR, Mehta Z, Rothwell PM, Bell PR. Carotid artery disease and stroke during coronary srtery bypass: a critical review of the literature. Eur J Vasc Endovasc Surg 2002; 23: 283–94.

59. Stamou SC, Hill PC, Dangas G et al. Stroke after coronary artery bypass: incidence, predictors, and clinical outcome. Stroke 2001; 32: 1508–13.

60. Barnes RW, Liebman PR, Marszalek PB, Kirk CL, Goldman MH. The natural history of asymptomatic carotid disease in patients undergoing cardiovascular surgery. Surgery 1981; 90: 1075–83.

61. Breslau PJ, Fell G, Ivey TD et al. Carotid arterial disease in patients undergoing coronary artery bypass operations. J Thorac Cardiovasc Surg 1981; 82: 765–7.

62. Brener BJ, Brief DK, Alpert J, Goldenkranz RJ, Parsonnet V. The risk of stroke in patients with asymptomatic carotid stenosis undergoing cardiac surgery: a follow-up study. J Vasc Surg 1987; 5: 269–79.

63. Schwartz LB, Bridgman AH, Kieffer RW et al. Asymptomatic carotid artery stenosis and stroke in patients undergoing cardiopulmonary bypass. J Vasc Surg 1995; 21: 146–53.

64. Mickleborough LL, Walker PM, Takagi Y et al. Risk factors for stroke in patients undergoing coronary artery bypass grafting. J Thorac Cardiovasc Surg 1996; 112: 1250–8.

65. Hill AB, Obrand D, O'Rourke K, Steinmetz OK, Miller N. Hemispheric stroke following cardiac surgery: a case-control estimate of the risk resulting from ipsilateral asymptomatic carotid artery stenosis. Ann Vasc Surg 2000; 14: 200–9.

66. Turnipseed WE, Berkoff HA, Belzer FD. Postoperative stroke in cardiac and peripheral vascular disease. Ann Surg 1980; 192: 365–8.

67. Gerraty RP, Gates PC, Doyle JC. Carotid stenosis and perioperative stroke risk in symptomatic and asymptomatic patients undergoing vascular or coronary surgery. Stroke 1993; 24: 1115–18.

68. Salasidis GC, Latter DA, Steinmetz OK, Blair JF, Graham AM. Carotid artery duplex scanning in preoperative assessment for coronary artery revascularization: the association between peripheral vascular disease, carotid artery stenosis, and stroke. J Vasc Surg 1995; 21(1): 154–62.

69. Vigneswaran WT, Sapsford RN, Stanbridge RD. Disease of the left main coronary artery: early surgical results and their association with carotid artery stenosis. Br Heart J 1993; 70(4): 342–5.

70. Durand DJ, Perler BA, Roseborough GS et al. Mandatory versus selective preoperative carotid screening: a retrospective analysis. Ann Thorac Surg 2004; 78: 159–66.

5

Diagnosis and clinical evaluation of patients with asymptomatic carotid artery stenosis

Richard E Temes and JP Mohr

Take-Home Messages

1. The rationale behind identification of patients with asymptomatic carotid artery stenosis (CAS) is that early treatment may reduce the incidence of cardiovascular and cerebrovascular events.
2. Screening for asymptomatic CAS should be limited to high-risk populations to avoid unnecessary cost and harm.
3. Duplex ultrasound should be the first choice for screening. However, clinicians should be aware of the various scenarios where the severity of carotid disease can be under- or overestimated by this technique.
4. Contrast-enhanced magnetic resonance angiography (MRA) is a safe and accurate imaging modality for confirmation of the diagnosis.
5. Computer tomographic angiography (CTA) is an emerging alternative to MRA, with the additional ability to identify carotid calcifications. The disadvantages of CTA are similar to those of traditional angiography (exposure to ionizing radiation and iodinated contrast).
6. Duplex ultrasound (DUS) and MRA, or CTA, often provide concordant results when performed in accredited laboratories. However, discrepancy among these techniques can occur. In these cases, traditional angiography is indicated, particularly if carotid revascularization is being considered.
7. Patients with 'asymptomatic' CAS should undergo detailed neurological evaluation.
8. Patients with asymptomatic CAS should undergo cardiac evaluation to identify and treat coronary artery disease and other cardiac causes of cerebral embolism.

INTRODUCTION

The rationale for identifying patients with asymptomatic carotid artery stenosis (CAS) is the expectation that early detection and treatment (including modification of risk factors) can reduce the risk of stroke.[1,2] Since these patients are by definition asymptomatic, they can only be identified through screening using various imaging modalities, particularly duplex ultrasound (DUS). As discussed in Chapter 4, screening the general population for asymptomatic CAS cannot be justified because of the low prevalence of this condition.[3,4] However, the prevalence of asymptomatic CAS can be as high as 30% in high-risk groups.[5,6]

Although some clinicians take the position that, in the absence of reliable community-based data, it is not clear whether any group can be identified as having a high enough prevalence to make screening cost-effective,[7] screening appropriate patients may provide certain benefits that are often overlooked. First, an awareness of the diagnosis may motivate patients to modify other risk factors (e.g. high blood pressure, smoking, physical inactivity). Secondly, the use of antiplatelet drugs not already part of the treatment plan for such patients may reduce stroke risk in asymptomatic individuals with CAS. No proof of such benefits currently exists, since the large, randomized trials comparing the effectiveness of interventions from the results of screening

> **Box 5.1** Senarios 1–3 in identification of patients with asymptomatic carotid artery stenoris
>
> *Carotid imaging in patients with symptomatic carotid stenosis who are found to have contralateral asymptomatic stenosis*
>
> One of the clinical scenarios where an asymptomatic carotid lesion may be identified is in patients who undergo carotid imaging during a work-up for an acute ischemic neurological event. Indeed, 63% of patients enrolled in the North American Symptomatic Carotid Endarterectomy Trial (NASCET) for a symptomatic carotid stenosis had contralateral asymptomatic stenoses ranging in severity from 0% to 99%.[8]
>
> Contralateral stenosis of 60–99% severity was found in 12% of this group. In the European Carotid Surgery Trial (ECST),[9] 127 out of 2295 patients (5.5%) had a contralateral asymptomatic stenosis ranging in severity from 70% to 99%. It has been demonstrated that patients with asymptomatic CAS who already had contralateral symptomatic carotid disease are in fact 'predisposed' for ischemic events emanating from the asymptomatic side.[10]
>
> *Carotid imaging in patients with incidentally found silent brain infarction*
>
> Many elderly patients undergo brain imaging for various reasons such as minor trauma or non-specific symptoms such as dizziness and headache. Occasionally, brain infarction is identified on these imaging studies without a clear history of ischemic neurological events: 'silent cerebral infarcts' (SCI). These findings often lead to initiating a work-up for ischemic stroke such as cardiac evaluation and carotid imaging.
>
> Although solid evidence for this practice is lacking, the rationale for this approach can certainly be supported. The presence of SCI has been shown to increase the risk of future stroke.[11,12] This risk appears to be independent of traditional risk factors for cerebrovascular disease.[13] The majority of patients with SCI in the general population do not have carotid occlusive disease. However, in selected high-risk patients the prevalence of carotid occlusive disease can be as high as 41%.[14] The clinical significance of SCI in patients with asymptomatic CAS will be discussed later in this chapter.
>
> *Carotid imaging in patients with non-specific visual or neurological symptoms*
>
> Many patients are referred to undergo carotid duplex imaging because of dizziness, vertigo, and non-specific visual disturbances. These symptoms are often mistakenly labeled as transient ischemic attacks (TIAs), even though they are rarely caused by cerebrovascular insufficiency.

among different patient populations are lacking. Thirdly, carotid revacularization has been shown to reduce future stroke risk in selected patients with asymptomatic carotid disease.

IDENTIFICATION OF PATIENTS WITH ASYMPTOMATIC CAROTID ARTERY STENOSIS

In the clinical setting, diagnosis of an asymptomatic carotid artery lesion is usually made in one of the following scenarios:

1. Carotid imaging in patients with asymptomatic carotid bruit detected on routine examination.

2. Carotid imaging in patients known to have high prevalence of asymptomatic CAS, such as patients with coronary or peripheral arterial disease.
3. Carotid imaging in patients undergoing cardiac or vascular surgery.
4. Carotid imaging in patients with symptomatic carotid stenosis who are found to have contralateral asymptomatic stenosis (see Box 5.1).
5. Carotid imaging in patients with incidentally found silent brain infarction on brain imaging (see Box 5.1).
6. Carotid imaging in patients with non-specific visual or neurological symptoms (see Box 5.1).

The first three clinical scenarios represent the most common pathway for identification of patients with asymptomatic CAS. These are discussed in detail in Chapter 4. A detailed discussion of the last three clinical scenarios (4–6) is shown in Box 5.1.

DIAGNOSTIC METHODOLOGIES FOR CAROTID OCCLUSIVE DISEASE

Duplex ultrasound

DUS examination is an integral part of the evaluation of the extracranial carotid circulation. Its creation as a technology was driven mainly by the perceived need to estimate stenosis non-invasively and by a widely known awareness that bruit alone was insufficient to settle the diagnois of stenosis. Doppler-derived velocity measurements criteria were established to provide a quantitative and reproducible tool to estimate the degree of carotid stenosis.[15] DUS has been found to be both accurate and reliable in the detection of carotid stenosis, both in the B-mode imaging and in the cross-sectional assessment achieved by the Doppler shift. Depending on the underlying population characteristics, the positive predictive value of DUS ranges from 82% to 97%.[16] A recent meta-analysis[17] of studies comparing DUS with carotid angiography demonstrated that for the diagnosis of 70–99% vs <70% stenosis, DUS had a pooled sensitivity of 86% (95% CI 84–89) and a pooled specificity of 87% (95% CI 84–90). For recognizing occlusion, DUS had a sensitivity of 96% (95% CI 94–98) and a specificity of 100% (95% CI 99–100).

Major Doppler studies do not agree on the cut-off velocity values for assessment of the degree of carotid stenosis despite efforts to standardize these criteria.[18] Reasons for the variability of Doppler velocity criteria for carotid stenosis include lack of standardized validation studies, variation in clinical and cerebrovascular hemodynamic characteristics of the population under study, variability in Doppler instrumentation, and potential variability in sonographer training. The sensitivity and specificity of DUS for detection of high-grade carotid stenosis may be as high as 85% in certified ultrasound laboratories that keep a rigorous quality control and assurance of ultrasound measurements and constant re-training of their sonographers. In clinical practice, however, sensitivity and specificity are more likely about 70%.

Because of Doppler velocity measurement variability, there are no generally accepted criteria for Doppler parameters of carotid stenosis that can be used in all clinical ultrasound laboratories and medical practices. Each carotid ultrasound laboratory must, therefore, develop its own criteria for high-grade carotid stenosis. These parameters must be validated with other imaging modalities and surgical findings and an ongoing quality control program must be in place. All of these are assured in the laboratories that are certified by ICAVL (Intersocietal Commission for Accreditation of Vascular Laboratories) or other accredited ultrasound associations.

The most important ultrasound parameters in the assessment of carotid stenosis are peak systolic velocity, end-diastolic velocity, and systolic velocity ratio (ICA/CCA ratio). These parameters must be evaluated in the prestenotic, stenotic, and poststenotic region. The degree of stenosis can also be assessed visually from gray-scale ultrasound images and cross-checked with color Doppler imaging. Doppler spectrum analysis of the blood flow velocities should always be cross-checked with the color Doppler image assessment of carotid stenosis. Color Doppler imaging can guide Doppler velocity determination in order to select the most critical site of stenosis for Doppler velocity measurements. DUS not only accurately depicts degree of stenosis but also provides additional information on plaque morphology that cannot be evaluated by angiography. A detailed discussion of ultrasonographic plaque morphology and its significance is addressed in detail in Chapter 8. DUS criteria for carotid stenosis used at the Stroke Division of the Department of Neurology at Columbia University (ICAVL accredited) are listed in Table 5.1.

It is very important for physicians to be aware of the potential pitfalls associated with estimating lesion severity with DUS. These pitfalls can be related to the patient, the operator, or the technique:

- Patient-related factors: (1) obese neck; (2) cervical spine immobility; (3) severe internal carotid artery tortuousity (may lead to overestimation of stenosis severity); and (4) high carotid bifurcation (the lesion cannot be interrogated).
- Operator-related factors: (1) mislabeling the study (right vs left); (2) mistaking the external for the internal carotid artery; (3) overestimating the maximal flow velocity due to improper angle; and (4) failure to set proper image settings (depth, gain, frame rate, etc.).
- Technology-related factors: (1) missing severe stenosis due to severe lesion calcifications; (2) diagnosis of a subocclusive stenosis as an occlusion; (3) underestimation of lesion severity in low-flow states (severe congestive heart failure, aortic stenosis, severe common carotid artery disease); and (4) overestimating lesion severity in bilateral carotid disease.

Magnetic resonance angiography

Magnetic resonance angiography (MRA) is an excellent imaging modality for diagnosis of carotid disease.

Table 5.1 Diagnostic Doppler criteria for carotid stenosis

Carotid stenosis	Peak systolic velocity (cm/s)	Peak diastolic velocity (cm/s)	Systolic velocity ICA/CCA ratio	Diastolic velocity ICA/CCA ratio	Spectral broadening (cm/s)
0%	<120	<40	<1.8	<2.4	<30
1–39%	<120	<40	<1.8	<2.4	<40
40–59%	<170	<40	<1.8	<2.4	<40
60–79%	>170	>40	>1.8	>2.4	>40
80–99%	>250	>100	>3.7	<5.5	>80
100% (occlusion)	N/A	N/A	N/A	N/A	N/A

Gray-scale imaging and color Doppler flow imaging (CDFI) are also included in the diagnostic criteria.

Gray-scale imaging provides anatomic information about the location and orientation of vessels as well as size, location, surface characteristics, and composition of atherosclerotic plaques. Plaques are classified as homogeneous (uniform echo pattern) or heterogeneous (complex echo pattern with mixed densities, sonolucent areas).

CDFI diagnostic criteria of the classification of carotid stenosis include three sources of information: (1) the Doppler frequency spectrum; (2) measurement of the residual vessel lumen; and (3) characteristic color flow patterns. Asymmetric blood flow patterns are considered.

Based on our own results (Meairs S, Steinke W, Mohr JP, Hennerici M. Ultrasound imaging and Doppler sonography. In: Barnett HJM, Mohr JP, Stein BM, Yatsu F, eds. Stroke: Pathophysiology, Diagnosis and Management. New York: Churchill Livingstone, 1998: 207–326.)

A recent meta-analysis[17] of studies comparing MRA and DUS to carotid angiography have shown that for the diagnosis of 70–99% vs <70% stenosis, MRA had a pooled sensitivity of 95% (95% CI 92–97) and a pooled specificity of 90% (95% CI 86–93). These numbers were 86% (95% CI 84–89) and 87% (95% CI 84–90) for DUS, respectively. For recognizing occlusion, MRA yielded a sensitivity of 98% (95% CI 94–100) and a specificity of 100% (95% CI 99–100), and DUS had a sensitivity of 96% (95% CI 94–98) and a specificity of 100% (95% CI 99–100).

Apart from its higher cost, MRA has several advantages over both DUS and CTA. With MRA, it is possible to acquire a three-dimensional (3D) data set that provides reproducible quantitative tissue information. MR techniques are not dependent on the angle of the imaging plane and are less dependent on the skill of the operator than DUS techniques, although proper imaging algorithms are instrumental. MRA is unique in that the modality can provide excellent contrast between the vessel wall and adjacent lumen by using flow-sensitive pulse sequences. These features of MR imaging provide important advantages as a means of non-invasive characterization of carotid plaque morphology.[19–21] MRA has shown additional benefit in the evaluation of collateral circulation in patients with asymptomatic CAS. With the use of MRA, individuals with asymptomatic CAS were found to have a higher prevalence of collateral circulation via the anterior portion of the circle of Willis and had higher anterior communicating artery diameters than controls.[22] How this information can be used to optimize patient management remains to be seen.

MRA imaging can be performed with and without intravenous (IV) contrast. Non-contrast MRA commonly overestimates the severity of carotid stenosis, but it can also underestimate stenosis severity because of poor image quality, and it can create other artifacts that may appear as a severe stenosis (Figure 5.1A). Contrast-enhanced MRA, on the other hand, is less subject to such effects and has excellent correlation with rotational angiography (Figure 5.1B).[23] Aside from the importance of contrast enhancement, there are continued efforts to optimize imaging sequences and algorithms,[24] which are beyond the scope of this chapter.

The safety and accuracy of contrast-enhanced MRA makes it an ideal alternative to conventional angiography for confirming the diagnosis of carotid disease. However, although MRA has a better discriminatory power compared with DUS in diagnosing 70–99% carotid stenosis, it should not be advocated as an initial screening test for carotid occlusive disease due to its high cost and limited availability.

Computed tomographic angiography

Computed tomographic angiography (CTA) is a new and minimally invasive technique consisting of an IV bolus injection of contrast solution followed by high-speed CT scanning and computer-assisted generation of images of large to medium-sized arteries in the region scanned. Modern CT angiography has been found to be an accurate estimator of stenosis in carotid disease.[25–27] A recent meta-analysis[28] of studies comparing CTA with carotid angiography demonstrated that the pooled sensitivity and specificity of CTA for detection of a 70–99% stenosis were 85% (95% CI 79–89%) and 93% (95% CI 89–96%),

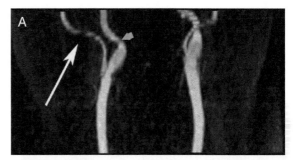
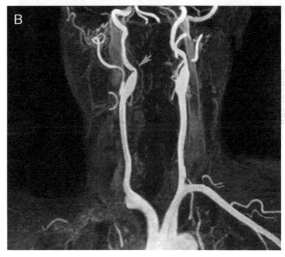

Figure 5.1 (A) Non-contrast carotid MRA (same projection and orientation as the contrast-enhanced MRA in Figure 5.1B). Note that the right ICA lesion (red arrow) is poorly defined because of partial volume averaging and lower spatial resolution. Also note the 'Stair-step' artifact that may simulate a stenosis (yellow arrow). (B) Contrast-enhanced MRA. The stenosis (red arrow) is much more clearly seen on this study because of the higher spatial resolution and absence of artifact. (See color plate section.)

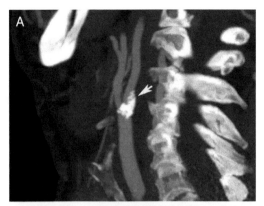

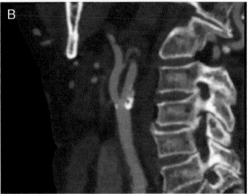

Figure 5.2 (A) Carotid CTA (same projection and orientation as Figure 5.2B). Note that the thick MIP image makes it look like the carotid artery is completely occluded by a bright calcified plaque (yellow arrow). (B) Carotid CTA. Note that the thin MIP image shows a razor thin plane through the lumen of the vessel and, subsequently, shows the stenosis to be much more mild. (See color plate section.)

respectively. For detection of an occlusion, the sensitivity and specificity were 97% (95% CI 93–99%) and 99% (95% CI 98–100%), respectively.

The accuracy of the frequently used maximum intensity projection (MIP) reconstructions may be limited by bone or calcifications that obscure the depiction of intraluminal contrast and thus the residual lumen (Figure 5.2A). This limitation can be overcome with the use of thin MIP imaging (Figure 5.2B). Paradoxically, the limitation of calcium imaging with respect to vessel lumen definition could have a unique application for this technology. Recent studies suggest that calcium detected by CTA may represent an independent risk marker for TIA and stroke that could be used for risk stratification and monitor the effects of therapy.[29] Other disadvantages of CTA that are shared by conventional angiography are the ionizing radiation and the need for intravenous iodinated contrast.

Carotid imaging sequence and management of discrepant findings

DUS should be the first screening tool for asymptomatic CAS because of its low cost and wide availability. No further confirmatory imaging is needed if the DUS study is normal. However, if carotid disease is identified (>50% stenosis), it is reasonable to confirm these findings by MRA, or CTA if the former is not available, because DUS can overestimate or underestimate lesion severity (see Duplex ultrasound section). Two clinical scenarios are particularly important: first, patients with large calcified plaque where DUS may underestimate lesion severity; and secondly, patients diagnosed with carotid occlusion, because DUS may mistake a subtotal stenosis for an occlusion.

DUS and MRA, or CTA, often provide concordant results when performed in experienced and accredited laboratories. However, discrepancy between DUS and MRA can occur in 15–20% of cases.[30] In these cases, digital subtraction angiography (DSA) is indicated, particularly if carotid revascularization is being considered.

CLINICAL EVALUATION OF PATIENTS WITH ASYMPTOMATIC CAROTID ARTERY STENOSIS

Does every patient with asymptomatic carotid artery stenosis need to be evaluated by a neurologist?

Once a patient with 'asymptomatic' CAS has been identified, the question that is often asked by non-neurologist physicians is whether the patient needs to be evaluated by a neurologist. The following are several reasons why a neurological evaluation should be considered for optimal management of these patients.

Importance of a complete neurological evaluation

Although the majority of patients with carotid occlusive disease who are labeled 'asymptomatic' are in fact truly asymptomatic, some may have had subtle neurological events that were not identified. The primary objective of a detailed neurological evaluation of patients with assumingly 'asymptomatic' CAS is to establish their freedom from prior neurological events and to illicit any present neurological deficits. Most patients (with and without carotid disease) are not familiar with the workings of their bodies, particularly their nervous system. Patients may attribute temporary motor, sensory, visual, or speech disturbance to a number of unrelated causes and may not even think of reporting it to their physicians. The neurological history and examination performed by non-neurologists is often incomplete and may not elucidate prior events or may even miss subtle neurological deficits, particularly those related to higher cortical function, oculomotor system, and gait. The literature is replete with studies demonstrating that a single or multiple questions regarding a history of TIA are not adequate to identify all patients with prior events. These strategies can under- or overcall cerebrovascular events. Bergmann and colleagues[31] evaluated the accuracy of using a single question about prior stroke and reported a true positive rate of 67%. Berger and colleagues[32] compared a single question with a multiple-item questionnaire of stroke symptoms in a general population and found increased accuracy using the multiple-item questionnaire (sensitivity of 89.5%). In the national prospective British Regional Heart Study of 7735 men aged 40–59 years, Walker and colleagues[33] reported a comparison between multiple-item questionnaire and medical record review for ascertainment of stroke/TIA history. In this study, patients tended to over-recall strokes more than they under-recalled them, 25% vs 11%. TIAs accounted for 57% of over-recalled strokes. In contrast, the general practice record review system tended to under-report events rather than to over-report them, 23% vs 5%. Patient recall of events should be used to complement rather than to supplant medical record data, but neither would be as good as a complete neurological history and examination.

Interpretation of brain imaging studies

Even with the most complete neurological evaluation, a prior cerebral ischemic injury can be missed – Silent Cerebral Infarct (SCI).[34] Silent infarcts differ from clinical strokes in that although there is damage to the brain, it is usually so strategically placed or so small that it does not cause symptoms or signs leading to a diagnosis of stroke.[35] The prevalence of SCI in the 'asymptomatic' general population ranges from 11%[36] to 28%,[37] depending on age, prevalence of hypertension, smoking, and other cardiovascular risk factors. Elderly people with SCI have an increased risk of dementia and a steeper decline in cognitive function, particularly in those with recurrent lesions.[38] SCIs are often lacunar but may also be cortical or subcortical and they vary in etiology and prognostic significance. For the purpose of this discussion we will focus on the relationship between SCI and carotid disease.

Although the relationship between cortical infarctions and infarctions in watershed territory and carotid disease is well established, the conventional wisdom has been that lacunar infarcts represent small-vessel disease.

Recently, however, several lines of evidence have suggested that lacunar infarcts can also be caused by atherosclerotic carotid disease.[14,39] The prevalence of SCI in patients with asymptomatic CAS is about 15%.[35] There remains a lack of agreement as to the prognostic significance of SCI in patients with asymptomatic CAS because of conflicting data. One view endorses the proposition that the presence of SCI in the setting of asymptomatic CAS is not related to thromboembolism from carotid disease, but more likely reflects small-vessel disease. This view is supported by findings from the Asymptomatic Carotid Atherosclerosis Study (ACAS),[35] which demonstrated that SCI were often small, evenly distributed between the ipsilateral and contralateral hemispheres, and unrelated to the severity of the stenosis.

Contrary to the above findings, however, an alternative view endorses the proposition that the presence of SCI in patients with asymptomatic CAS indicates a causative link and has a prognostic value. The association between SCI and asymptomatic CAS was demonstrated by several studies.[40,41] Norris and colleagues[40] performed brain CT imaging on 137 patients with asymptomatic CAS. Thirty percent of these patients were found to have SCI, the majority of which were ipsilateral to the stenosis, and the highest prevalence was among patients with >75% stenosis. These investigators, however, did not perform multivariate analysis to exclude the effect of potential confounders. Another study by Sabetai and colleagues[41] in 218 patients with asymptomatic CAS demonstrated that carotid plaque echogenicity, and not severity, predicted the incidence of silent non-lacunar infarcts as demonstrated by brain CT imaging.

The prognostic value of SCI in patients with asymptomatic CAS has also been suggested by various studies.[8,42] In a subanalysis of patients with contralateral asymptomatic CAS in NASCET, Inzitari and colleagues[8] demonstrated that SCI is an independent predictor of future larger artery ischemic stroke. Similarly, Tegos and colleagues[42] also demonstrated that the presence of discrete cortical or subcortical SCI on brain CT in patients with carotid disease increases their risk of future stroke by about 4-fold (Figure 5.3).

These previous findings, which are based on brain CT imaging, have also been corroborated by MR imaging. Diffusion-weighted imaging (DWI), in particular, is very sensitive to small-volume lesions or multiple lesions that may be missed by brain CT. Recent studies have clearly illustrated that different lesion patterns on MRI can predict causal categories defined by the TOAST classification.[43] Therefore, despite the lack of consensus on this issue, the presence of ipsilateral SCI in patients with asymptomatic CAS, particularly when discrete and cortical, may be indicative of higher

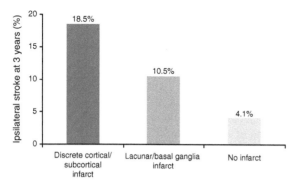

Figure 5.3 Impact of silent brain infarct type by CT scan on future risk of stroke in patients with carotid occlusive disease. (Modified from Tegos et al.[42])

risk for future stroke. Therefore, these findings should be considered in clinical decision-making.

Risk stratification of patients with asymptomatic carotid artery stenosis

A third reason for patients to be evaluated by a neurologist is to assess the need for further dedicated testing to assess patient future risk for neurological ischemic events. This will be covered in detail in the risk stratification section of this book.

Does every patient with asymptomatic carotid artery stenosis need a cardiovascular evaluation?

It is routine practice to refer patients with symptomatic carotid occlusive disease for detailed cardiac evaluation to rule out cardiac causes of embolism. However, despite the recognition that there is a strong association between coronary artery disease (CAD) and asymptomatic CAS, it is not currently a routine practice to evaluate these patients for the presence of cardiac disease.[44,45] However, every patient with a diagnosis of asymptomatic CAS should undergo a detailed cardiac evaluation for the following reasons.

Patients with asymptomatic carotid artery stenosis are at high risk for future cardiac morbidity and mortality

It is estimated that 40–50% of patients with asymptomatic CAS have ischemic heart disease.[46,47] Moreover, about one-third of patients with asymptomatic CAS and no history of CAD have inducible myocardial ischemia on stress testing.[46] The presence of ischemic heart disease in these patients increases the risk of cardiac morbidity and mortality more than that of stroke.[46–48]

Chimowitz and colleagues[47] reported that among patients with asymptomatic CAS in the Veterans Affairs Cooperative Study, the 4-year risk of coronary events was significantly higher (40%) among patients with a history of CAD than patients without a history of CAD (33%). However, a subgroup of patients with carotid stenosis and no history of CAD who have coexistent intracranial occlusive disease, diabetes, or peripheral vascular disease have a risk of cardiac events similar to that of patients with a history of CAD. Of course, the high frequency of coronary events in this study should not be generalized to all other patients with asymptomatic CAS since these patients were all men with very high prevalence of smoking (~90%), peripheral arterial disease (~60%), and diabetes, all known to increase the risk of cardiac events. Nonetheless, cardiac disease remains one of the leading causes of morbidity and mortality, even for lower-risk patients with asymptomatic CAS.[49] Therefore, all patients with asymptomatic CAS should be screened for CAD and, if present, intensive medical therapy should be implemented as well as coronary revascularization when needed.

Cardiac disease increases the risk of ischemic stroke in patients with asymptomatic carotid artery stenosis

It has been clearly demonstrated that not all strokes that occur in the distribution of an asymptomatic CAS are due to the carotid lesion. Cardiac diseases such as coronary heart disease, congestive heart failure, valvular heart disease, and atrial fibrillation are well-known causes of ischemic stroke. The most detailed analysis of the frequency and etiology of ipsilateral ischemic strokes in patients with asymptomatic CAS was reported by Inzitari and colleagues.[8] These investigators reported on the 5-year incidence of ischemic stroke ipsilateral to the asymptomatic carotid stenosis in patients enrolled in NASCET. In this study, a large number of strokes in the territory of the asymptomatic carotid artery had causes other than large-artery disease (Figure 5.4). Among patients with an asymptomatic CAS of 60–99%, the risk of lacunar stroke at 5 years was approximately two-thirds the risk of large-artery stroke. The risk of cardioembolic stroke was less than one-quarter the risk of large-artery stroke. The combined risk of stroke with a lacunar or cardioembolic cause approached the risk of a large-artery stroke (8.1% vs 9.9%). Risk factors for cardioembolic stroke were a history of myocardial infarction or angina and hypertension.

Therefore, early identification and treatment of cardiac disease in patients with asymptomatic CAS is instrumental for optimal reduction of ischemic stroke in these patients.

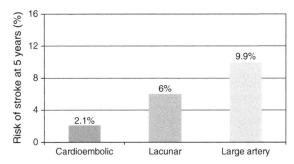

Figure 5.4 The 5-year risk of first ipsilateral stroke of cardioembolic, lacunar, or large-artery origin in patients with asymptomatic carotid disease (60–99% stenosis). (Modified from Inzitari et al.[8])

SUMMARY

The rationale behind identification of asymptomatic CAS is that early treatment can reduce the incidence of cardiovascular and cerebrovascular events. Selection of appropriate populations at risk is mandatory to avoid unnecessary cost and harm. Various non-invasive diagnostic techniques are available, each with their individual strengths and flaws. Duplex ultrasound is the most commonly used test because of its wide availability, low cost, and ease of use. However, it is crucial for clinicians to be aware of the potential pitfalls of DUS in specific clinical scenarios and the variability in diagnostic accuracy among various laboratories. MRA is a safe and accurate imaging modality for confirmation of the diagnosis. The use of CTA has generated interest in its ability to detect carotid calcifications, which have been found to be an independent risk factor for TIA and stroke. Conventional angiography should only be used in cases of discrepancy between two non-invasive modalities or in patients undergoing carotid artery stenting.

All patients with asymptomatic CAS should undergo detailed neurological and cardiac evaluation to confirm their 'asymptomatic' status and to identify any subclinical cerebrovascular or cardiovascular disease. Early identification and management of cardiac disease are critical for optimal care of these patients.

REFERENCES

1. Executive Committee for the Asymptomatic Carotid Atherosclerosis Study. Endarterectomy for asymptomatic carotid stenosis. JAMA 1995; 273: 1421–8.
2. MRC Asymptomatic Carotid Surgery Trial (ACST) Collaborative Group. Prevention of disabling and fatal strokes by successful carotid endarterectomy in patients without recent neurological symptoms: randomized controlled trial. Lancet 2004; 363: 1491–502.
3. Jungquist G, Hanson BS, Isacsson SO et al. Risk factors for carotid artery stenosis: an epidemiological study of men aged 69 years. J Clin Epidemiol 1991; 44(4–5): 347–53.
4. O'Leary DH, Anderson KM, Wolf PA, Evans JC, Poehlman HW. Cholesterol and carotid atherosclerosis in older persons: the Framingham Study. Ann Epidemiol 1992; 2(1–2): 147–53.
5. Komorovsky R, Desideri A, Coscarelli S, Cortigiani L, Celegon L. Impact of carotid arterial narrowing on outcomes of patients with acute coronary syndromes. Am J Cardiol 2004; 93: 1552–5.
6. Cina CS, Safar HA, Maggisano R, Bailey R, Clase CM. Prevalence and progression of internal carotid artery stenosis in patients with peripheral arterial occlusive disease. J Vasc Surg 2002; 36: 75–82.
7. Whitty CJ, Sudlow CL, Warlow CP. Investigating individual subjects and screening populations for asymptomatic carotid stenosis can be harmful. J Neurol Neurosurg Psychiatry 1988; 64(5): 619–23.
8. Inzitari D, Eliasziw M, Gates P et al. The causes and risk of stroke in patients with asymptomatic internal-carotid-artery stenosis. North American Symptomatic Carotid Endarterectomy Trial Collaborators. N Engl J Med 2000; 342: 1693–1700.
9. The European Carotid Surgery Trialists Collaborative Group. Risk of stroke in the distribution of an asymptomatic carotid artery. Lancet 1995; 345(8944): 209–12.
10. Rothwell PM, Villagra R, Gibson R, Donders RCJM, Warlow CP. Evidence of a chronic systemic cause of instability of atherosclerotic plaques. Lancet 2000; 355: 19–24.
11. EAFT Study Group European Atrial Fibrillation Trial. Silent brain infarction in nonrheumatic atrial fibrillation. Neurology 1996; 46: 159–65.
12. Bernick C, Kuller L, Dulberg C et al. Silent MRI infarcts and the risk of future stroke: the cardiovascular health study. Neurology 2001; 57: 1222–9.
13. Vermeer SE, Hollander M, van Dijk EJ et al. Rotterdam Scan Study. Silent brain infarcts and white matter lesions increase stroke risk in the general population: the Rotterdam Scan Study. Stroke 2003; 34(5): 1126–9.
14. Uehara T, Tabuchi M, Mori E. Risk factors for silent cerebral infarcts in subcortical white matter and basal ganglia. Stroke 1999; 30: 378–382.
15. Faught WE, Mattos MA, van Bemmelen PS et al. Color-flow duplex scanning of carotid arteries: new velocity criteria based on receiver operator characteristic analysis for threshold stenoses used in the symptomatic and asymptomatic carotid trials. J Vasc Surg 1994; 19: 818–27.
16. Zwiebel WJ. Duplex sonography of the cerebral arteries: efficacy, limitations, and indications. Am J Radiol 1992; 158: 29–36.
17. Nederkoorn PJ, van der Graaf Y, Hunink MG. Duplex ultrasound and magnetic resonance angiography compared with digital subtraction angiography in a carotid artery stenosis: a systematic review. Stroke 2003; 34: 1324–32.
18. Grant EG, Benson CB, Moneta GL et al. Carotid artery stenosis: Gray-Scale and Doppler US diagnosis – Society of Radiologists in Ultrasound Consensus Conference. Radiology 2003; 229: 340–6.
19. Yuan C, Murakami JW, Hayes CE et al. Phased-array magnetic resonance imaging of the carotid artery bifurcation: preliminary results in healthy volunteers and a patient with atherosclerotic disease. J Magn Reson Imaging 1995; 5: 561–5.
20. Yuan C, Beach KW, Smith LH Jr, Hatsukami TS. Measurement of atherosclerotic carotid plaque size in vivo using high resolution magnetic resonance imaging. Circulation 1998; 98: 2666–71.
21. Hatsukami TS, Ross R, Polissar NL, Yuan C. Visualization of fibrous cap thickness and rupture in human atherosclerotic carotid plaque in vivo with high-resolution magnetic resonance imaging. Circulation 2000; 102: 959–64.

22. Hendrikse J, Eikelboom BC, van der Grond J. Magnetic resonance angiography of collateral compensation in asymptomatic and symptomatic internal carotid artery stenosis. J Vasc Surg 2002; 36(4): 1–7.

23. Anzalone N, Scomazzoni F, Castellano R et al. Carotid artery stenosis: intraindividual correlations of 3D time-of-flight MR angiography, contrast-enhanced MR angiography, conventional DSA, and rotational angiography for detection and grading. Radiology 2005; 236(1): 204–13.

24. Benjamin MS, Gillams AR, Carter AP. Carotid MRA – what advantages do the turbo field-echo and 3D phase-contrast sequences offer? Neuroradiology 1997; 39(7): 469–73.

25. Sugahara T, Korogi Y, Hirai T et al. CT angiography in vascular intervention for steno-occlusive diseases: role of multiplanar reconstruction and source images. Br J Radiol 1998; 71: 601–61.

26. Magarelli N, Scarabino T, Simeone AL et al. Carotid stenosis: a comparison between MR and spiral CT angiography. Neuroradiology 1998; 40: 367–73.

27. Randoux B, Marro B, Koskas F et al. Carotid artery stenosis: prospective comparison of CT, three-dimensional gadolinium-enhanced MR, and conventional angiography. Radiology 2001; 220: 179–85.

28. Koelemay MJ, Nederkoorn PJ, Reitsma JB, Majoie CB. Systematic review of computed tomographic angiography for assessment of carotid artery disease. Stroke 2004; 35: 2306–12.

29. Nandalur KR, Baskurt E, Hagspiel KD et al. Carotid artery calcification on CT may independently predict stroke risk. AJR Am J Roentgenol 2006; 186(2): 547–52.

30. Nederkoorn PJ, Mali WP, Eikelboom BC et al. Preoperative diagnosis of carotid artery stenosis: accuracy of noninvasive testing. Stroke 2002; 33: 2003–8.

31. Bergmann MM, Byers T, Freedman DS, Mokdad A. Validity of self-reported diagnoses leading to hospitalization: a comparison of self-reports with hospital records in a prospective study of American adults. Am J Epidemiol 1998; 147: 969–77.

32. Berger K, Hense HW, Rothdach A, Weltermann B, Keil U. A single question about prior stroke versus a stroke questionnaire to assess stroke prevalence in populations. Neuroepidemiology 2000; 19: 245–57.

33. Walker MK, Whincup PH, Shaper AG, Lennon LT, Thomson AG. Validation of patient recall of doctor-diagnosed heart attack and stroke: a postal questionnaire and record review comparison. Am J Epidemiol 1998; 148: 355–61.

34. Chodosh EH, Foulkes MA, Kase CS et al. Silent stroke in the NINCDS Stroke Data Bank. Neurology 1988; 38: 1674–9.

35. Brott T, Tomsick T, Feinberg W et al. Baseline silent cerebral infarction in the Asymptomatic Carotid Atherosclerosis Study. Stroke 1994; 25: 1122–9.

36. Howard G, Wagenknecht LE, Cai J et al. Cigarette smoking and other risk factors for silent cerebral infarction in the general population. Stroke 1998; 29: 913–17.

37. Price TR, Manolio TA, Kronmal RA et al. Silent brain infarction on magnetic resonance imaging and neurological abnormalities in community-dwelling older adults. The Cardiovascular Health Study. CHS Collaborative Research Group. Stroke 1997; 28: 1158–64.

38. Vermeer SE, Prins ND, den Heijer T et al. Silent brain infarcts and the risk of dementia and cognitive decline. N Engl J Med 2003; 348: 1215–22.

39. Tejada J, Díez-Tejedor E, Hernández-Echebarría L, Balboa O. Does a relationship exist between carotid stenosis and lacunar infarction? Stroke 2003; 34: 1404–11.

40. Norris JW, Zhu CZ. Silent stroke and carotid stenosis. Stroke 1992; 23: 483–5.

41. Sabetai MM, Tegos TJ, Clifford C et al. Carotid plaque echogenicity and types of silent CT-brain infarcts. Is there an association in patients with asymptomatic carotid stenosis? Int Angiol 2001; 20(1): 51–7.

42. Tegos TJ, Kalodiki E, Nicolaides AN et al. Brain CT infarction in patients with carotid atheroma. Does it predict a future event? Int Angiol 2001; 20(2): 110–17.

43. Kang DW, Chalela JA, Ezzeddine MA, Warach S. Association of ischemic lesion patterns on early diffusion-weighted imaging with TOAST stroke subtypes. Arch Neurol 2003; 60: 1730–4.

44. Tanaka H, Nishino M, Ishida M. Progression of carotid atherosclerosis in Japanese patients with coronary artery disease. Stroke 1992; 23: 946–51.

45. Crouse JR 3rd. Carotid and coronary atherosclerosis. What are the connections? Postgrad Med 1991; 90: 175–9.

46. Love BB, Grover-McKay M, Biller J, Rezai K, McKay CR. Coronary artery disease and cardiac events with asymptomatic and symptomatic cerebrovascular disease. Stroke 1992; 23: 939–45.

47. Chimowitz MI, Weiss DG, Cohen SL, Starling MR, Hobson RW 2nd. Cardiac prognosis of patients with carotid stenosis and no history of coronary artery disease. Veterans Affairs Cooperative Study Group 167. Stroke 1994; 25(4): 759–65.

48. Hedblad B, Janzon L, Jungquist G, Ogren M. Factors modifying the prognosis in men with asymptomatic carotid artery disease. J Intern Med 1998; 243(1): 57–64.

49. Norris JW, Zhu CZ, Bornstein NM, Chambers BR. Vascular risks of asymptomatic carotid stenosis. Stroke 1991; 22: 1485–90.

6

Medical treatment for patients with asymptomatic carotid artery stenosis

Michael R Jaff

Take-Home Messages

1. Medical and behavioral therapy of traditional cardiovascular risk factors (hypertension, dyslipidemia, diabetes mellitus, smoking cessation) should always be the first-line treatment for patients with asymptomatic carotid artery stenosis (CAS) to reduce global risks of cardiovascular and cerebrovascular events.
2. Treatment of hypertension is the most effective therapy to reduce global stroke risk, primarily due to reduction of lacunar and hemorrhagic strokes. Whether blood pressure reduction reduces stroke specifically related to carotid artery disease in unclear.
3. The magnitude of benefit from statin therapy in reducing global stroke risk depends on the presence or absence of concomitant comorbidities such as hypertension, diabetes mellitus, and coronary artery disease (CAD). Statin therapy for an average of 5 years results in 8 fewer strokes per 1000 CAD patients treated, compared with 5 fewer strokes per 1000 patients without CAD.
4. Intensive glycemic control in patients with type 1 diabetes mellitus results in significant reduction in cardiovascular and cerebrovascular events.
5. The role of aspirin in primary prevention of stroke depends on gender and concomitant comorbidities. Aspirin therapy for an average of 6.4 years results in 2 fewer strokes per 1000 women treated (but not men).
6. Among patients with asymptomatic CAS, carotid revascularization combined with usual medical care further reduces ischemic ipsilateral neurological events.

INTRODUCTION

Over the course of time, time-honored medical therapies occasionally develop in the absence of solid clinical data. In the modern era of prospective randomized controlled trials demonstrating major advances in therapy for coronary artery disease (CAD), for example, physicians have come to expect a more robust evidence base in cerebrovascular disease. Unfortunately, the body of literature is limited, specifically in the area of therapy for patients with asymptomatic extracranial carotid artery stenosis (CAS).

In 2000, the American Heart Association estimated that there were 500 000 initial strokes, 200 000 stroke recurrences, and 4 700 000 stroke survivors in the United States, many of whom required chronic care.[1] Because 75% of strokes are first-time events, there exists an opportunity to reduce the risk of stroke in patients felt to be at increased risk of a cerebrovascular event. However, stroke can be hemorrhagic or ischemic in origin; ischemic stroke can be caused by small-vessel occlusive disease, large-vessel occlusive disease (extracranial carotid disease), or embolism (heart, aortic arch, cryptogenic brain infarction) (Figure 6.1). Unfortunately, the majority of clinical trials addressing the impact of medical therapy on prevention of ischemic stroke have not adequately defined the etiology of ischemic stroke or the presence or absence of extracranial carotid disease. Therefore, although medical

Embolism
- Arterial atheroembolism (carotid atherosclerosis)
- Cardiac
  - Atrial fibrillation
  - Myocardial infarction
  - Cardiomyopathy
  - Prosthetic valves
  - Paradoxical (DVT)

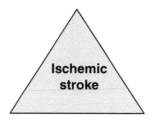

Small-vessel occlusive disease	Large-vessel occlusive disease
• Lacunar	• Carotid atherothrombosis
• Arteritis	• Arteritis
• Drug induced	• Dissection

Figure 6.1 Types and etiologies of ischemic stroke.

management of traditional cardiovascular risk factors (dyslipidemia, hypertension, diabetes mellitus, smoking cessation) should always be first-line therapy for all at-risk patients, the evidence that medical therapy alone is sufficient for optimal reduction of ischemic stroke risk in patients with asymptomatic CAS remains elusive. The purpose of the forthcoming discussion is 2-fold:

1. To review the class I evidence regarding the impact of medical therapy alone vs medical therapy and carotid endarterectomy on incidence of cardiovascular and cerebrovasculat events in patients with asymptomatic CAS.
2. To review the impact of individual risk factor modification on global risk of ischemic stroke.

EVIDENCE FROM PROSPECTIVE RANDOMIZED CLINICAL TRIALS OF MEDICAL THERAPY ALONE vs MEDICAL THERAPY AND CAROTID ENDARTERECTOMY

There are three class I studies that compared medical therapy alone to medical therapy and carotid endarterectomy (CE) in patients with asymptomatic CAS: the Veterans Affairs Study,[2] the Asymptomatic Carotid Atherosclerosis Study (ACAS),[3] and the Asymptomatic Carotid Surgery Trial (ACST).[4] Two other studies were incomplete[5,6] and not included in this analysis. A common

criticism of all of these randomized trials was the lack of 'current day' optimal medical therapy, raising the question of the modern applicability of these data sets, except perhaps for the ACST trial.[4]

In the Veterans Affairs Study,[2] CE reduced the overall incidence of ipsilateral neurological events – transient ischemic attack (TIA) and stroke – compared with medical therapy alone, but there was no significant influence on the combined incidence of stroke and death. The major criticism of this trial was the small sample size, rendering meaningful conclusions limited.

The second randomized controlled trial to address the role of medical therapy vs CE was ACAS.[3] This study randomized 1662 patients with asymptomatic CAS of varying degrees of severity to medical therapy alone vs medical therapy + CE. The study was halted after a median follow-up of 2.7 years because of a projected 5-year absolute risk reduction of 5.9% favoring CE. The 5-year projected rate of ipsilateral stroke was 11.0% for the medically treated patients and 5.1% for the surgically treated patients (53% relative risk reduction, $p < 0.004$). Interestingly, in this trial, there was no significant reduction in rates of major ipsilateral stroke among the surgically treated cohort.

The most modern data applicable to current clinical practice are that derived from the ACST trial.[4] In this trial, 3120 patients were randomized to medical therapy alone vs medical therapy + CE. At randomization, there was widespread use of antiplatelet and antihypertensive drugs, and increasing use of lipid-lowering drugs (17% in 1993–1996, 58% in 2000–2003). After randomization, the use of all three types of drug increased still further. At last follow-up in 2002–2003, more than 90% of the survivors were on antiplatelet therapy, 81% were on antihypertensives, and 70% were on lipid-lowering treatment. The use of these drugs (and the mean blood pressure) was similar in both treatment groups not only at randomization but also during follow-up, so the trial is one of surgery against a background of appropriate medical management for most patients. The absolute benefit gained was significant for those with and without high cholesterol, with or without high blood pressure, and with or without hyperlipidemia, hypertension, diabetes mellitus, and prior myocardial infarction (MI). Combining the perioperative events (stroke and death within 30 days) and the non-perioperative strokes, the 5-year risks were 6.4% (immediate CE) vs 11.8% (deferred CE) for all strokes ($p < 0.0001$) and 3.5% vs 6.1% for fatal or disabling strokes ($p < 0.004$). The gain mostly involved non-perioperative carotid territory ischemic strokes: 2.7% vs 9.5%; gain of 6.8% (4.8–8.8), $p < 0.0001$. The benefit was seen in both contralateral and ipsilateral carotid territory strokes. Subgroup analyses demonstrated stroke reduction in men ($n = 2044$) and women ($n = 1076$) and for those younger than 65 years of age or between 65 and 74 years. The benefit was uncertain for those older than 75 years.

In summary, all prospective controlled randomized clinical trials of medical therapy alone vs medical therapy + revascularization demonstrated the additional benefit of revascularization in reducing ipsilateral neurological events. Of course, these findings do not diminish the importance of medical therapy but merely imply that medical therapy alone may not be sufficient to optimally reduce stroke risk in all patients with asymptomatic CAS. In clinical practice, all patients with asymptomatic CAS should receive intensive risk factor intervention and antiplatelet therapy in combination with selective carotid revascularization, particularly those with a favorable risk to benefit ratio (see Risk stratification section).

GLOBAL STROKE PREVENTION THROUGH RISK FACTOR MANAGEMENT

Despite the decline in mortality rates from stroke over the last three decades in the United States and other industrialized nations, the incidence and lifetime risk of stroke remain unchanged over the past 50 years. Although part of the decline in death rate may be due to a reduction in stroke severity, it is likely that improved detection and treatment of the atherosclerotic cardiovascular risk factors is also instrumental to this decline. Risk factor modification to reduce the

incidence of global stroke risk includes reducing elevated blood pressure, cessation of cigarette smoking[7], treating high-risk individuals with HMG CoA reductase inhibitors, achieving better control of blood sugar in diabetics, increasing physical activity,[8,9] and adhering to a healthy diet. It is also likely that prevention and treatment of predisposing cardiac diseases such as coronary heart disease (CHD), congestive heart failure, valvular heart disease, and atrial fibrillation would also reduce stroke occurrence. In the forthcoming discussion we will focus on the role of management of hypertension, dyslipidemia, diabetes mellitus, and antiplatelet therapy in primary prevention of stroke, specifically in patients with asymptomatic CAS whenever data are available.

Management of hypertension in patients with asymptomatic carotid artery stenosis

Is hypertension a risk factor for stroke in asymptomatic carotid artery stenosis?

Hypertension is the most common and most powerful precursor of global ischemic and hemorrhagic stroke. It is in fact a much stronger risk factor for stroke than for CAD.[10] The stroke risk is related to both systolic[11–13] and diastolic blood pressure.[14,15] A prospective follow-up of a Framingham cohort of 5209 men and women over 18 years demonstrated that hypertensive patients are seven times more likely to develop atherothrombotic brain infarction than normotensive patients, with the risk proportional to the blood pressure throughout the spectrum.[16] Although stroke risk is clearly more directly related to systolic pressure, diastolic pressure is also a critical determinant of this risk. Indeed, a combined analysis of nine prospective observational studies of 420 000 individuals[10] demonstrated that the incidence of stroke increased 46% and CHD increased 29% with each 7.5 mmHg increase in diastolic blood pressure.

The most common stroke type in hypertensive individuals are lacunar strokes and intracranial hemorrhage which are typically located in the basal ganglia, thalamus, internal capsule, brainstem, or cerebellum. However, the extent to which hypertension contributes to the risk of stroke from an asymptomatic carotid artery plaque remains unknown.

Prevalence and etiology of hypertension in patients with carotid artery stenosis

Hypertension is common in patients with symptomatic and asymptomatic carotid stenosis. The prevalence of hypertension in ACAS[3] and ACST[4] was 64% and 65%

of patients, respectively. Although primary hypertension is the most common type in the general population as well as patients with CAS, secondary hypertension is common in patients with CAS. Spence[17] studied 170 patients with carotid stenosis in the North American Symptomatic Carotid Endarterectomy Trial (NASCET) and the ACAS trial: 145 (85.3%) were hypertensive, 16.6% of whom had renovascular hypertension and 8.3% had adrenocortical hypertension. Furthermore, the prevalence of renovascular hypertension was even higher among the 79 patients with resistant hypertension (25.3%). The blood pressure was significantly higher in patients with renovascular and adrenocortical hypertension than in patients with primary hypertension.

Treatment of hypertension in patients with carotid artery stenosis

All patients with hypertension, regardless of the presence or absence of carotid artery disease, should be treated with antihypertensive therapy to reduce the global risk of stroke and cardiovascular morbidity and mortality.[18–21] There is debate as to whether specific antihypertensive agents are preferable to reduce cerebrovascular events. The Losartan Intervention For Endpoint (LIFE) trial[22] showed that patients randomized to losartan had significantly better outcomes, with about 25% RRR for stroke, compared with patients randomized to atenolol, despite identical blood pressure reduction. The Study on Cognition and Prognosis in the Elderly (SCOPE)[23] also showed a significant reduction of non-fatal stroke with candesartan vs alternative therapies. The Heart Outcomes Prevention Evaluation (HOPE) study[24] provided evidence that treatment with the angiotensin-converting enzyme (ACE) inhibitor ramipril can further reduce the risk of stroke in high-risk patients by mechanisms other than lowering blood pressure. In this study, patients were normotensive at baseline. Therefore, for the first time, in a patient population without left ventricular dysfunction, the effects of an ACE inhibitor ramipril on reducing stroke risk were demonstrated. Ramipril 10 mg achieved a significant 33% reduction in stroke among patients with diabetes. However, these results were not reproduced in other trials such as ALLHAT[25] (Antihypertensive and Lipid-Lowering treatment to prevent Heart Attack Trial), which reported superior results in patients randomized to diuretics. Current guidelines for treatment of hypertension are shown in Table 6.1.[26,27]

It is worth noting that despite medical treatment, the long-term risk of ischemic stroke, MI, and death for hypertensive patients remains higher than that of normotensive individuals.[28] This is of course not surprising, since hypertensive patients are continuously exposed to atherosclerotic risk and target organ damage both prior to and during therapy. The impact of risk factor exposure during long-term follow-up is exemplified by the fact that smoking and diabetes are significantly predictive of stroke in this population.

Is it safe to significantly lower blood pressure in patients with severe carotid artery stenosis?

It has been suggested that there is a J-shaped relationship between blood pressure control and the risk of stroke in treated hypertensive patients.[29] Although this remains an unproven hypothesis, some clinicians have been particularly concerned that lowering blood pressure in patients with severe carotid stenosis may reduce cerebral perfusion. In the presence of hemodynamically significant carotid stenosis, blood pressure falls distal to the stenosis when it narrows the lumen by $\geq 70\%$ or when the residual lumen diameter drops to ≤ 2 mm.[30] In the absence of sufficient collateral circulation, low cerebral perfusion pressure can cause ischemia in the 'watershed', poorly collateralized zones between cerebral vessels. Furthermore, the collateral circulation to the brain may be impaired because of an incomplete or hypofunctional circle of Willis[31] or significant disease of either the contralateral carotid artery or the posterior circulation (vertebrobasilar system). In cases of severe carotid atherosclerosis, cerebral ischemia is more likely to arise when blood pressure proximal to the stenosis is within the normotensive range and inadvertently lowered. Finally, regardless of treatment status, patients with high blood pressure have a diminished capacity to autoregulate cerebral blood flow,[32,33] making them more vulnerable to the potentially harmful effects of an excessive or too rapid decline in perfusion pressure. This issue is further compounded by the loss of the normal autoregulatory capacity of the cerebral circulation and dependency of cerebral blood flow on perfusion pressure in patients with a carotid occlusion or severe bilateral carotid stenosis.[34–37]

Although there are no published data with regard to the relationship between blood pressure control and ischemic stroke in patients with asymptomatic CAS, some data exist in patients with symptomatic CAS. In a review of the NASCET, European Carotid Surgery Trial (ECST), and the UK-TIA trials, Rothwell and colleagues[38] demonstrated that the risk of subsequent stroke increased as blood pressure increased for patients with unilateral CAS > 70% (Figure 6.2A). However, patients with severe bilateral carotid stenosis or severe stenosis and contralateral occlusion (3% of patients) appeared to have a lower risk of hypertension-related stroke. In these patients, stroke risk declined as blood pressure increased (Figure 6.2B). This protection was abolished by revascularization.

Table 6.1 Classification and treatment of blood pressure[26]

Classification	Systolic blood pressure (mmHg)		Diastolic blood pressure (mmHg)	No compelling indication*	With compelling indication*
Normal	<120	and	<80	No antihypertensive drug	No antihypertensive drug
Prehypertension	120–139	or	80–90	No antihypertensive drug	Drugs for the compelling indication
Stage 1 hypertension	140–159	or	90–99	Thiazide-type diuretics for most. May consider ACEIs, ARBs, β-blockers, calcium channel blockers, or combination	Drugs for the compelling indication. Other drugs (diuretics, ACEIs, ARBs, β-blocks, calcium channel blockers) as needed
Stage 2 hypertension	≥160	or	≥100	Two-drug combination for most† (usually thiazide-type diuretic and ACEI or ARB or β-blocker or calcium channel blocker)	Drugs for the compelling indication. Other drugs (diuretics, ACEIs, ARBs, β-blockers, calcium channel blockers) as needed

ACEIs, angiotensin-converting enzyme inhibitors; ARBs, angiotensin type 1 receptor blockers.

*Lifestyle modifications are encouraged for all and include (1) weight reduction if overweight, (2) limitation of ethyl alcohol intake, (3) increased aerobic physical activity (30–45 minutes daily), (4) reduction of sodium intake (<2.34 g), (5) maintenance of adequate dietary potassium (≥ 120 mmol/day), (6) smoking cessation, and (7) DASH diet (rich in fruit, vegetables, and low-fat dairy products and reduced in saturated and total fat). Compelling indications include (1) congestive heart failure, (2) myocardial infarction, (3) diabetes, (4) chronic renal failure, and (5) prior stroke.

†Initial combined therapy should be used cautiously in those at risk for orthostatic hypotension.

From JNC 7.[27]

It is prudent to avoid severe hypotension in patients with severe bilateral carotid disease, regardless of their symptom status.

Management of dyslipidemia in patients with asymptomatic carotid artery stenosis

Are blood lipids a risk factor for ischemic stroke?

Epidemiological data relating blood lipids and the risk of a first ischemic stroke in populations free of vascular disease at baseline have provided conflicting results. Some studies have shown that serum cholesterol is positively associated with the risk of ischemic stroke, although the strength of this association is considerably weaker than that observed for coronary heart disease.[39–42] Sacco and associates[43] demonstrated a protective effect of high-density lipoprotein cholesterol (HDL-C), after risk factor adjustment, for first stroke in the northern Manhattan study. The protective effect of a higher HDL-C level was dose-dependent, was significant among participants aged ≥75 years old, was more potent for the atherosclerotic stroke subtype, and was present in all three racial or ethnic groups studied. Other studies, however, failed to show a relationship between total serum cholesterol and ischemic stroke.[44]

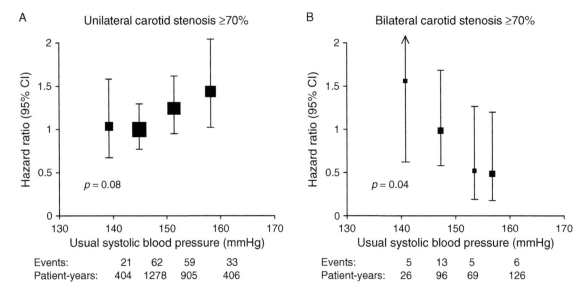

Figure 6.2 Relationships between usual systolic blood pressure and stroke risk in patients from NASCET and European Carotid Surgery Trial (ECST) stratified according to severity of carotid disease. (A) Unilateral carotid stenosis. (B) Bilateral carotid stenosis. Hazard ratios are derived from a Cox model and adjusted for age, sex, and previous ischemic heart disease and stratified by study. (Adapted from Rothwell et al.[38])

The reasons for these inconsistencies are not entirely clear. Several points are worth noting:

- the relationship between serum cholesterol and ischemic stroke may be dependent on other risk factors that are unmeasured or unknown
- none of the studies have considered the relationship between serum cholesterol as a continuous variable and the risk of stroke in a high-risk cohort
- there is a weak inverse association between cholesterol and hemorrhagic stroke risk, particularly among individuals with higher blood pressure.[40,41]

Compounding the cholesterol and stroke risk paradox is a recent subanalysis from the PROGRESS (Perindopril Protection Against Recurrent Stroke Study) trial[45] which failed to demonstrate an association between blood lipids and recurrent stroke in patients with established cerebrovascular disease, confirming the findings of a previous study.[46]

Statins and stroke prevention

Before the statin era, reducing total blood cholesterol levels failed to significantly reduce the incidence of stroke.[47] Currently, there are no prospective randomized trials examining the role of statins compared with placebo or usual care in preventing ischemic stroke in patients with asymptomatic CAS. Therefore, we must rely on statin studies in patients at high risk for cardiovascular events or those with established CAD. Typically, the primary endpoint of these studies has been combined cardiovascular events, with stroke as a secondary endpoint.

As shown in Table 6.2,[48-53] only 2 out of 6 clinical trials comparing statins with placebo or usual care in patients with cardiovascular risk factors have demonstrated a significant reduction in rates of ischemic stroke. The largest absolute risk reduction (ARR) in stroke (1.3%) was observed in the CARDS (Collaborative Atorvastatin Diabetes Study) trial,[52] which included patients with type 2 diabetes mellitus. Conversely, 6 out of 8 clinical trials that compared statins with placebo or usual care in patients with established CAD revealed a significant reduction in incidence of ischemic stroke (Table 6.3).[54-61] Whether intensive lipid reduction (compared with moderate lipid lowering) provides even greater reduction in stroke risk remains debatable.[61,62]

These findings from individual clinical trials were also confirmed in a recent meta-analysis of 65 138 participants in nine clinical trials of statins that reported stroke as an endpoint.[62] There were 2282 strokes. Hemorrhagic strokes accounted for 9%; 69% were confirmed to be ischemic and 22% were 'cryptogenic'. Overall, there was a 17% RRR of first stroke of any type (statin 3.0% vs control 3.7%, $p < 0.0001$); 22% RRR in ischemic stroke (RR = 0.78, 99% CI 0.70–0.87; $p < 0.0001$); and 12% RRR in cryptogenic stroke

Table 6.2 Randomized controlled primary prevention statin trials: stroke secondary endpoint

Trials	Population	No of patients (follow-up years)	Treatment	LDL reduction	Stroke		ARR	p value
					Control	Statin		
WOSCOP[49]	Hypercholesterolemia	6595 (4.9)	Placebo vs pravastatin	26%	1.6%	1.6%	–	NS
PROSPER[50]*	Elderly (>70 years)	5804 (3.0)	Placebo vs pravastatin	27%	4.5%	4.7%	–	NS
ASCOT-LLA[51]	Hypertensives	10,305 (3.0)	Placebo vs atorvastatin	35%	2.4%	1.7%	0.7%	<0.05
CARDS[52]	Diabetes mellitus	2838 (4.0)	Placebo vs atorvastatin	40%	2.8%	1.5%	1.3%	<0.05
ALLHAT-LLT[53]	Hypertensives	10,355 (4.8)	Usual care vs pravastatin	28%	4.5%	4.1%	0.4%	NS
KLIS[54]	Hypercholesterolemia	3853 (5.0)	Usual care vs pravastatin	20%	2.5%	2.1%	0.4%	NS

ARR, absolute risk reduction; LDL, low-density lipoprotein.

*Included patients with prior cardiovascular (44%) or cerebrovascular (11%) events.

Table 6.3 Randomized controlled statin trials in patients with established CAD: stroke secondary endpoint

Trials	Population	No of patients (follow-up years)	Treatment	LDL reduction	Stroke		ARR	p value
					Control	Statin		
SSSS[55]	CAD	4444 (5.0)	Placebo vs simvastatin	35%	4.3%	2.7%	1.6%	NSa[*]
CARE[56]	CAD	4159 (5.4)	Placebo vs pravastatin	32%	3.7%	2.5%	1.2%	<0.05
LIPID[57]	CAD	9014 (6.0)	Placebo vs pravastatin	23%	4.5%	3.7%	0.8%	<0.05
HPS[58]	CAD/CVA	20,536 (6.0)	Placebo vs simvastatin	–	5.7%	4.3%	1.4%	<0.05[†]
MIRACL[59]	CAD	3086 (0.35)	Placebo vs atorvastatin (80 mg)	–	1.6%	0.8%	0.8%	0.04
GREACE[60]	CAD	1600 (3.0)	Usual care vs atorvastatin	46%	2.1%	1.1%	1.0%	<0.05
TNT[61]	CAD	10,001 (4.9)	10 mg vs 80 mg atorvastatin	35%	3.1%	2.3%	0.8%	0.02
IDEAL[62]	CAD	8888 (4.8)	Simvastatin 20 vs atorvastatin 80	23%	3.9%	3.4%	0.5%	0.2

CAD, coronary artery disease; CVA, cerebrovascular accident; ARR, absolute risk reduction; LDL, low-density lipoprotein.
*No significant difference for stroke.
†No difference in patients with prior stroke (n = 3280).

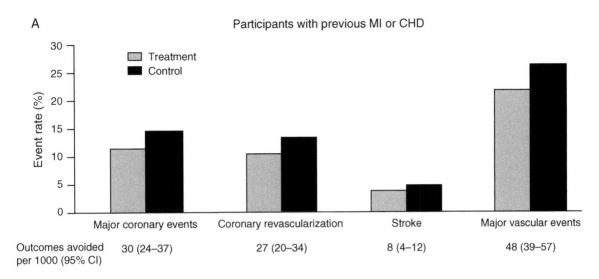

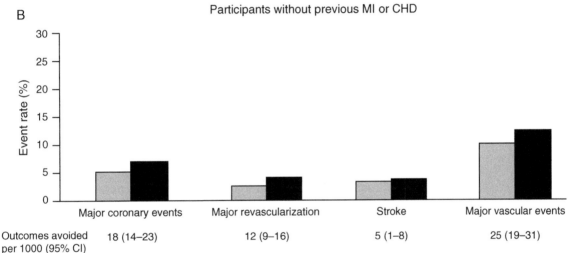

Figure 6.3 Five-year absolute benefits on particular vascular outcomes per mmol/L low-density lipoprotein (LDL-C) reduction in participants with (A) and without (B) previous myocardial infarction (MI) or coronary heart disease (CHD). Many participants had more than one type of outcome, so the sum of absolute differences the for separate outcomes exceeds the total number of participants avoiding at least one major vascular event. (Modified from Baigent et al.[62])

(RR = 0.88, 99% CI 0.75–1.02; p = 0.03) per mmol/L reduction in low-density lipoprotein cholesterol (LDL-C). There was no reduction in risk of hemorrhagic stroke. Following the first year after enrollment, there were significant reductions (20–25% RRR/year) during each of the subsequent 3 years and only a favorable trend thereafter. During an average of 5 years of treatment, the reduction in the overall incidence of stroke translated into 8 fewer participants having any stroke per 1000 among those with pre-existing CHD at baseline

(Figure 6.3A), compared with 5 fewer per 1000 among participants with no such history (Figure 6.3B).

Several hypotheses have been proposed to explain the potential mechanisms of benefit of statins in preventing stroke:

- reduction of cholesterol levels[63]
- cardioprotective effects through reducing the incidence of MI, with subsequent reduction of incidence of left ventricular thrombus and cardiogenic embolism[58]

- direct impact on carotid plaque by slowing progression or even inducing regression[64–70]
- carotid plaque stabilization (pleiotropic effects)[71–73]
- improving endothelial function and cerebral vasoreactivity.[74]

In summary, despite the absence of dedicated randomized clinical trials of statin therapy in patients with asymptomatic CAS, the preponderance of evidence points to the benefit of statins in reducing the incidence of ischemic stroke in high-risk populations (mainly patients with CAD diabetes mellitus, or hypertension). Therefore, until more specific data become available it would be prudent to follow the latest National Cholesterol Education Program (NCEP) update and treat patients with carotid stenosis >50% with statins, irrespective of symptom status.[75]

Management of diabetes mellitus in patients with asymptomatic carotid artery stenosis

Patients with diabetes mellitus, with or without carotid stenosis, are at an increased risk of ischemic stroke. In fact, recent data suggest that diabetes confers a 3-fold increase in the risk of ischemic stroke. It is believed that diabetes should be considered second only to hypertension as a risk factor for ischemic stroke. Although it has been shown for many years that intensive insulin therapy in recent-onset insulin-dependent diabetic patients reduces microvascular complications,[76] a positive impact on incidence of ischemic stroke has just recently been demonstrated. In the Diabetes Control and Complications Trial (DCCT),[77] in type 1 diabetic patients who received intensive glycemic control (as compared to those who received conventional therapy), the risk of any cardiovascular disease was reduced by 42%, and that of non-fatal MI, stroke, or death from cardiovascular disease was reduced by 57%. The vast majority of this benefit was due to reduction in glycosylated hemoglobin. Interestingly, aggressive glycemic control in type 1 and type 2 diabetic patients in the UK Prospective Diabetes Study[78] failed to decrease stroke incidence over 9 years of follow-up.

However, diabetic patients have higher prevalence of other cardiovascular risk factors such as hypertension, and this combination has been shown to be particularly hazardous in terms of elevated stroke risk.[79] In fact, it has been proposed that a significant proportion of the risk of stroke assumed to be related to hypertension may be attributable to concomitant diabetes. In the Syst-Eur (Systolic Hypertension in Europe) trial,[20] control of isolated systolic hypertension with a calcium channel blocker led to a 42% reduction in stroke incidence

compared with placebo after a mean of 2 years of follow-up. Interestingly, the magnitude of stroke reduction was significantly higher in diabetic patients (73%) than in the overall population.[80] These findings were later confirmed by the UK Prospective Diabetes Study Group who demonstrated that stringent diastolic blood pressure control in diabetic patients resulted in a 44% RRR in stroke compared with less stringent control.[81] Similarly, the effects of statin therapy is also more pronounced in diabetic patients in terms of primary prevention of ischemic stroke than in non-diabetic patients.[48–53]

Antiplatelet therapy in patients with asymptomatic carotid artery stenosis

Primary prevention of stroke in the general population

Aspirin

There are many published guidelines arguing for and against routine use of aspirin for primary prevention of cardiovascular and cerebrovascular events in the general population. These guidelines, as expected, have evolved over time with the emergence of new data. In 1998, the European Society of Cardiology recommended low-dose aspirin for men at particularly high risk for coronary heart disease, but not for all persons at high risk.[82] In 2002, The US Preventive Services Task Force[83] and the American Heart Association[84] took the position that aspirin therapy is effective in decreasing the incidence of CHD in adults of both sexes who are deemed to be at increased risk. Subsequently, guidelines from the American Heart Association on the primary prevention of cardiovascular disease in women recommended use of low-dose aspirin therapy in women whose 10-year risk of a first coronary event exceeds 20% and consideration of aspirin use in women whose 10-year risk is 10–20%.[85]

Evidence-based data on the exact role of aspirin in the primary prevention of cardiovascular and cerebrovascular events in men and women continue to emerge. Although the benefits of aspirin therapy for reducing the risk of MI, stroke, and vascular death among individuals with pre-existing cardiovascular disease are well established[86–88] the role of aspirin in primary prevention of cardiovascular events in general and stroke in particular is less clear. The popular notion that an aspirin a day will keep the cardiologist away, at least as far as reduction in incidence of MI is concerned, may not be universally applicable to stroke and cardiovascular mortality.

A recent meta-analysis[89] (Figure 6.4) of six prospective randomized controlled trials[90–95] of aspirin therapy in participants without cardiovascular disease with

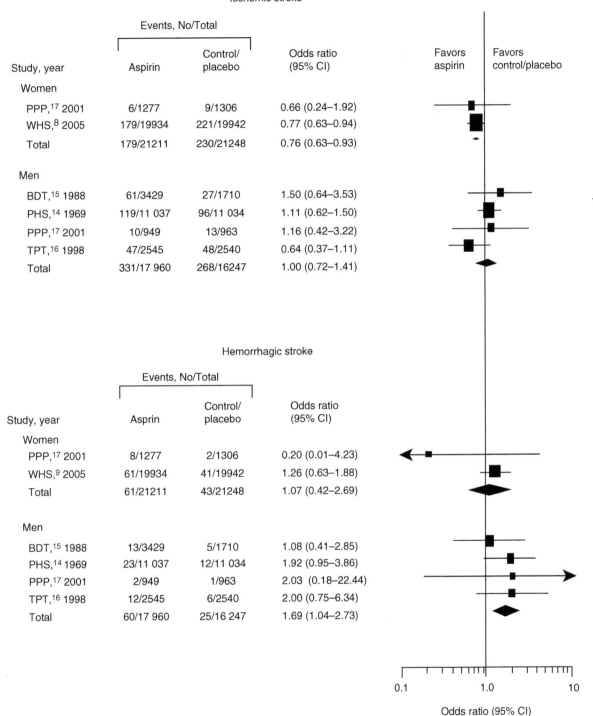

Figure 6.4 Meta-analysis of effect of aspirin treatment on the primary prevention of ischemic and hemorrhagic stroke. Size of data markers are proportional to the amount of data contributed by each trial. Test for heterogeneity for ischemic stroke: women, $p = 0.82$; men, $p = 0.81$. Test for heterogeneity for hemorrhagic stroke: women, $p = 0.25$; men, $p = 0.78$. CI indicates confidence interval. (Modified from Berger et al.[89])

a total of 95 456 individuals has been reported. This meta-analysis demonstrated that aspirin therapy is associated with a significant reduction in the risk of cardiovascular events in men and women. However, the specific types of benefit differ in important ways between women and men. In women, aspirin therapy significantly reduces the risk of ischemic stroke, without effect on the risk of MI. Conversely, aspirin therapy in men significantly reduces the risk of MI, with an insignificant increase in the risk of hemorrhagic stroke. These data are consistent with a recent epidemiological study by Nelson and colleagues.[96] In patients >70 years old without known cardiovascular disease, any benefits of low-dose aspirin on risk of cardiovascular disease were offset by adverse events.

In summary, for primary prevention of first stroke in low-risk patients, aspirin therapy for an average of 6.4 years results in an absolute benefit of approximately 2 fewer strokes per 1000 women (but not men). By contrast, aspirin therapy reduces the risk of MI corresponding to an absolute benefit of approximately 8 fewer events per 1000 men (but not women) treated for 6.4 years. In terms of side effects, aspirin therapy for an average of 6.4 years results in an absolute increase of approximately 2.5 major bleeding events caused per 1000 women and 3 major bleeding events per 1000 men.[89] Therefore, both the beneficial and harmful effects of antiplatelet therapy should be considered by the physician and patient before initiating this therapy for the primary prevention of cerebrovascular and cardiovascular events.

Clopidogrel

The efficacy of clopidogrel in secondary prevention of cardiovascular ischemic events has been established in the Clopidogrel vs Aspirin in Patients at Risk of Ischemic Events (CAPRIE) study.[97] Therefore, clopidogrel can be considered a reasonable alternative to aspirin for secondary prevention in patients with aspirin intolerance. The available evidence, however, does not support the addition of clopidogrel to aspirin in the absence of other indications for secondary prevention of stroke.[98]

There are no head-to-head trials comparing aspirin to clopidogrel for primary prevention of stroke in patients with asymptomatic CAS. Among high-risk patients with stable cardiovascular disease (including patients with asymptomatic CAS), dual antiplatelet therapy with aspirin + clopidogrel was not associated with a difference in the primary composite endpoint of cardiovascular death, MI, or stroke compared with monotherapy.[99]

Primary prevention of stroke in patients with asymptomatic carotid artery stenosis

Aspirin

Although it may be tempting to extrapolate results of the aspirin primary prevention trials to patients with asymptomatic CAS, this extrapolation is difficult. Patients with asymptomatic CAS are at higher risk for cardiovascular and cerebrovascular events than those included in the above primary prevention trials. It has been shown that the cardioprotective benefit of aspirin is related to the cardiovascular risk in the population studied.[100]

The evidence for aspirin benefit in patients with asymptomatic CAS is conflicting. A post-hoc analysis of the Veterans Affairs Study[101] demonstrated that patients with significant asymptomatic CAS who were intolerant of aspirin had a higher incidence of neurological events than those patients able to tolerate the drug (37.8% vs 17.3%, $p < 0.05$). Conversely, a subsequent prospective placebo-controlled randomized trial failed to confirm these findings. In the Asymptomatic Cervical Bruit Study,[102] 372 neurologically asymptomatic patients (divided almost equally between men and women) with carotid stenosis >50% were randomized to aspirin vs placebo and were followed up to a median of 2.3 years. The annual rate of all ischemic events and death from any cause was 12.4% for the placebo group and 10.9% for the aspirin group ($p = 0.61$) (Table 6.4). Of course, this trial is limited by the small number of patients and shorter follow-up duration.

In summary, there is consensus that aspirin should be used in patients with asymptomatic CAS, unless contraindicated, because aspirin was used in all of the surgery vs medical therapy trials as an antiplatelet drug except in the surgical arm of one study, in which there was a higher rate of MI in those who were not given aspirin.[27]

SUMMARY

All patients with asymptomatic carotid artery disease should be screened for other treatable causes of stroke, and intensive medical therapy of all identified risk factors should be pursued.[27] The magnitude of stroke reduction with medical therapy, however, may vary according to the presence or absence of concomitant comorbidities. For example, the extent of stroke reduction from blood pressure control is significantly greater in patients with concomitant hypertension and diabetes mellitus than in patients with hypertension alone. Similarly, the benefit of statins in stroke reduction is greater in patients with diabetes mellitus or coronary artery disease than in patients without either condition. The most contemporary evidence with regard to the value of carotid revascularization in addition to usual medical care indicates that carotid endarterectomy offers additional benefits in stroke prevention to selected patients with asymptomatic carotid artery disease.

Table 6.4 Clinical outcomes associated with aspirin vs placebo in patients with asymptomatic carotid artery disease

End point	Aspirin group		Placebo group	
	No. of patients N (%)	Annual rate (%)	No. of patients N (%)	Annual rate (%)
Transient ischemic attack	16 (8.5)	3.5	23 (12.5)	5.3
Stroke	11 (5.8)	2.4	10 (5.4)	2.3
Myocardial infarction	7 (3.7)	1.5	4 (2.2)	0.9
Unstable angina	5 (2.7)	1.1	4 (2.2)	0.9
Death from vascular causes	10 (5.3)	2.2	7 (3.8)	1.6
Death from non-vascular causes	1 (0.5)	0.2	6 (3.3)	1.4
Total	50 (26.5)	11.0	54 (29.4)	12.3

Modified from the Asymptomatic Cervical Bruit Study.[104]

REFERENCES

1. American Heart Association. Heart Disease and Stroke Statistics – 2005 Update. Dallas: American Heart Association, 2004: 16–20.
2. Hobson RW, Weiss DG, Fields WS et al. Efficacy of carotid endarterectomy for asymptomatic carotid stenosis. N Engl J Med 1993; 328: 221–7.
3. Executive Committee for the Asymptomatic Carotid Atherosclerosis Study. Endarterectomy for asymptomatic carotid stenosis. JAMA 1995; 273: 1421–8.
4. MRC Asymptomatic Carotid Surgery Trial (ACST) Collaborative Group. Prevention of disabling and fatal strokes by successful carotid endarterectomy in patients without recent neurological symptoms: randomized controlled trial. Lancet 2004; 363: 1491–502.
5. Mayo Asymptomatic Carotid Endarterectomy Study Group. Effectiveness of carotid endarterectomy for asymptomatic carotid stenosis: design of a clinical trial. Mayo Clin Proc 1992; 64: 897–904.
6. The CASANOVA Study Group. Carotid surgery versus medical therapy in asymptomatic carotid stenosis. Stroke 1991; 22: 1229–35.
7. Kawachi I, Colditz GA, Stampfer MJ et al. Smoking cessation and decreased risk of stroke in women. JAMA 1993; 269(2): 232–6.
8. Rodriguez CJ, Sacco RL, Sciacca RR et al. Physical activity attenuates the effect of increased left ventricular mass on the risk of ischemic stroke: The Northern Manhattan Stroke Study. J Am Coll Cardiol 2002; 39(9): 1482–8.
9. Pitsavos C, Panagiotakos DB, Chrysohoou C et al. Seven Countries Study (the Corfu Cohort). Physical activity decreases the risk of stroke in middle-age men with left ventricular hypertrophy: 40-year follow-up (1961–2001) of the Seven Countries Study (the Corfu cohort). J Hum Hypertens 2004; 18(7): 495–501.
10. MacMahon S, Rodgers A. The epidemiologic association between blood pressure and stroke: implications for primary and secondary prevention. Hypertens Res 1994; 17: S23.
11. Iso H, Jacobs DR, Wentworth D, Neaton JD, Cohen JD. Serum cholesterol levels and six-year mortality from stroke in 350,977 men screened for the Multiple Risk Factor Intervention Trial. N Engl J Med 1989; 320: 904–10.
12. Rutan GH, Kuller LH, James PH. Mortality associated with diastolic hypertension and isolated systolic hypertension among men screened for the Multiple Risk Factor Intervention Trial. Hypertension 1988; 77: 504–14.
13. Nielsen WB, Vestbo J, Jensen GB. Isolated systolic hypertension as a major risk factor for stroke and myocardial infarction and an unexploited source of cardiovascular prevention: a prospective population-based study. J Hum Hypertens 1995; 9: 175–80.
14. MacMahon S, Peto R, Cutler J et al. Blood pressure, stroke, and coronary heart disease. Part 1, Prolonged differences in blood pressure: prospective observational studies corrected for the regression dilution bias. Lancet 1990; 335(8692): 765–74.
15. Rodgers A, MacMahon S, Gamble G et al. Blood pressure and risk of stroke in patients with cerebrovascular disease. The United Kingdom Transient Ischaemic Attack Collaborative Group. BMJ 1996; 313(7050): 147.
16. Kannel WB, Dawber TR, Sorlie P, Wolf PA. Stroke. Components of blood pressure and risk of atherothrombotic brain infarction: the Framingham study. 1976; 7(4): 327–31.
17. Spence JD. Management of resistant hypertension in patients with carotid stenosis: high prevalence of renovascular hypertension. Cerebrovasc Dis 2000; 10(4): 249–54.
18. Systolic Hypertension in the Elderly Program (SHEP) Cooperative Research Group. Prevention of stroke by antihypertensive drug treatment in older persons with isolated systolic hypertension. JAMA 1991; 265: 3255–64.
19. Staessen JA, Fagard R, Thijs L et al for the Systolic Hypertension in Europe (Syst-Eur) Trial Investigators. Randomised double-blind comparison of placebo and active treatment for older patients with isolated systolic hypertension. Lancet 1997; 350: 757–64.
20. Hansson L, Zanchetti A, Carruthers SG et al. Effects of intensive blood-pressure lowering and low-dose aspirin in patients with hypertension: principal results of the Hypertension Optimal Treatment (HOT) randomized trial. HOT Study Group. Lancet 1998; 351: 1755–62.
21. Blood Pressure Lowering Treatment Trialists' Collaboration. Effects of ACE inhibitors, calcium antagonists, and other blood pressure lowering drugs: results of prospectively designed overview on randomized trials. Lancet 2000; 356: 1955–64.
22. Dahlof B, Devereux RB, Kjeldsen SE et al. LIFE Study Group. Cardiovascular morbidity and mortality in the Losartan Intervention For Endpoint reduction in hypertension study (LIFE): a randomised trial against atenolol. Lancet 2002; 359(9311): 995–1003.

23. Lithell H, Hansson L, Skoog I et al; SCOPE Study Group. The Study on Cognition and Prognosis in the Elderly (SCOPE): principal results of a randomized double-blind intervention trial. J Hypertens 2003; 21(5): 875–86.

24. Lonn E, Shaikholeslami R, Yi Q et al. Effects of ramipril on left ventricular mass and function in cardiovascular patients with controlled blood pressure and with preserved left ventricular ejection fraction: a substudy of the Heart Outcomes Prevention Evaluation (HOPE) Trial. J Am Coll Cardiol 2004; 43(12): 2200–6.

25. The ALLHAT Officers and Coordinators for the ALLHAT Collaborative Research Group. Major outcomes in high-risk hypertensive patients randomised to angiotensin-converting enzyme inhibitor or calcium channel blocker vs diuretic. The Antihypertensive and Lipid-Lowering treatment to prevent Heart Attack Trial (ALLHAT). JAMA 2002; 288: 2981–97.

26. Chobanian AV, Bakris GL, Black HR et al. National Heart, Lung, and Blood Institute Joint National Committee on Prevention, Detection, Evaluation, and Treatment of High Blood Pressure; National High Blood Pressure Education Program Coordinating Committee. The Seventh Report of the Joint National Committee on Prevention, Detection, Evaluation, and Treatment of High Blood Pressure: the JNC 7 report. JAMA 2003; 289: 2560–72.

27. Goldstein LB, Adams R, Alberts MJ et al. Primary prevention of ischemic stroke. A guideline from the American Heart Association/American Stroke Association Stroke Council: Cosponsored by the Atherosclerotic Peripheral Vascular Disease Interdisciplinary Working Group; Cardiovascular Nursing Council; Clinical Cardiology Council; Nutrition, Physical Activity, and Metabolism Council; and the Quality of Care and Outcomes Research Interdisciplinary Working Group. Stroke 2006; 37: 1583–633.

28. Almgren T, Persson B, Wilhelmsen L, Rosengren A, Andersson K. Stroke and coronary heart disease in treated hypertension – a prospective cohort study over three decades. J Intern Med 2005; 257: 496–502.

29. Voko Z, Bots ML, Hofman A et al. J-shaped relation between blood pressure and stroke in treated hypertensives. Hypertension 1999; 34: 1181–5.

30. Kistler JP, Ropper AH, Heros RC. Therapy of ischemic cerebral vascular disease due to atherothrombosis, part 1. N Engl J Med 1984; 311: 27–34.

31. Schomer DF, Marks MP, Steinberg GK et al. The anatomy of the posterior communicating artery as a risk factor for ischemic cerebral infarction. N Engl J Med 1994; 330: 1565–70.

32. Strandgaard S. Autoregulation of cerebral blood flow in hypertensive patients: the modifying influence of prolonged antihypertensive treatment on the tolerance of acute drug-induced hypotension. Circulation 1973; 53: 720–7.

33. Benetos A, Safar ME, Laurent S et al. Common carotid blood flow in patients with hypertension and stenosis of the internal carotid artery. J Clin Hypertens 1986; 2(1): 44–54.

34. Powers WJ. Cerebral hemodynamics in ischemic cerebrovascular disease. Ann Neurol 1991; 29: 231–40.

35. Van der Grond J, Balm R, Kappelle J, Eikelboom BC, Mali WP. Cerebral metabolism of patients with stenosis or occlusion of the internal carotid artery. Stroke 1995; 26: 822–8.

36. Grubb RL Jr, Derdeyn CP, Fritsch SM et al. Importance of hemodynamic factors in the prognosis of symptomatic carotid occlusion. JAMA 1998; 280: 1055–60.

37. Vernieri F, Pasqualetti P, Passarelli F, Rossini PM, Silvestrini M. Outcome of carotid artery occlusion is predicted by cerebrovascular reactivity. Stroke 1999; 30: 593–8.

38. Rothwell PM, Howard SC, Spence D. Relationship between blood pressure and stroke risk in symptomatic carotid occlusive disease. Stroke 2003; 34: 2583–90.

39. Iso H, Jacobs DR Jr, Wentworth D, Neaton JD, Cohen JD. Serum cholesterol levels and six-year mortality from stroke in 350,977 men screened for the multiple risk factor intervention trial. N Engl J Med 1989; 320: 904–10.

40. The Asia Pacific Cohort Studies Collaboration. Cholesterol, coronary heart disease and stroke in the Asia Pacific region. Int J Epidemiol 2003; 32: 563–72.

41. Lindenstrom E, Boysen G, Nyboe J. Influence of total cholesterol, high density lipoprotein cholesterol, and triglycerides on risk of cerebrovascular disease: the Copenhagen City Heart Study. BMJ 1994; 309: 11–15.

42. Wannamethee SG, Shaper AG, Ebrahim S. HDL-cholesterol, total cholesterol, and the risk of stroke in middle-aged British men. Stroke 2000; 31: 1882–8.

43. Sacco RL, Benson RT, Kargman DE et al. High-density lipoprotein cholesterol and ischemic stroke in the elderly: the Northern Manhattan Stroke Study. JAMA 2001; 285(21): 2729–35.

44. Prospective Studies Collaboration. Cholesterol, diastolic blood pressure, and stroke: 13,000 strokes in 450,000 people in 45 prospective cohorts. Prospective Studies Collaboration. Lancet 1995; 346: 1647–53.

45. Patel A, Woodward M, Campbell DJ et al. Plasma lipids predict myocardial infarction, but not stroke, in patients with established cerebrovascular disease. Eur Heart J 2005; 26: 1910–15.

46. Heart Protection Study Collaborative Group. Effects of cholesterol lowering with simvastatin on stroke and other major vascular events in 20 536 people with cerebrovascular disease or other high-risk conditions. Lancet 2004; 363: 757–67.

47. Atkins D, Psaty BM, Koepsell TD, Longstreth WT Jr, Larson EB. Cholesterol reduction and the risk for stroke in men. A meta-analysis of randomized, controlled trials. Ann Intern Med 1993; 119(2): 136–45.

48. Shepherd J, Cobbe SM, Ford I et al. Prevention of coronary heart disease with pravastatin in men with hypercholesterolemia. West of Scotland Coronary Prevention Study Group. N Engl J Med 1995; 333(20): 1301–7.

49. Shepherd J, Blauw GJ, Murphy MB et al. On behalf of the PROSPER study group. Pravastatin in elderly individuals at risk of vascular disease (PROSPER): a randomised controlled trial. Lancet 2002; 360: 1623–30.

50. Sever PS, Dahlof B, Poulter NR et al; ASCOT investigators. Prevention of coronary and stroke events with atorvastatin in hypertensive patients who have average or lower-than-average cholesterol concentrations, in the Anglo-Scandinavian Cardiac Outcomes Trial – Lipid Lowering Arm (ASCOT-LLA): a multicentre randomised controlled trial. Lancet 2003; 361(9364): 1149–58.

51. Colhoun HM, Betteridge DJ, Durrington PN et al; CARDS investigators. Primary prevention of cardiovascular disease with atorvastatin in type 2 diabetes in the Collaborative Atorvastatin Diabetes Study (CARDS): multicentre randomised placebo-controlled trial. Lancet 2004; 364: 685–96.

52. ALLHAT Officers and Coordinators for the ALLHAT Collaborative Research Group. The Antihypertensive and Lipid-Lowering Treatment to Prevent Heart Attack Trial. Major outcomes in moderately hypercholesterolemic, hypertensive patients randomized to pravastatin vs usual care: The Antihypertensive and Lipid-Lowering Treatment to Prevent Heart Attack Trial (ALLHAT-LLT). JAMA 2002; 288(23): 2998–3007.

53. The Kyushu Lipid Intervention Study Group. Pravastatin use and risk of coronary events and cerebral infarction in Japanese men with moderate hypercholesterolemia: the Kyushu Lipid Intervention Study. J Atheroscler Thromb 2000; 7(2): 110–21.

54. The Scandinavian Simvastatin Survival Study Group. Randomised trial of cholesterol lowering in 4444 patients with

coronary heart disease: the Scandinavian Simvastatin Survival Study (4S). Lancet 1994; 344(8934): 1383–9.

55. Sacks FM, Pfeffer MA, Moye LA et al. The effect of pravastatin on coronary events after myocardial infarction in patients with average cholesterol levels. Cholesterol and Recurrent Events Trial investigators. N Engl J Med 1996; 335(14): 1001–9.

56. The Long-Term Intervention with Pravastatin in Ischaemic Disease (LIPID) Study Group. Prevention of cardiovascular events and death with pravastatin in patients with coronary heart disease and a broad range of initial cholesterol levels. N Engl J Med 1998; 339(19): 1349–57.

57. Heart Protection Study Collaborative Group. MRC/BHF Heart Protection Study of cholesterol lowering with simvastatin in 20,536 high-risk individuals: a randomised placebo-controlled trial. Lancet 2002; 360(9326): 7–22.

58. Schwartz GG, Olsson AG, Ezekowitz MD, et al; Myocardial Ischemia Reduction with Aggressive Cholesterol Lowering (MIRACL) Study Investigators. Effects of atorvastatin on early recurrent ischemic events in acute coronary syndromes: the MIRACL study: a randomized controlled trial. JAMA 2001; 285(13): 1711–8.

59. Athyros VG, Papageorgiou AA, Mercouris BR et al. Treatment with atorvastatin to the National Cholesterol Educational Program goal versus 'usual' care in secondary coronary heart disease prevention. The GREek Atorvastatin and Coronary-heart-disease Evaluation (GREACE) study. Curr Med Res Opin 2002; 18(4): 220–8.

60. LaRosa JC, Grundy SM, Waters DD et al. for the Treating to New Target (TNT) Investigators. Intensive lipid lowering with atorvastatin in patients with stable coronary disease. N Engl J Med 2005; 352: 1425–1435.

61. Pedersen TR, Faergeman O, Kastelein JJ et al; Incremental Decrease in End Points Through Aggressive Lipid Lowering (IDEAL) Study Group. High-dose atorvastatin vs usual-dose simvastatin for secondary prevention after myocardial infarction: the IDEAL study: a randomized controlled trial. JAMA 2005; 294(19): 2437–45.

62. Baigent C, Keech A, Kearney PM et al; Cholesterol Treatment Trialists' (CTT) Collaborators. Efficacy and safety of cholesterol-lowering treatment: prospective meta-analysis of data from 90,056 participants in 14 randomised trials of statins. Lancet 2005; 366(9493): 1267–78.

63. Corvol JC, Bouzamondo A, Sirol M et al. Differential effects of lipid-lowering therapies on stroke prevention: a meta-analysis of randomized trials. Arch Intern Med 2003; 163(6): 669–76.

64. Furberg CD, Adams HP Jr, Applegate WB et al. Effect of lovastatin on early carotid atherosclerosis and cardiovascular events. Asymptomatic Carotid Artery Progression Study (ACAPS) Research Group. Circulation 1994; 90(4): 1679–87.

65. Adams HP, Byington RP, Hoen H et al. Effect of cholesterol-lowering medication on progression of mild atherosclerotic lesions of the carotid arteries and on the risk of stroke. Cerebrovasc Dis 1995; 5: 171–7.

66. Crouse JR 3rd, Byington RP, Bond MG et al. Pravastatin, Lipids, and Atherosclerosis in the Carotid Arteries (PLAC-II). Am J Cardiol 1995; 75(7): 455–9.

67. Salonen R, Nyyssonen K, Porkkala E et al. Kuopio Atherosclerosis Prevention Study (KAPS). A population-based primary preventive trial of the effect of LDL lowering on atherosclerotic progression in carotid and femoral arteries. Circulation 1995; 92(7): 1758–64.

68. MacMahon S, Sharpe N, Gamble G et al. Effects of lowering average of below-average cholesterol levels on the progression of carotid atherosclerosis: results of the LIPID Atherosclerosis Substudy. LIPID Trial Research Group. Circulation 1998; 97(18): 1784–90.

69. Smilde TJ, van Wissen S, Wollersheim H et al. Effect of aggressive versus conventional lipid lowering on atherosclerosis progression in familial hypercholesterolaemia (ASAP): a prospective, randomised, double-blind trial. Lancet 2001; 357(9256): 577–81.

70. Taylor AJ, Kent SM, Flaherty PJ et al. Arterial Biology for the Investigation of the Treatment Effects of Reducing Cholesterol: a randomized trial comparing the effects of atorvastatin and pravastatin on carotid intima medial thickness. Circulation 2002; 106(16): 2055–60.

71. Takemoto M, Liao JK. Pleiotropic effects of 3-hydroxy-3-methylglutaryl coenzyme a reductase inhibitors. Arterioscler Thromb Vasc Biol 2001; 21(11): 1712–9.

72. Crisby M, Nordin-Fredriksson G, Shah PK et al. Pravastatin treatment increases collagen content and decreases lipid content, inflammation, metalloproteinases, and cell death in human carotid plaques: implications for plaque stabilization. Circulation 2001; 103(7): 926–33.

73. Cortellaro M, Cofrancesco E, Arbustini E et al. Atorvastatin and thrombogenicity of the carotid atherosclerotic plaque: the ATROCAP study. Thromb Haemost 2002; 88(1): 41–7.

74. Sterzer P, Meintzschel F, Rosler A et al. Pravastatin improves cerebral vasomotor reactivity in patients with subcortical small-vessel disease. Stroke 2001; 32(12): 2817–20.

75. Grundy SM, Cleeman JI, Merz CN et al; National Heart, Lung, and Blood Institute; American College of Cardiology Foundation; American Heart Association. Implications of recent clinical trials for the National Cholesterol Education Program Adult Treatment Panel III guidelines. Circulation 2004; 110(2): 227–39.

76. The Diabetes Control and Complications Trial Research Group. The effect of intensive diabetes therapy on the development and progression of neuropathy. Ann Intern Med 1995; 122(8): 561–8.

77. The Diabetes Control and Complications Trial/Epidemiology of Diabetes Interventions and Complications (DCCT/EDIC) Study Research Group. Intensive diabetes treatment and cardiovascular disease in patients with type 1 diabetes. N Engl J Med 2005; 353: 2643–53.

78. UK Prospective Diabetes Study (UKPDS) Group. Intensive blood-glucose control with sulphonylureas or insulin compared with conventional treatment and risk of complications in patients with type 2 diabetes (UKPDS 33). Lancet 1998; 352(9131): 837–53.

79. Hu G, Sarti C, Jousilahti P et al. The impact of history of hypertension and type 2 diabetes at baseline on the incidence of stroke and stroke mortality. Stroke 2005; 36: 2538–43.

80. Curb JD, Pressel SL, Cutler JA et al. Effect of diuretic-based antihypertensive treatment on cardiovascular disease risk in older diabetic patients with isolated systolic hypertension. Systolic Hypertension in the Elderly Program Cooperative Research Group. JAMA 1996; 276(23): 1886–92.

81. UK Prospective Diabetes Study Group. Tight blood pressure control and risk of macrovascular and microvascular complications in type 2 diabetes: UKPDS 38. BMJ 1998; 317(7160): 703–13.

82. Prevention of coronary heart disease in clinical practice: recommendations of the Second Joint Task Force of European and other Societies on Coronary Prevention. Eur Heart J 1998; 19: 1434–503.

83. US Preventive Services Task Force. Aspirin for the primary prevention of cardiovascular events: recommendation and rationale. Ann Intern Med 2002; 136: 157–160.

84. Pearson TA, Blair SN, Daniels SR et al; American Heart Association Science Advisory and Coordinating Committee. AHA guidelines for primary prevention of cardiovascular disease and stroke: 2002 update: consensus panel guide to comprehensive risk reduction for adult patients without coronary or other

atherosclerotic vascular diseases. Circulation 2002; 106: 388–391.

85. Mosca L, Appel LJ, Benjamin EJ et al; American Heart Association. Evidence-based guidelines for cardiovascular disease prevention in women. Circulation 2004; 109: 672–93.

86. Antiplatelet Trialists' Collaboration. Collaborative overview of randomised trials of antiplatelet therapy: prevention of death, myocardial infarction, and stroke by prolonged antiplatelet therapy in various categories of patients. BMJ 1994; 308: 81–106.

87. Antiplatelet Trialists' Collaboration. Collaborative meta-analysis of randomised trials of antiplatelet therapy for prevention of death, myocardial infarction, and stroke in high risk patients. BMJ 2002; 324: 71–86.

88. Patrono C, Coller B, FitzGerald GA, Hirsh J, Roth G. Platelet-active drugs: the relationships among dose, effectiveness, and side effects: the Seventh ACCP Conference on Antithrombotic and Thrombolytic Therapy. Chest 2004; 126: 234S–64S.

89. Berger JS, Roncaglioni MC, Avanzini F et al. Aspirin for the primary prevention of cardiovascular events in women and men: a sex-specific meta-analysis of randomized controlled trials. JAMA 2006; 295(3): 306–13.

90. Ridker PM, Cook NR, Lee IM et al. A randomized trial of low-dose aspirin in the primary prevention of cardiovascular disease in women. N Engl J Med 2005; 352(13): 1293–304.

91. Steering Committee of the Physicians' Health Study Research Group. Final report on the aspirin component of the ongoing Physicians' Health Study. N Engl J Med 1989; 321: 129–35.

92. Peto R, Gray R, Collins R, et al. Randomised trial of prophylactic daily aspirin in British male doctors. Br Med J (Clin Res Ed) 1988; 296: 313–16.

93. The Medical Research Council's General Practice Research Framework. Thrombosis prevention trial: randomised trial of low-intensity oral anticoagulation with warfarin and low-dose aspirin in the primary prevention of ischaemic heart disease in men at increased risk. Lancet 1998; 351: 233–41.

94. Hansson L, Zanchetti A, Carruthers SG et al. Effects of intensive blood-pressure lowering and low-dose aspirin in patients with hypertension: principal results of the Hypertension Optimal Treatment (HOT) randomized trial. Lancet 1998; 351: 1755–62.

95. Collaborative Group of the Primary Prevention Project. Low-dose aspirin and vitamin E in people at cardiovascular risk: a randomised trial in general practice. Lancet 2001; 357: 89–95.

96. Nelson MR, Liew D, Bertram M, Vos T. Epidemiological modelling of routine use of low dose aspirin for the primary prevention of coronary heart disease and stroke in those aged > or = 70. BMJ 2005; 330(7503): 1306.

97. CAPRIE Steering Committee. A randomized blinded trial of clopidogrel vs aspirin in patients at risk of ischemic events (CAPRIE). Lancet 1996; 348: 1329–1339.

98. Diener HC, Bogousslavsky J, Brass LM et al; MATCH investigators. Aspirin and clopidogrel compared with clopidogrel alone after recent ischaemic stroke or transient ischaemic attack in high-risk patients (MATCH): randomised, double-blind, placebo-controlled trial. Lancet 2004; 364(9431): 331–7.

99. Bhatt DL, Fox KA, Hacke W, et al. Clopidogrel and aspirin versus aspirin alone for the prevention of atherothrombotic events. N Engl J Med 2006; 354: 1706–17.

100. Patrono C, Coller B, FitzGerald GA, Hirsh J, Roth G. Platelet-active drugs: the relationships among dose, effectiveness, and side effects: the Seventh ACCP Conference on Antithrombotic and Thrombolytic Therapy. Chest 2004; 126: 234S–264S.

101. Hobson RW 2nd, Krupski WC, Weiss DG. Influence of aspirin in the management of asymptomatic carotid artery stenosis. VA Cooperative Study Group on Asymptomatic Carotid Stenosis. J Vasc Surg 1993; 17: 257–65.

102. Cote R, Battista RN, Abrahamowicz M et al. Lack of effect of aspirin in asymptomatic patients with carotid bruits and substantial carotid narrowing. The Asymptomatic Cervical Bruit Study Group. Ann Intern Med 1995; 123(9): 649–55.

RISK STRATIFICATION SECTION

Section Editors:
Issam D Moussa and JP Mohr

Introduction: Selection of patients with asymptomatic carotid artery disease for carotid revascularization: the case for risk stratification

Issam D Moussa and JP Mohr – Section Editors

INTRODUCTION

It is inarguable that primary prevention is the best option for reducing the burden of stroke in individual patients and society. Most strokes that occur in patients with asymptomatic carotid artery stenosis (CAS) are not preceded by warning transient ischemic attacks (TIAs),[1] and even when TIAs occur many patients don't seek timely medical attention.[2] Therefore, the argument that carotid revascularization should be withheld in these patients waiting for a warning clinical sign is unacceptable because the first presenting symptom in the majority of patients will be a complete stroke. For each patient, clinicians should balance the net benefits of a given preventive therapy (medical, endovascular, or surgical), against its associated risks and costs. Where possible, these assessments should be based on the results of randomized clinical trials.

In the case of patients with asymptomatic CAS, prospective randomized clinical trials comparing medical therapy alone to medical therapy and carotid endarterectomy (CEA) have shown that CEA is superior in preventing stroke.[3,4] The largest and most contemporary of these trials is ACST,[4] which supports and extends the results of ACAS.[3] The ACST showed a statistically significant reduction in 5-year risk of stroke (5.3%, 95% CI 3.0–7.8%) and a small but definite reduction in the risk of disabling or fatal stroke with surgery (2.5%, 95% CI 0.8–4.3%) compared with medical therapy alone.

Despite this class IA evidence, recommendations regarding treatment of patients with asymptomatic CAS vary from endorsement of carotid revascularization for selected patients (e.g. based on patient age, life expectancy, concomitant illnesses, etc.) with moderate to severe stenosis (60–99% or 80–99%) in whom the procedure can be performed with a low (i.e. <3%) complication rate to advising that this procedure not be performed in patients without ipsilateral neurological symptoms.

WHY THE SKEPTICISM REGARDING CAROTID REVASCULARIZATION?

At the crux of the conflicting attitudes toward management of patients with asymptomatic CAS are two major issues:

1. The assertion that the number of patients with asymptomatic CAS who need to be treated with CEA (NNT) to prevent 1 stroke is too high (Table R1). Proponents of this argument assert, despite the

Table R1 The number of patients with asymptomatic carotid artery stenosis who need to be treated (NNT) with carotid endarterectomy to prevent 1 stroke at 2, 3, and 5 years

When	NNT to prevent 1 stroke
At 2 years[5]	67 patients
At 3 years[6]	53 patients
At 5 years[5]	16–20 patients
	40 patients (for disabling or fatal stroke)

absence of prospective evidence, that stand-alone intensive medical therapy is sufficient for stroke reduction. Therefore, it would be insightful to compare the number of neurologically asymptomatic patients who need to be treated with statins or aspirin, for example, to prevent 1 stroke at 5 years (Table R2). It is clear from these data that while primary prevention with medical therapy is efficacious, a significantly larger number of patients will need to be treated to prevent a single event.

2. There is lack of confidence in the generalizability of the CEA trials because the complication rate after CEA in clinical trials has not been reproduced

in the community. Rothwell et al[7] compared the operative risks in ACAS with the results of a meta-analysis of 46 surgical case series that published operative risks for asymptomatic CAS during ACAS and the 5 years after publication.[10] The operative mortality was 8 × higher than in ACAS (1.11% vs 0.14%; $p < 0.01$), and the risk of stroke and death was about 3 × higher among comparable studies in which outcome was assessed by a neurologist (4.3% vs 1.5%; $p < 0.001$) (Figure R1). The higher perioperative complication rate after CEA in the community can significantly diminish the long-term efficacy of this operation (Table R3).

Table R2 The number of patients with asymptomatic CAS who need to be treated (NNT) with carotid endarterectomy (CEA), statins, or aspirin to prevent 1 stroke at 5 years

Treatment	Study	NNT to prevent 1 stroke at 5 years
CEA + usual medical care	ACST[4]	16–20 patients
Statins	Primary prevention trials[8]	200 patients
Aspirin*	Primary prevention trials[9]	500 patients

*Follow-up 6.4 years; no stroke reduction in men.

Table R3 Projected impact of operative risk on 5-year efficacy of carotid endarterectomy in patients with asymptomatic carotid artery disease[3]

Operative risk (%)	ACAS 60–99%	
	ARR at 5 years	NNT at 5 years
0	8.2%	12
2	6.2%	16
4	4.2%	24
6	2.2%	45
8	0.2%	500
10	n/a	n/s

ACAS, Asymptomatic Carotid Atherosclerosis Study; ARR, absolute risk reduction; NNT, number needed to treat. From Reference 3.

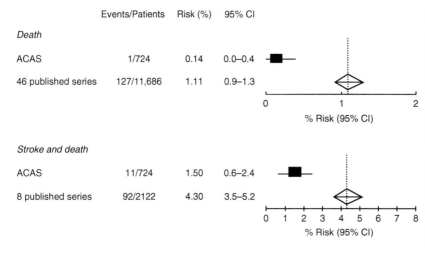

	Events/Patients	Risk (%)	95% CI
Death			
ACAS	1/724	0.14	0.0–0.4
46 published series	127/11,686	1.11	0.9–1.3
Stroke and death			
ACAS	11/724	1.50	0.6–2.4
8 published series	92/2122	4.30	3.5–5.2

Figure R1 The overall results of a meta-analysis of the operative risk of death (top) from all studies published between 1990 and 2000 inclusive that reported risks of carotid endarterectomy (CEA) for asymptomatic stenosis and the operative risk of stroke and death in those studies in which outcome was assessed by a neurologist (bottom) compared with the same risks in the Asymptomatic Carotid Atherosclerosis Study (ACAS). (Adapted from Rothwell et al.[7])

This issue is certainly of real clinical significance and it is one of the underlying reasons for the emergence of lesser-invasive techniques of carotid revascularization (i.e. carotid stenting). In any case, institution-specific assessment of the risk of carotid intervention, including endarterectomy and stenting, should be a prime consideration in clinical decision-making regarding carotid revascularization in patients with asymptomatic CAS.

RISK STRATIFICATION OF PATIENTS WITH ASYMPTOMATIC CAROTID ARTERY STENOSIS

Most experts agree that there are patients with asymptomatic CAS who are at high risk for stroke and who may derive significant benefit from carotid revascularization. Identifying those patients, however, has been elusive in clinical trials. Risk stratification of patients with asymptomatic CAS is particularly important among patients with 60–79% stenosis, in whom the appropriate management is more uncertain. Identifying high-risk patients will certainly lead to better resource utilization for both medical and revascularization therapies for patients with asymptomatic CAS.

In the following chapters we review the current state of knowledge regarding the various risk stratification strategies to improve patient selection for carotid revascularization:

- Chapter 7 addresses the impact of patient demographics and clinical comorbidities
- Chapter 8 reviewes the role of carotid plaque quantitative and qualitative parameters
- Chapter 9 addresses the utility of identifying asymptomatic microembolic signals with transcranial Doppler (TCD)

- Chapter 10 reviews the role of cerebrovascular reserve in predicting stroke risk
- Chapter 11 addresses the potential future use of inflammatory biomarkers for this purpose.

REFERENCES

1. Mackey AE, Abrahamowicz M, Langlois Y et al. Outcome of asymptomatic patients with carotid disease. Neurology 1997; 48: 896–903.
2. Giles MF, Flossman E, Rothwell PM. Patient behavior immediately after transient ischemic attack according to clinical characteristics, perception of the event, and predicted risk of stroke. Stroke 2006; 37; 1254–60.
3. Executive Committee for the Asymptomatic Carotid Atherosclerosis Study. Endarterectomy for asymptomatic carotid stenosis. JAMA 1995; 273: 1421–8.
4. Halliday A, Mansfield A, Marro J et al; MRC Asymptomatic Carotid Surgery Trial (ACST) Collaborative Group. Prevention of disabling and fatal strokes by successful carotid endarterectomy in patients without recent neurological symptoms: randomised controlled trial. Lancet 2004; 363: 1491–502.
5. Barnett HJ, Meldrum HE, Eliasziw M; North American Symptomatic Carotid Endarterectomy Trial (NASCET) collaborators. The appropriate use of carotid endarterectomy. CMAJ 2002; 166: 1169–79.
6. Chambers BR, You RX, Donnan GA. Carotid endarterectomy for asymptomatic carotid stenosis. Cochrane Database Syst Rev 2003; 1: 1–15.
7. Rothwell PM, Goldstein LB. Carotid endarterectomy for asymptomatic carotid stenosis: asymptomatic carotid surgery trial. Stroke 2004; 35: 2425–7.
8. Baigent C, Keech A, Kearney PM et al; Cholesterol Treatment Trialists' (CTT) Collaborators. Efficacy and safety of cholesterol-lowering treatment: prospective meta-analysis of data from 90,056 participants in 14 randomised trials of statins. Lancet 2005; 366(9493): 1267–78.
9. Berger JS, Roncaglioni MC, Avanzini F et al. Aspirin for the primary prevention of cardiovascular events in women and men: a sex–specific meta-analysis of randomized controlled trials. JAMA 2006; 295(3): 306–13.
10. Bond R, Rerkasem K, Rothwell PM. High morbidity due to endarterectomy for asymptomatic carotid stenosis. Cerebrovasc Dis 2003; 16(Suppl): 65.

7

Risk stratification of patients with asymptomatic carotid artery stenosis: demographic and clinical considerations

Issam D Moussa and JP Mohr

Take-Home Messages

1. There is lack of consensus on how to best select patients with asymptomatic coronary artery stenosis (CAS) who would benefit the most from carotid revascularization in terms of stroke prevention and have the least procedural complications.
2. Patients older than 80 years of age are at higher risk of stroke from carotid disease as well as from other causes. They are also at higher risk of complications after carotid revascularization. The decision to proceed with carotid revascularization should be made on a case by case basis using a strict risk stratification process to select those at highest risk for ischemic stroke and lowest risk for overall mortality.
3. The natural history of conservatively treated asymptomatic CAS is more favorable in women than men.
4. Complications after carotid endarterectomy (CEA) are higher in women than men. There is no evidence of a gender difference in outcome after carotid artery stenting.
5. The risk of stroke after cardiac surgery in patients with asymptomatic CAS increases with bilateral as opposed to unilateral disease and for the more severe degrees of unilateral stenosis.
6. CEA in patients with asymptomatic CAS undergoing cardiac surgery is associated with a 10–12% 30-day major adverse cardiovascular event whether done in a staged or synchronous fashion. Carotid artery stenting may be an alternative option.
7. Among patients with severe asymptomatic CAS, the presence of renal insufficiency and a history of contralateral neurological symptoms significantly increase the risk of future stroke. These patients should be strongly considered for carotid revascularization.

INTRODUCTION

Several prospective randomized clinical trials have established that medical therapy combined with carotid endarterectomy (CEA) is superior to medical therapy alone in treatment of patients with asymptomatic carotid artery stenosis (CAS).[1–3] However, there remains significant discord among individual physicians as to how to select patients with asymptomatic CAS who stand to gain the most from carotid revascularization in terms of stroke prevention and have the least procedural complications. When physicians encounter patients with asymptomatic CAS, they typically have access to a limited set of clinical information as well as carotid imaging data – ultrasound or magnetic resonance angiography/computed tomographic angiography (MRA/CTA). The purpose of this chapter is to review the relevant demographic and clinical data that need to be considered in the process of clinical decision-making regarding carotid revascularization in patients with asymptomatic CAS.

DEMOGRAPHIC FACTORS

Age

In patients with asymptomatic CAS, the most challenging age group with respect to clinical decision-making regarding carotid revascularization comprises those patients older than 80 years of age (octogenarians). They have the highest prevalence of asymptomatic CAS in the general population,[4] but their natural history presents the physician with a dilemma. The prevalence of ischemic stroke from asymptomatic CAS[5] as well as from other causes[6,7] is known to increase with advancing age in men and women (Figure 7.1). Stroke becomes the second leading cause of death by 85 years of age[8] as well as a leading cause of disability.[9] The economic impact of stroke on an individual is difficult to define with precision because of the many variables involved, but it is clear that strokes are very expensive.[10] These epidemiological observations provide theoretical support for utilization of carotid revascularization to reduce the incidence of stroke in this population. Stroke prevention among the elderly almost certainly will assume even more importance in the future because current predictions indicate that the proportion of the US population aged ≥75 years old will double from approximately 5% in 1990 to nearly 10% by 2030.[11]

Contrary to the above logic, however, it may be argued that the advisability of carotid revascularization in very elderly patients with asymptomatic CAS is questionable for two reasons:

1. Octogenarian patients have short life expectancy and hence any benefit from carotid revascularization may be of limited duration.
2. Carotid revascularization in octogenarian patients is associated with a higher periprocedural complication rate.

With regard to the issue of life expectancy among octogenarians with asymptomatic CAS, it must be remembered that longevity varies according to the presence or absence of coronary artery disease (CAD) as well as other comorbidities. According to US census data, life expectancy at the age of 80 years is 7.2 years for men and 9.1 years for women. By the age of 85 years, men can expect 5.3 additional years of life, and women, 6.5 years.[12] For many patients, these additional years are relatively healthy. However, stroke can be a devastating event, particularly for the very elderly, resulting in loss of function and independence.[13]

With regard to the issue of periprocedural complications among octogenarians with asymptomatic CAS undergoing carotid revascularization, CEA and carotid artery stenting need to be addressed separately. With CEA, the perioperative stroke and death rate in ACST[3] was 2.6% in patients <75 years of age and 3.7% in patients >75 years of age. These findings are consistent with prior studies.[14,15] Similarly, carotid artery stenting in patients over the age of 80 years is also associated with higher periprocedural death and stroke rate than in patients <80 years of age.[16–18] The question whether the periprocedural complication rate in octogenarians is higher with CEA or carotid artery stenting will be discussed in the carotid revascularization section of this book. Briefly, the SAPPHIRE trial,[19] which included asymptomatic patients >80 years of age, demonstrated that carotid artery stenting is as effective as CEA for stroke prevention but is associated with lower periprocedural myocardial infarction (MI).

Unfortunately, evidence-based data comparing carotid revascularization to medical therapy alone in octogenarians are limited. Among the three prospective randomized clinical trials that compared CEA to medical therapy,[1–3] only the ACST trial[3] included patients older than 79 years of age. In this trial, older patients (>75 years of age) did not benefit from CEA compared with medical therapy; however, the lack of significant net benefit may have been due to the lack of statistical power (only 650 patients in both groups). There are no prospective randomized clinical trials comparing carotid artery stenting to medical therapy in patients with carotid occlusive disease.

Therefore, until a more definitive answer becomes available, age alone should not exclude otherwise-qualified candidates from consideration for carotid revascularization.

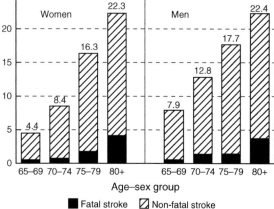

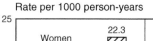

Figure 7.1 Stroke incidence in the general population according to age and gender. (Adapted from Manolio et al.[6])

The decision to proceed with carotid revascularization in octogenarians should be made on a case by case basis by implementing a strict risk stratification process to select those at highest risk for ischemic stroke and lowest risk for overall mortality. Furthermore, other factors such as mental health, functional capacity, and the extent of other comorbidities should be considered.

Gender

The effect of gender on outcome of patients undergoing carotid revascularization (CEA in particular) for asymptomatic CAS remains controversial despite numerous studies that have addressed this topic. The ACAS trial[2] was the first study to highlight the potential perioperative risk differential between women and men undergoing CEA for asymptomatic CAS. The incidence of perioperative stroke or death in this trial was nearly twice as high for women as for men (3.6% vs 1.7%, $p = 0.12$). Subsequently, the 5-year relative stroke risk reduction was only 17% for women vs 66% for men ($p = 0.10$). Although this difference was not statistically significant, it was clinically important, and it set the stage for a series of retrospective cohort studies the

results of which either supported[20,21] or contradicted ACAS findings.[22] The conflicting results of these studies most likely reflected differing patient risk profiles. The results of the ACST trial,[3] the largest prospective randomized clinical trial comparing CEA to medical therapy in asymptomatic CAS, certainly added much needed clarification to the controversy. In this trial, women (one-third of patients) had slightly a higher rate of perioperative complications (3.6% vs 2.5%, $p = $ NS); however, they did realize net benefit from CEA at 5-year follow-up. Nonetheless, the absolute risk reduction of 5-year risk of non-operative ischemic stroke was twice as high in men (8.21%; 95% CI 5.64–10.78, $p < 0.0001$) as in women (4.08%; 95% CI 0.74–7.41, $p = 0.02$). Therefore, it is reasonable to state that properly selected women with asymptomatic CAS may benefit from CEA; however, the magnitude of benefit is less than that in men (Figure 7.2).[23]

The underlying cause of this benefit differential from CEA between men and women, aside from the higher perioperative risk in women, is probably the more favorable natural history of asymptomatic CAS in women who are treated conservatively (Figure 7.3).[24] The lower rate of ischemic stroke in women vs men with asymptomatic CAS was also apparent in the

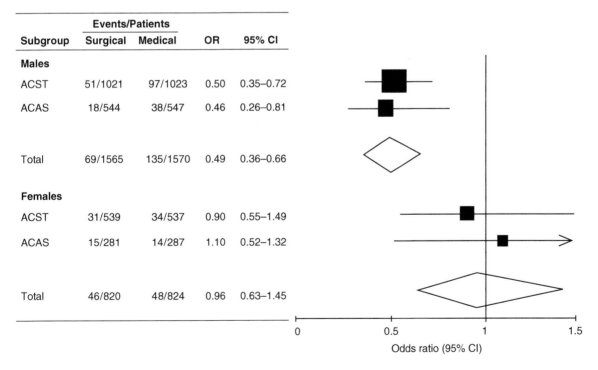

Subgroup	Events/Patients		OR	95% CI
	Surgical	Medical		
Males				
ACST	51/1021	97/1023	0.50	0.35–0.72
ACAS	18/544	38/547	0.46	0.26–0.81
Total	69/1565	135/1570	0.49	0.36–0.66
Females				
ACST	31/539	34/537	0.90	0.55–1.49
ACAS	15/281	14/287	1.10	0.52–1.32
Total	46/820	48/824	0.96	0.63–1.45

Odds ratio (95% CI)

Figure 7.2 The effect of endarterectomy for asymptomatic carotid stenosis on the risk of any stroke and operative death by sex in ACST3 and ACAS. (Adapted from Rothwell and Goldstein.[23])

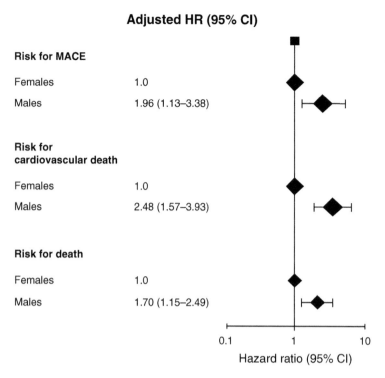

Figure 7.3 Adjusted hazard ratios for major adverse cardiovascular, cerebral, and peripheral vascular events (MACE), vascular mortality, and all-cause mortality in 525 patients with asymptomatic high-grade carotid artery stenosis undergoing conservative medical treatment. (Modified from Dick et al.[24])

medical treatment arms of both the ACAS and ACST trials. The 5-year risk of ipsilateral ischemic stroke was lower for women than men in ACAS (8.7% vs 12.1%)[2] and ACST (7.5% vs 10.6%).[3]

Although the reasons for this difference are not entirely clear, it is worth noting that:

- Men have higher carotid plaque burden than women for the same degree of carotid stenosis, and plaque burden is an independent predictor of stroke.[25]
- The asymptomatic carotid plaque in men have significantly higher fat and lower smooth muscle cell content,[26] a finding consistent with prior observations suggesting that plaque burden is related to plaque phenotype and instability.[27]

Whether the differential in the risk to benefit ratio between men and women after CEA is also applicable to carotid artery stenting remains a subject of investigation. As of this writing, there is no evidence for a gender effect on clinical outcome after carotid artery stenting.[17,28] Convincing data, however, will need to await the results of the ongoing prospective randomized clinical trials comparing carotid stenting to CEA in patients with asymptomatic CAS (CREST and ACT 1 trials).

Therefore, until further evidence is available, selected women with asymptomatic CAS should be considered

for carotid revascularization. However, there are two caveats:

1. The threshold for carotid revascularization should be higher in women than that in men.
2. Proper patient counseling should emphasize the differential in net benefit between men and women undergoing CEA, a differential that is not apparent with carotid artery stenting.

COMORBID CONDITIONS

Physicians caring for patients with asymptomatic CAS need to be aware of the numerous disease states, aside from the traditional cardiovascular risk factors, that are known to increase the risk of ischemic stroke. The role of systemic and metabolic disorders such as sleep apnea, thyroid disease, nutritional deficiencies, and other related conditions are beyond the scope of this chapter. In the forthcoming discussion we will focus on disease states that are relatively common in patients with asymptomatic CAS and which need to be considered in the process of triaging these patients to medical therapy alone vs medical therapy + carotid revascularization.

Coronary artery disease

Almost half of patients with asymptomatic CAS have underlying CAD.[29,30] The presence of CAD increases the risk of ischemic stroke[31] as well as the risk of cardiovascular mortality.[32] However, the effect of CAD on mortality is modifiable through medical therapy and coronary revascularization in selected patients. The increased stroke risk in patients with concomitant CAD and asymptomatic CAS is probably due to several mechanisms:

- Patients with CAD have a higher prevalence of risk factors known to increase stroke risk such as hypertension, diabetes, and smoking.
- Patients with CAD have a higher risk of myocardial infarction as well as other cardiac morbidities that are known to increase stroke risk such as atrial fibrillation and congestive heart failure.[6]
- The magnitude of increased stroke risk in patients with CAD is partially related to the acuity of coronary disease.[31] The association between coronary and carotid plaque instability and subsequent increase in stroke risk has also been studied at the pathological level.[33] Specifically, it has been demonstrated that carotid plaques (obtained by CEA) from patients with unstable angina, compared with those from patients with stable angina, have a significantly greater amount of inflammatory infiltrate (macrophages and T lymphocytes) and a stronger expression of interleukin-6 and C-reactive protein.

Evidence-based data regarding the management of patients with concomitant CAD and severe asymptomatic CAS do not exist. Management of these patients should be guided by the acuity of coronary disease

presentation. Most experts agree that patients with symptomatic CAD (acute coronary syndrome or stable angina) should receive optimal medical therapy and, if needed, coronary revascularization if it can be achieved percutaneously before considering carotid revascularization. However, management of patients with concomitant CAD and asymptomatic CAS is most controversial among those undergoing coronary artery bypass graft (CABG) surgery. Although these patients are at higher risk for perioperative ischemic stroke, there is no consensus on a standard approach to their management.

Carotid revascularization prior to coronary artery bypass graft surgery

Is asymptomatic carotid artery stenosis a risk factor for ischemic stroke after coronary artery bypass graft surgery?

Although the incidence of post-CABG stroke is rather low (about 1.5–2%), its impact on patient morbidity and mortality is substantial; almost a quarter of these patients die during the same hospitalization.[34] In a meta-analysis of relevant studies, Naylor and colleagues[34] found that there is considerable variability in the frequency of post-CABG stroke according to age and severity of carotid disease (Table 7.1).

Although it is often difficult to pin down the etiology of post-CABG stroke in a particular patient, the causes of this event are often multifactorial and interlinked.[35-40] Factors predictive of an increased risk of post-CABG stroke include:

- advanced age
- development of atrial fibrillation
- the presence of a carotid bruit

Table 7.1 Incidence of post-cardiac surgery stroke according to age and presence and severity of carotid occlusive disease

Post-cardiac surgery stroke by age		Post-cardiac surgery stroke by degree of carotid disease	
Age (years)	Stroke	Carotid disease	Stroke
<50	<0.5%	No disease	1.9%
50–60	1–1.5%	Unilateral 50–99%	3%
60–70	2–3%	Bilateral 50–99%	5%
70–80	4–7%	Carotid occlusion	7–11%
>80	8–9%	–	–

From Naylor et al.[34]

- neurologically symptomatic as opposed to asymptomatic patients
- the presence of severe carotid artery disease.

Indeed, much of the debate regarding the etiology and prevention of operative stroke in these patients has focused on the relevance of carotid artery disease, partly because it is correctable.

Which patients with asymptomatic carotid artery stenosis should undergo carotid revascularization before coronary artery bypass graft surgery?

The optimum management of patients with combined carotid and coronary artery disease undergoing CABG is the subject of ongoing debate. To date, no Level 1 evidence exists to guide practice. In reality, however, the vast majority of patients with asymptomatic CAS can safely undergo cardiac surgery. In practice, therefore, only a relatively small minority of patients require the clinician to consider carotid revascularization prior to CABG. Since there are no conclusive data to guide clinical decision-making in these patients, physicians need to use clinical judgment and rely on the current state of knowledge in managing these patients. Most agree that post-CABG stroke risk increases for asymptomatic patients with bilateral as opposed to unilateral disease and for the more severe degrees of unilateral stenosis.[34] However, it is also known that only a minority of these patients will suffer a stroke related to the carotid stenosis. Since the postulated mechanism of carotid origin post-CABG stroke is cerebral hemodynamic insufficiency, it would be intuitive to risk stratify these patients based on the severity of carotid disease and the state of their cerebrovascular reserve (Chapter 10). Although prospective evidence validating this approach is lacking, evaluation of cerebrovascular reserve in these patients may help select those at high risk for cerebral hemodynamic compromise and subsequent ischemic stroke perioperatively.[41] Of course, a universally accepted approach will not be adopted until it is validated in a prospective randomized trial.

When and how should carotid revascularization be performed?

Once a decision has been made to perform carotid revascularization two questions arise:

(1) Should carotid revascularization be performed by CEA or carotid artery stenting?

The only prospective randomized clinical trial of CEA vs carotid artery stenting that included patients with concomitant CAD and carotid occlusive disease is the SAPPHIRE trial.[19] More than 80% of patients included in this trial had ischemic heart disease, the majority of whom were neurologically asymptomatic. Specific data on patients who underwent subsequent CABG, however, are not available. This study has demonstrated that carotid artery stenting is not inferior to CEA in stroke prevention, albeit, with a better safety profile with regard to associated cardiac morbidity. Dedicated prospective clinical trials comparing CEA to carotid artery stenting in patients with concomitant CAD and asymptomatic CAS prior to CABG do not exist.

The use of carotid artery stenting as an alternative to CEA before cardiac surgery has been proposed as a less-risky carotid revascularization strategy. The literature on carotid stenting contains numerous case series in which stenting is performed as an alternative to CEA in 'high-risk' patients outside of randomized trials. The more specific literature highlighting those patients in whom the 'high-risk' indication for stenting was imminent cardiac surgery is limited to only a few published case series with a small number of patients.[42-45] The results of these case series were favorable is some studies[42,43,45] and unfavorable in others.[44] The variation in outcome among these studies is probably the result of the small number of patients, and variability in using nitinol self-expandable stents, distal protection devices, and antiplatelet therapy protocols. Until further evidence is available, the use of carotid artery stenting to revascularize patients with asymptomatic CAS prior to cardiac surgery should be performed only in the context of prospective registries or clinical trials.

(2) Should carotid revascularization be performed prior to or synchronously with CABG?

- CEA

There has been much controversy regarding the timing of CEA in relation to cardiac surgery, with no Level 1 evidence to guide clinical practice. Three potential sequences can be adopted for surgical revascularization of the carotid and coronary vessels: (1) staged operations with CEA preceding CABG; (2) reverse staged operations with CABG preceding CEA; and (3) synchronous CEA and CABG. Naylor and colleagues[46] reported a systematic review of 97 published studies following 8972 staged or synchronous operations (50–60% of patients with asymptomatic CAS) (Table 7.2). Overall, 10–12% of patients undergoing staged or synchronous procedures suffered death or major cardiovascular morbidity (stroke, MI) within 30 days of surgery, with no difference between either strategy.

The American Heart Association (AHA) has published guidelines regarding the appropriateness of synchronous CABG with CEA in CABG patients with asymptomatic CAS. The consensus view is that synchronous CEA with CABG is 'acceptable but not proven' in patients

Table 7.2 Perioperative major adverse cardiovascular events in patients with concomitant carotid and coronary artery disease undergoing staged or synchronous CEA–CABG

	Operative mortality	Any stroke	Ipsilateral stroke	Myocardial infarction
Synchronous CEA/CABG	4.6%	4.6%	3.0%	3.6%
Staged CEA–CABG	3.9%	2.7%	2.5%	6.5%
Staged CABG–CEA	2.0%	6.3%	5.8%	0.9%

CEA, carotid endarterectomy; CABG, coronary artery bypass graft.
From Naylor et al.[46]

with unilateral >60% asymptomatic stenosis where there is a proven operative stroke and death risk of <3%. In those facilities with an operative stroke and death risk >3%, the guidelines qualified the appropriateness of synchronous procedures as 'uncertain'.[47]

• Cartoid artery stenting

Once a decision has been made to proceed with carotid artery stenting, the question that arises is how long should cardiac surgery be delayed to allow sufficient duration for dual antiplatelet therapy? The answer to this question, in the absence of any conclusive evidence-based data, should be primarily based on the acuity of CAD presentation. Patients who have chronic stable angina should wait 30 days before undergoing cardiac surgery to allow optimal dual antiplatelet therapy.[48]

However, different strategies are needed in patients who need cardiac surgery more urgently (within days). Addressing this scenario, Abraham et al[45] reported on 37 patients who had concomitant surgical CAD and significant carotid artery disease who underwent carotid artery stenting before CABG. In this case series, all patients underwent carotid artery stenting with intravenous heparin to maintain an activated clotting time of 200–250 seconds along with GpIIb/IIIa inhibitor eptifibatide for up to 6 hours before CABG. All patients had CABG within 48 hours after carotid artery stenting during the same hospitalization. Antiplatelet treatment with aspirin and clopidogrel were started immediately after the CABG. There were no neurovascular complications, including transient ischemic attacks (TIAs), minor or major strokes, up to 30-days postoperatively.

Chronic renal insufficiency

Patients with elevated serum creatinine concentration are at an increased risk of all major stroke events even after adjustment for confounding factors, such as diabetes mellitus, blood pressure, antihypertensive therapy, and prior stroke.[49] More specifically, it has been demonstrated

that high serum creatinine levels are predictive of lacunar infarcts along with age, diabetes, blood pressure, and carotid stenosis.[50] Although the precise reason for the independent association between chronic renal insufficiency (CRI) and stroke remains unclear, several studies have shown that these patients have a higher prevalence of carotid, peripheral, and coronary plaque burden than age- and risk factors-matched controls.[51–54]

Prospective data regarding the impact of CRI on prognosis of patients with documented asymptomatic CAS are limited. The ACSRS prospective observational registry[55] followed 1101 patients with asymptomatic CAS for up to 7 years. This observational study demonstrated that high serum creatinine, along with contralateral neurological symptoms and carotid stenosis severity, is an independent predictor of ipsilateral ischemic neurological events. In fact, a serum creatinine concentration >85 μmol/L increased the risk of ipsilateral stroke by 2.1-fold (Figure 7.4). This finding can certainly be used to support the argument for utilization of carotid revascularization in these patients to optimize stroke prevention.

However, an opposing argument to carotid revascularization in these patients can also be proposed because of the following:

1. CRI has an independent and graded association with increased risk of death and cardiovascular events,[56] which may limit the duration of potential benefit from stroke prevention after carotid revascularization.
2. Patients with CRI have a higher incidence of perioperative complication rate after CEA.[57,58] Whether renal insufficiency increases the risk of complications after carotid artery stenting remains the subject of ongoing investigation. A study from Cleveland Clinic[59] has implicated CRI as a risk factor for post-carotid artery stenting complications; however, patients with renal insufficiency in this study were significantly older than those without renal insufficiency. Other studies have not confirmed these findings.[16,17,28] The ongoing prospective randomized

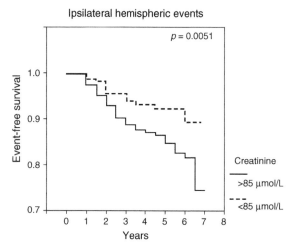

Figure 7.4 The ipsilateral hemispheric event-free cumulative survival rate in relation to the creatinine plasma level. In view of the small number of patients that have been followed for 7 years ($n = 27$), the abrupt drop in the survival curve should be ignored. (Adapted from Nicolaides et al.[55])

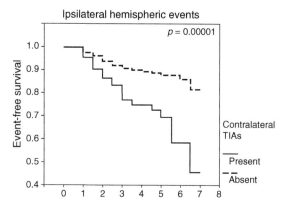

Figure 7.5 The ipsilateral hemispheric event-free cumulative survival rate in relation to the presence or absence of a history of contralateral transient ischemic attacks (TIAs) 6 months or more before admission to the study. (Adapted from Nicolaides et al.[55])

clinical trials of CEA vs carotid stenting will provide much needed insight into periprocedural and long-term outcome of patients with CRI. Until then, the presence of renal insufficiency should not exclude patients from consideration for carotid revascularization but they need to be informed about the potential for an increased periprocedural complication rate, particularly with CEA.

Contralateral neurological symptoms

There is evidence to suggest that patients with asymptomatic CAS with prior history of contralateral symptomatic carotid disease are at an increased risk of future ischemic neurological events on the asymptomatic side. Indeed, in NASCET[60] 8% of patients were found to have a contralateral asymptomatic CAS (>60%). Over 5 years of follow-up, the annual risk of ischemic stroke in patients treated with medical therapy was 3.2%, the majority of which were attributed to large-artery disease. Importantly, 80% of first strokes were not preceded by TIAs. In ECST,[61] the annual risk of ischemic stroke on the contralateral asymptomatic side in patients treated with medical therapy was 3.3% for stenoses of 80–89% and 4.8% for stenoses of 90–99%. These stroke rates are 1.5–2.0 times higher than the stroke risk in studies of bilaterally asymptomatic patients.

These findings were also corroborated by the results of the ACAS[2] and ACST[3] trials. In ACAS,[2] 30% of patients presented with a history of neurological symptoms in one carotid artery and were enrolled in the study because a contralateral asymptomatic stenosis was discovered. In this subgroup, the 5-year risk of stroke or death from the asymptomatic side was 12.6% in the medical cohort and 4.5% in the surgical cohort. Similar findings were also reported in the ACST trial where the ipsilateral stroke rate in the control group was double in those with a history of contralateral symptoms than those without such a history.[3] These observations were also confirmed in the prospective ACSRS registry that followed 1101 patients with asymptomatic CAS for up to 7 years.[55] This study also showed that the presence of contralateral neurological symptoms, along with high serum creatinine and carotid stenosis severity, is an independent predictor of ischemic neurological events on the asymptomatic side. In fact, a history of contralateral TIAs increased the risk of ipsilateral stroke by 3-fold (Figure 7.5).

It appears that patients with asymptomatic CAS who already had contralateral symptomatic carotid disease are in fact 'predisposed' for ischemic events, which is consistent with the concept of a 'vulnerable patient'. This clinical observation has in fact been corroborated by angiographic and pathological studies. In an analysis of 5393 carotid bifurcation angiograms from 3007 symptomatic patients in the ECST trial, Rothwell and colleagues[62] demonstrated that patients with angiographic plaque surface irregularity in a symptomatic carotid artery are more likely to have irregular plaques in the asymptomatic carotid artery. Furthermore, these patients were more likely than patients with smooth plaques to have had a previous MI and are more likely to die from cardiovascular causes. Further support for this hypothesis came from observations by Fisher and colleagues,[63] who demonstrated that an asymptomatic carotid plaque in patients with contralateral ischemic neurological events had a higher incidence of ulcers and thrombus than one in those patients without prior neurological symptoms.

It seems appropriate, therefore, to consider these patients at higher risk for future ischemic stroke and to strongly consider carotid revascularization for stroke prevention.

HOW VALUABLE IS CLINICAL STRATIFICATION IN PREDICTING FUTURE ISCHEMIC STROKE AND MORTALITY IN PATIENTS WITH ASYMPTOMATIC CAROTID ARTERY STENOSIS?

Clinical risk stratification for prediction of future ischemic stroke

Although most experts agree that age, gender, and certain comorbidities put patients with asymptomatic CAS at higher risk for future neurological ischemic events, prospective studies to validate the utility of this information are needed before clinicians can consistently rely on it. In the largest prospective observational study to date, the ACSRS[55] followed 1101 patients with asymptomatic CAS for up to 7 years. Among the various demographic and clinical risk factors (age, gender, cardiac symptoms, hypertension, diabetes, smoking, and fasting total lipid profile, etc.), only two clinical risk factors, aside from lesion severity, were associated with an increased overall stroke rate: history of contralateral TIAs and creatinine levels. The rate of ipsilateral hemispheric neurological events increased proportionally to the number of risk factors.

These investigators constructed a risk stratification model based on the combination of all three risk factors – stenosis severity, history of contralateral TIAs, and creatinine level. This model allowed identification of a high-risk group with a 26% cumulative stroke rate at 7 years (4.3% annual stroke rate) and a low-risk group with a 4.2% cumulative stroke rate at 7 years (0.7% annual stroke rate). The patients at highest risk (6.3% annual stroke rate) were those with 80–99% stenoses, history of contralateral TIAs, and creatinine concentration >85 μmol/L. However, highlighting the difficulty in predicting the future behavior of an individual patient, only 54% of the strokes occurred in the high-risk group while the rest occurred in the low-risk group. This indicates that the above risk stratification model lacks the adequate sensitivity to identify many patients who are at risk of future neurological events. Other risk stratification modalities (see subsequent chapters) should complement this model to better target more at-risk patients.

Clinical risk stratification for prediction of future mortality

The results of the largest prospective randomized clinical trials of CEA vs medical therapy in patients with asymptomatic CAS[2,3] have demonstrated that about 20 operations need to be performed to prevent 1 stroke for a 5-year follow-up and suggest that patients are unlikely to benefit from surgery if they do not live for 5 years. Therefore, a key goal of clinical decision-making is to identify patients with asymptomatic CAS who are at high risk for future ipsilateral stroke and low risk of mortality over the next 5–10 years. Although factors that affect mortality in these patients are well known, a quantitative model is lacking. To that end, the ACSRS natural history study[64] followed 1101 patients with asymptomatic CAS for 6–84 months (mean 38 months). Six factors were identified as independent predictors of cardiovascular mortality: age, male gender, cardiac failure, left ventricular hypertrophy, myocardial ischemia, and an internal carotid artery (ICA) stenosis >80%. Based on these risk factors, the investigators identified a high-risk group consisting of one-third of the population with a 40% cumulative cardiovascular death rate and a 66% all-cause death rate at 7 years. The remaining two-thirds consisted of a low-risk group with a 10% cumulative cardiovascular death rate and a 21% all-cause death rate at 7 years. Accordingly, one can identify a subgroup of patients who are at high risk for future stroke (annual stroke risk 2–6%) who have a reasonable chance of surviving beyond 5 years (annual mortality risk <5%) (Figure 7.6). This and other models for patient selection need to be evaluated in future randomized clinical trials of conservative vs interventional therapy for asymptomatic CAS.

SUMMARY

The decision to utilize carotid revascularization in patients with asymptomatic CAS in an attempt to reduce the possibility of a future stroke can be a difficult one for patients and physicians alike. The automatic extrapolation of outcomes from population-based studies to an individual patient can be problematic. Consideration of specific demographics and clinical comorbidities of patients is paramount to clinical decision-making. Specific factors considered during the consultation with the patient include the risks of the natural history of the condition vs the risks of the procedure in similar patients. Further complicating the process of 'risk stratification' is the consideration of less-objective features such as the life expectancy of the patient and the patient's tolerance for 'active' (intervention) vs 'passive' (natural history) risk taking.

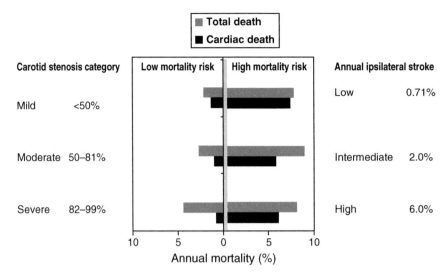

Figure 7.6 Stratification of patients with asymptomatic carotid disease according to their risk of ipsilateral stroke and mortality based on age, gender, lesion severity, and presence or absence of cardiac failure, left ventricular hypertrophy, and myocardial ischemia. (Modified from Kakkos et al.[64])

REFERENCES

1. Hobson RW, Weiss DG, Fields WS et al. Efficacy of carotid endarterectomy for asymptomatic carotid stenosis. N Engl J Med 1993; 328: 221–7.
2. Executive Committee for the Asymptomatic Carotid Atherosclerosis Study. Endarterectomy for asymptomatic carotid stenosis. JAMA 1995; 273: 1421–8.
3. Halliday A, Mansfield A, Marro J et al. MRC Asymptomatic Carotid Surgery Trial (ACST) Collaborative Group. Prevention of disabling and fatal strokes by successful carotid endarterectomy in patients without recent neurological symptoms: randomised controlled trial. Lancet 2004; 363: 1491–502.
4. Fabris F, Zanocchi M, Bo M et al. Carotid plaque, aging, and risk factors: a study of 457 subjects. Stroke 1994; 25(6): 1133–40.
5. Moore DJ, Miles RD, Gooley NA, Sumner DS. Noninvasive assessment of stroke risk in asymptomatic and nonhemispheric patients with suspected carotid disease. Five-year follow-up of 294 unoperated and 81 operated patients. Ann Surg 1985; 202(4): 491–504.
6. Manolio TA, Kronmal RA, Burke GL et al. Short-term predictors of incident stroke in older adults. The Cardiovascular Health Study. Stroke 1996; 27: 1479–86.
7. Sacco RL. Risk factors, outcomes, and stroke subtypes for ischemic stroke. Neurology 1997; 49(5 Suppl 4): S39–44.
8. Robbins M, Baum HM. National survey of stroke incidence. Stroke 1981; 121(Suppl 1): 45–7.
9. Kammersgaard LP, Jorgensen HS, Reith J et al. Short- and long-term prognosis for very old stroke patients. The Copenhagen Stroke Study. Age Ageing 2004; 33: 149–54.
10. Cronenwett JL, Birkmeyer JD, Nackman GB et al. Cost-effectiveness of carotid endarterectomy in asymptomatic patients. J Vasc Surg 1997; 25: 298–311.
11. Manton KG, Stallard E. Cross-sectional estimates of active life expectancy for the U.S. elderly and oldest-old populations. J Gerontol 1991; 46(3): S170–82.
12. National Center for Health Statistics. Vital statistics of the United States 1991; Vol II, Mortality, Part A, Sec 6 life tables, Table 6-4. Washington: Public Health Service, 1996: 16.
13. Katz S, Branch LG, Branson MH et al. Active life expectancy. N Engl J Med 1983; 309: 1218–24.
14. Goldstein LB, Samsa GP, Matchar DB et al. Multicenter review of preoperative risk factors for endarterectomy for asymptomatic carotid artery stenosis. Stroke 1998; 29: 750–3.
15. Rothwell PM, Slattery J, Warlow CP. Clinical and angiographic predictors of stroke and death from carotid endarterectomy: systematic review. BMJ 1997; 315: 1571–7.
16. Howard G, Hobson RW, Brott T et al. Does the stroke risk in stenting increase at older ages? Thirty-day stroke-death rates in the CREST lead-in phase. Stroke 2004; 35: 258.
17. Kastrup A, Groschel K, Schulz JB, Nagele T, Ernemann U. Clinical predictors of transient ischemic attack, stroke, or death within 30 days of carotid angioplasty and stenting. Stroke 2005; 36: 787–91.
18. Grey WA, Wholey M, Yadav S et al. CAPTURE II Registry. Presented at the American College of Cardiology Scientific Sessions. Atlanta, GA 2006.
19. Yadav JS, Wholey MH, Kuntz RE et al. Stenting and Angioplasty with Protection in Patients at High Risk for Endarterectomy Investigators. Protected carotid-artery stenting versus endarterectomy in high-risk patients. N Engl J Med 2004; 351(15): 1493–501.
20. Hertzer NR, O'Hara PJ, Mascha EJ et al. Early outcome assessment for 2228 consecutive carotid endarterectomy procedures: the Cleveland Clinic experience from 1989 to 1995. J Vasc Surg 1997; 26: 1–10.
21. Rigdon EE. Racial and gender differences in outcome after carotid endarterectomy. Am Surg 1998; 64: 527–32.
22. Schneider JR, Droste JS, Golan JF. Carotid endarterectomy in women versus men: patient characteristics and outcomes. J Vasc Surg 1997; 25: 890–8.
23. Rothwell PM, Goldstein LB. Carotid endarterectomy for asymptomatic carotid stenosis: asymptomatic carotid surgery trial. Stroke 2004; 35: 2425–7.
24. Dick P, Sherif C, Sabeti S et al. Gender differences in outcome of conservatively treated patients with asymptomatic high grade carotid stenosis. Stroke 2005; 36: 1178–83.
25. Iemolo F, Martiniuk A, Steinman DA, Spence JD. Sex differences in carotid plaque and stenosis. Stroke 2004; 35: 477–81.

26. Van den Broek T, Velema E, Schoneveld AH et al. Risk factors for atherosclerosis and plaque phenotype. Eur Heart J 2004; 25. Abstract supplement 102.

27. Pasterkamp G, Schoneveld AH, van der Wal AC et al. Relation of arterial geometry to luminal narrowing and histologic markers for plaque vulnerability: the remodeling paradox. J Am Coll Cardiol 1998; 32: 655–62.

28. Roubin GS, New G, Iyer SS et al. Immediate and late clinical outcomes of carotid artery stenting in patients with symptomatic and asymptomatic carotid artery stenosis. A 5-year prospective analysis. Circulation 2001; 103: 532–7.

29. Hertzer NR, Young JR, Beven EG et al. Coronary angiography in 506 patients with extracranial cerebrovascular disease. Arch Intern Med 1985; 145: 849–52.

30. Love BB, Grover-McKay M, Biller J, Rezai K, McKay CR. Coronary artery disease and cardiac events with asymptomatic and symptomatic cerebrovascular disease. Stroke 1992; 23: 939–45.

31. Kannel WB, Wolf PA, Verter J. Manifestations of coronary disease predisposing to stroke. The Framingham Study. JAMA 1983; 250: 2942–6.

32. Hedblad B, Janzon L, Jungquist G, Ogren M. Factors modifying the prognosis in men with asymptomatic carotid artery disease. J Intern Med 1998; 243(1): 57–64.

33. Sangiorgi G, Mauriello A, Trimarchi S et al. Does carotid plaque inflammatory infiltrate differ between patients affected by stable or unstable angina? Eur Heart J 2000; 19 (Suppl): Abstract.

34. Naylor AR, Mehta Z, Rothwell PM, Bell PR. Carotid artery disease and stroke during coronary artery bypass: a critical review of the literature. Eur J Vasc Endovasc Surg 2002; 23: 283–94.

35. Brener BJ, Brief DK, Alpert J, Goldenkranz RJ, Parsonnet V. The risk of stroke in patients with asymptomatic carotid stenosis undergoing cardiac surgery: a follow-up study. J Vasc Surg 1987; 5: 269–79.

36. Schwartz LB, Bridgman AH, Kieffer RW et al. Asymptomatic carotid artery stenosis and stroke in patients undergoing cardiopulmonary bypass. J Vasc Surg 1995; 21: 146–53.

37. Mickleborough LL, Walker PM, Takagi Y et al. Risk factors for stroke in patients undergoing coronary artery bypass grafting. J Thorac Cardiovasc Surg 1996; 112: 1250–8.

38. Hill AB, Obrand D, O'Rourke K, Steinmetz OK, Miller N. Hemispheric stroke following cardiac surgery: a case–control estimate of the risk resulting from ipsilateral asymptomatic carotid artery stenosis. Ann Vasc Surg 2000 14: 200–9.

39. Turnipseed WE, Berkoff HA, Belzer FD. Postoperative stroke in cardiac and peripheral vascular disease. Ann Surg 1980; 192: 365–8.

40. Gerraty RP, Gates PC, Doyle JC. Carotid stenosis and perioperative stroke risk in symptomatic and asymptomatic patients undergoing vascular or coronary surgery. Stroke 1993; 24: 1115–18.

41. Griffiths PD, Gaines P, Cleveland T et al. Assessment of cerebral hemodynamics and vascular reserve in patients with symptomatic carotid artery occlusion: an integrated MR method. Neuroradiology 2005; 47: 175–82.

42. Babatasi G, Massetti M, Theron J, Khayat A. Asymptomatic carotid stenosis in patients undergoing major cardiac surgery: can percutaneous carotid angioplasty be an alternative? Eur J Cardiothorac Surg 1997; 11: 547–53.

43. Lopes DK, Mericle RA, Lanzino G et al. Stent placement for the treatment of occlusive atherosclerotic carotid artery disease in patients with concomitant coronary artery disease. J Neurosurg 2002; 96: 490–6.

44. Randall MS, McKevitt FM, Cleveland TJ, Gaines PA, Venables GS. Is there any benefit from staged carotid and coronary revascularization using carotid stents? A single-center experience highlights the need for a randomized controlled trial. Stroke 2006; 37: 435–9.

45. Abraham J, Kramer J, Jones P. Carotid artery stenting prior to CABG: a better alternative to treat concomitant coronary and carotid disease. Poster presentation ACP Chicago, IL, November 2005.

46. Naylor AR, Cuffe RL, Rothwell PM, Bell PR. A systematic review of outcomes following staged and synchronous carotid endarterectomy and coronary artery bypass. Eur J Vasc Endovasc Surg 2003; 25: 380–9.

47. Biller J, Feinberg WM, Castaldo JE et al. Guidelines for carotid endarterectomy: A statement for healthcare professionals from a Special Writing Group of the Stroke Council, American Heart Association. Circulation 1998; 97: 501–9.

48. McKevitt FM, Randall MS, Cleveland TJ et al. The benefits of combined anti-platelet treatment in carotid artery stenting. Eur J Vasc Endovasc Surg 2005; 29: 522–7.

49. Wannamethee SG, Shaper AG, Perry IJ. Serum creatinine concentration and risk of cardiovascular disease. A possible marker for increased risk of stroke. Stroke 1997; 28: 557–63.

50. Longstreth WT Jr, Bernick C, Manolio TA et al. Lacunar infarcts defined by magnetic resonance imaging of 3660 elderly people: the Cardiovascular Health Study. Arch Neurol 1998; 55: 1217–25.

51. Leskinen Y, Lehtimäki T, Loimaala A et al. Carotid atherosclerosis in chronic renal failure – the central role of increased plaque burden. Atherosclerosis 2003; 171: 295–302.

52. Rossi A, Bonfante L, Giacomini A et al. Carotid artery lesions in patients with nondiabetic chronic renal failure. Am J Kidney Dis 1996; 27: 58–66.

53. Savage T, Clarke AL, Giles M, Tomson CR, Raine AE. Calcified plaque is common in the carotid and femoral arteries of dialysis patients without clinical vascular disease. Nephrol Dial Transplant 1998; 13: 12.

54. Pascazio L, Bianco F, Giorgini A et al. Echo color Doppler imaging of carotid vessels in hemodialysis patients: evidence of high levels of atherosclerotic lesions. Am J Kidney Dis 1996; 28: 713–20.

55. Nicolaides AN, Kakkos S, Griffin M, Geroulakos G, Ioannidou E. Severity of asymptomatic carotid stenosis and risk of ipsilateral hemispheric ischaemic events: results from the ACSRS study. Eur J Vasc Endovasc Surg 2005; 30: 275–84.

56. Go AS, Chertow GM, Fan D, McCulloch CE, Hsu CY. Chronic kidney disease and the risks of death, cardiovascular events, and hospitalization. N Engl J Med 2004; 351: 1296–305.

57. O'Hara PJ, Hertzer NR, Mascha EJ et al. Carotid endarterectomy in octogenarians: early results and late outcome. J Vasc Surg 1998; 27: 860–7.

58. Hamdan AD, Pomposelli FB Jr, Gibbons GW, Campbell DR, LoGerfo FW. Renal insufficiency and altered postoperative risk in carotid endarterectomy. J Vasc Surg 1999; 29: 1006–11.

59. Saw J, Gurm HS, Fathi RB et al. Effect of chronic kidney disease on outcomes after carotid artery stenting. Am J Cardiol 2004; 94: 1093–6.

60. Inzitari D, Eliasziw M, Gates P et al. The causes and risk of stroke in patients with asymptomatic internal-carotid-artery stenosis. N Engl J Med 2000; 342: 1693–1700.

61. The European Carotid Surgery Trialists Collaborative Group. Risk of stroke in the distribution of an asymptomatic carotid artery. Lancet 1995; 345(8944): 209–12.

62. Rothwell PM, Villagra R, Gibson R, Donders RC, Warlow CP. Evidence of a chronic systemic cause of instability of atherosclerotic plaques. Lancet 2000; 355: 19–24.

63. Fisher M, Paganini-Hill A, Martin et al. Carotid plaque pathology: thrombosis, ulceration, and stroke pathogenesis. Stroke 2005; 36: 253–7.

64. Kakkos SK, Nicolaides AN, Griffin M et al; the Asymptomatic Carotid Stenosis and Risk of Stroke (ACSRS) Study Group. Factors associated with mortality in patients with asymptomatic carotid stenosis: results from the ACSRS Study. Int Angiol 2005; 24(3): 221–30.

8

Risk stratification of patients with asymptomatic carotid artery stenosis: evaluation of carotid stenosis severity, progression, and morphology by duplex ultrasound

Bernardo Liberato and Tatjana Rundek

Take-Home Messages

1. Carotid plaque quantitative and qualitative characteristics determined by duplex ultrasound are important parameters for assessing the risk of future stroke and other vascular events in patients with asymptomatic carotid artery stenosis (CAS).
2. The important quantitative ultrasonographic carotid plaque parameters are carotid stenosis severity and carotid stenosis progression. The important qualitative parameters are plaque ulceration and plaque echogenicity.
3. The higher the degree of carotid stenosis in neurologically asymptomatic individuals, the higher the risk of stroke and transient ischemic attack (TIA). Most experts agree that a critical threshold of >80% stenosis is associated with a rise of ipsilateral ischemic neurological events and should trigger an evaluation for carotid revascularization.
4. Among patients with asymptomatic CAS, the risk of stroke and TIA is 3 times greater in patients with carotid stenosis progression to 80% stenosis or more than in patients without such progression.
5. Plaque echogenicity is a descriptive and subjective ultrasonographic morphological feature. Novel computerized ultrasound technologies such as the gray-scale median analyses of plaque echogenicity are more objective methods and their validation is currently underway.
6. Data on the prognostic significance of carotid plaque qualitative parameters in neurologically asymptomatic patients are either lacking (plaque ulceration) or conflicting (plaque echogenicity). Some studies have shown that echolucent carotid plaques are associated with a 2–5- fold increased risk for stroke; however, the clinical utility of these observations for triaging patients to carotid revascularization await prospective confirmation.

INTRODUCTION

The evaluation of patients harboring significant carotid atherosclerotic disease entails a careful evaluation of the likely mechanism(s) leading to the increased risk of future stroke. This will facilitate clinical decision-making in terms of triaging patients to medical therapy alone vs medical therapy and carotid revascularization.

The atherosclerotic carotid artery plaque may cause cerebral ischemia by one or a combination of the following mechanisms:

- artery-to-artery embolization from the carotid plaque to the intracerebral vessels;
- direct occlusion with propagation of thrombus from the external portion of the carotid artery plaque to its intracranial branches;

- hemodynamic compromise, with low-flow state downstream producing cerebral perfusion failure.

Artery-to-artery embolization has been largely based on inference since scant clinical and pathological studies are available to precisely document such a mechanism. The areas of focal arterial occlusion compatible with recent embolization are difficult to document by conventional digital subtraction or magnetic resonance angiography (MRA), which are often used in clinical practice. Regardless of the lack of clinical confirmation, however, artery-to-artery embolization in the absence of cardiac embolic source, is the most likely underlying pathophysiological mechanism responsible for stroke.

Recent studies provide evidence that cerebral ischemia in patients with high-grade carotid stenosis is frequently the result of a cerebral embolization from a 'vulnerable' carotid plaque. This is especially true in patients with cortical infarcts. Transcranial Doppler (TCD) studies have shown a higher rate of cerebral microemboli in patients with severe carotid stenosis if they present with cortical infarctions than in patients who present with a watershed, subcortical pattern of ischemia.[1] Also, a higher rate of microembolic signals (MES) was observed in recently symptomatic patients with carotid stenosis than in asymptomatic patients.[1,2] The risk of future embolization is significantly higher in asymptomatic patients with present MES detected by

TCD monitoring than in those without MES.[3,4] These results, however, have not been consistently reproduced.[5] Chapter 9 of this book is dedicated to the assessment of cerebral embolization by TCD.

In this chapter, we focus on carotid plaque quantitative and qualitative characterization using duplex ultrasound and how these parameters can be used to augment other clinical and physiological parameters in risk stratification of patients with asymptomatic carotid artery stenosis (CAS).

CAROTID PLAQUE QUANTITATIVE PARAMETERS (STENOSIS SEVERITY, STENOSIS PROGRESSION, AND PLAQUE SIZE)

Carotid stenosis severity

The majority of the studies that evaluated the impact of carotid stenosis severity on vascular outcomes have relied on duplex ultrasound (Figure 8.1). It has been shown that carotid ultrasound assessment of the degree of carotid stenosis is comparable to other non-invasive and invasive methods.[6]

The association between carotid stenosis severity and risk of future stroke is well documented in symptomatic patients.[7–10] This association, however,

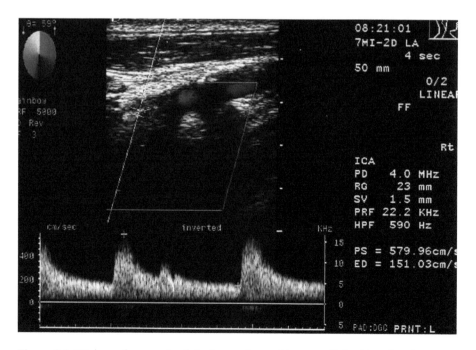

Figure 8.1 High-grade stenosis of the internal carotid artery. Color Doppler shows 80-99% stenosis of the internal carotid artery. (See color plate section.)

remains the subject of debate in asymptomatic patients. Chambers and Norris[11] have clearly shown an increased risk of stroke/TIA at 1-year follow-up with increasing carotid stenosis severity (2% with 0–29% stenosis, 6% with 30–74% stenosis, and 20% with >75% stenosis). In the Asymptomatic Cervical Bruit Study,[12] 357 patients with asymptomatic carotid stenosis >50% were prospectively followed for up to 6 years (mean 3.1 years). While the annual rate of ipsilateral stroke and combined stroke/TIA in the total population was 1.4% and 4.2%, respectively, this rate increased to 2.8% and 7.5% in patients with an 80–99% stenosis. In multivariate analysis, severity of carotid stenosis was the strongest predictor of neurological and other vascular events.

However, the inclusion of strokes in the contralateral carotid artery territory distribution in some reports can falsely overestimate the risk of stroke due to ipsilateral carotid stenosis. In a study by Bock and associates,[13] the annual rate of risk of TIA and stroke among patients with 80–99% stenosis was 21%, while among those with carotid stenosis <80% it was 5%. However, only 5% of these events occurred in the carotid distribution affected by the stenosis. Contrary to previous natural history studies that showed an association between carotid stenosis severity and stroke risk, the Asymptomatic Carotid Surgery Trial (ACST) failed to confirm these findings.[14] The reasons for this discrepancy are not entirely clear. Part of the explanation may be that measurement of the exact degree of stenosis is less

accurate with Doppler ultrasound scanning than with catheter angiography. Another explanation is that near-occlusions were not identified in ACST, a condition known to be associated with a low risk of stroke during medical treatment and no proven benefit from endarterectomy. The high prevalence of near-occlusions with increasing lesion severity may dilute the potential benefit of endarterectomy in severely occluded vessels as determined by duplex ultrasound. Furthermore, it is noteworthy to point out that the duplex ultrasound criteria used in the ACST trial were only locally validated, but neither the velocity criteria nor the imaging criteria were prespecified.

The largest natural history study to evaluate the association between carotid stenosis severity and future stroke risk in patients with asymptomatic CAS is the Asymptomatic Carotid Stenosis and Risk of Stroke (ACSRS) study.[15] This was a prospective observational natural history study of 1101 patients with asymptomatic CAS who were followed up to 7 years. In this study, previously validated duplex ultrasound criteria were used and outcomes were reported according to European Carotid Surgery Trial (ECST) and North American Symptomatic Carotid Endarterectomy Trial (NASCET) stenosis categories (Table 8.1). The risk of ipsilateral ischemic hemispheric events was found to rise with increased severity of carotid stenosis, confirming the findings of previous natural history studies (see Chapter 1). These investigators identified three groups with variable risk of future stroke (Figure 8.2): (a) a low-risk group (50–69% ECST,

Table 8.1 Duplex velocity criteria selected for highest accuracy*

Angiographic diameter stenosis		Duplex velocity criteria				
N (%)	E (%)	PSV_{IC}	EDV_{IC}	PSV_{IC}/PSV_{CC}	PSV_{IC}/EDV_{CC}	EDV_{IC}/EDV_{CC}
12	50	<120	<40	<1.5	<7	
30	60					<2.6
47	70	120–150	40–80	1.5–2	7–10	
60	77		80–130	2–3.2		
65	80	150–250				
70	83		>130	3.2–4	10–20	2.6–5.5
82	90	>250		>4	20–30	
90	95				>30	>5.5
99	99			Trickle flow		

N, NASCET; E, ECST; PSV, peak systolic velocity; EDV, end-diastolic velocity; IC, internal carotid;
CC, common carotid.
*Minimum false-positive and false-negative tests.
(Adapted from Nicolaides et al.[15])

equivalent to 12–46% NASCET) with a 7-year cumulative event rate of 8%; (b) a moderate-risk group (70–89% ECST, equivalent to 47–81% NASCET) with a 7-year cumulative event rate of 18%; and (c) a high-risk group (90–99% ECST, equivalent to 82–99% NASCET) with a

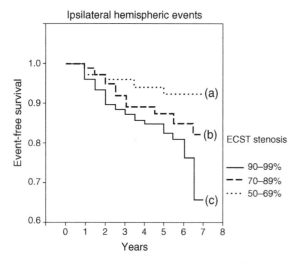

Figure 8.2 The ipsilateral hemispheric event-free cumulative survival rate in relation to the ECST % stenosis of the internal carotid artery: group a 50–69%, *n* = 101; group b 70–89%, *n* = 593; group c 90–99%, *n* = 328. Overall log rank: 11.7, *p* = 0.0026; 50–69 vs 70–89%, *p* = 0.045; 79–89 vs 90–99%, *p* = 0.020; 50–69 vs 90–99%, *p* = 0.0014. (Modified from Nicolaides et al.[15])

7-year cumulative event rate of 35%. Interestingly, the relationship between stenosis severity and event rate was linear when expressed as ECST % stenosis (Figure 8.3A), and was S-shaped when expressed as NASCET % stenosis (Figure 8.3B). Nonetheless, again highlighting the difficulty in predicting a specific individual's risk of stroke, a considerable number of events occurred at low grades of stenosis. In fact, 34% of all ipsilateral ischemic hemispheric events occurred in patients with stenosis <60%.

In summary, the preponderance of evidence points to the central role of stenosis severity (>80% stenosis) in predicting increased risk of ipsilateral stroke. Furthermore, it appears that the predictive ability of the baseline carotid stenosis severity does not diminish with time. Lewis et al[16] demonstrated that the baseline stenosis severity remains a significant independent predictor of ipsilateral neurological events during the first 4 years of follow-up, with an increase of approximately 50% in risk associated with each successive category of stenosis.

Carotid stenosis progression

Most natural history studies addressing this topic reported an association between carotid disease progression and neurological events (see Chapter 1). Roederer and associates[17] found that in asymptomatic patients who initially presented with <80% carotid stenosis, progression to carotid stenosis >80% was associated with a high incidence of stroke, TIA, or progression to carotid occlusion. Alternatively, only 1.5% of patients whose plaques remained stable developed symptoms over a 12-month follow-up.

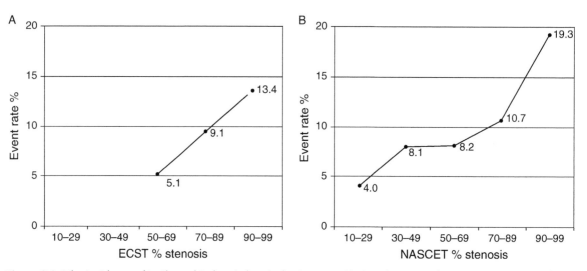

Figure 8.3 The incidence of ipsilateral ischemic hemispheric events (A) in relation to the ECST % stenosis of the internal carotid artery and (B) in relation to the NASCET % stenosis of the internal carotid artery. (Adapted from Nicolaides et al.[15])

In the largest study to date on the impact of carotid disease progression on neurological events, Lewis et al[16] reported on 3664 duplex ultrasonographic examinations done in 714 asymptomatic patients over 2285 patient-years. Patients whose carotid stenosis progressed to stenosis >80% from the baseline examination had a 3 times greater risk of stroke or TIA than patients without carotid stenosis progression (Table 8.2). Although lack of disease progression has a very high negative predictive value for occurrence of ischemic neurological events, the positive predictive value remains low (Table 8.3). This is probably because carotid disease progression is only one of many other factors that can lead to an ischemic neurological event in an individual patient. More recently, Sabeti et al[18] confirmed previous observations in a prospective follow-up study of 1268 patients with asymptomatic CAS where progressive disease was associated with a 2.9-fold increased adjusted risk of ipsilateral neurological events (Figure 8.4).

Progression of asymptomatic carotid stenosis toward occlusion can also be fraught with consequences. At the time of occlusion, strokes were reported to occur in up to 20% of patients[19] and with an addition of 2–6% of patients with stroke annually thereafter. The majority of neurological events associated with carotid disease progression occur within 6 months of diagnosis.[17] It remains controversial, however, whether carotid disease progression precedes[17] or occurs concurrently with neurological events.[12,13]

In summary, most experts agree that carotid stenosis progression beyond an 80% stenosis threshold is associated with higher risk of ischemic ipsilateral stroke and it should trigger an evaluation for carotid revascularization.

Carotid plaque size

Carotid plaque size measured by duplex ultrasound is usually expressed as one of the following parameters: maximal carotid plaque thickness, plaque area, or

---

Table 8.2 Adjusted relative risk for transient ischemic attack (TIA) or stroke associated with carotid stenosis progression in asymptomatic individuals*

Initial carotid stenosis severity	Degree of progression	Relative risk of TIA/stroke (95% CI)	p value
<50%	Progression to >50%	2.0 (0.7–5.8)	NS
<80%	Progression to ≥80%	3.0 (1.3–6.7)	<0.01

*Relative risk for progression estimated by Cox proportional hazards model for all participants, adjusted for initial lesion severity and baseline risk factors (age, sex, heart disease, hypertension, hyperlipidemia, diabetes, claudication, smoking, and use of aspirin). CL, confidence interval.
(Modified from Lewis et al.[16])

Table 8.3 Estimated ability of stenosis progression to predict transient ischemic attack (TIA) or stroke within 2 years

Initial carotid stenosis severity	Progression in the previous 2 years	Ability of stenosis progression to predict TIA/stroke within 2 years	
		PPV (%)	NPV (%)
<50%	To ≥ 50%	10	95
50–79%	To ≥ 80%	16	95
<80%	To ≥ 80%	17	94

PPV, positive predictive value; NPV, negative predictive value.
(Modified from Lewis et al.[16])

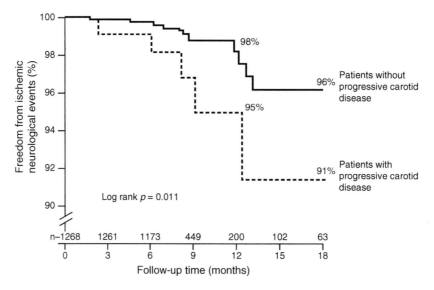

Figure 8.4 Kaplan–Meier estimates of freedom from ischemic neurological events in patients with and without progression of atherosclerotic carotid disease. (Adapted from Sabeti et al.[18])

plaque volume. Plaque size has a direct correlation with degree of stenosis, but it is also an independent predictor of future ischemic events.[20] Large population-based studies have shown that carotid plaque size is an independent predictor of future stroke, myocardial infarction (MI), and vascular death, even in individuals with a low degree of carotid stenosis.[9,21] Also, there may be an important sex difference regarding plaque size and the risk of future vascular events. It has been reported that at any given degree of carotid stenosis, men have a larger plaque burden than women, predisposing them to worse vascular outcomes.[22] However, definite confirmation of these findings warrants more research.

In patients who present with a carotid plaque without significant stenosis, carotid plaque size measured by any of the duplex ultrasound parameters (thickness, area, or volume) should be evaluated because plaque size is an important marker of subclinical atherosclerosis and a reliable predictor of future vascular events.

CAROTID PLAQUE QUALITATIVE (MORPHOLOGICAL) PARAMETERS

It has been suggested that carotid plaque morphology assessed by duplex ultrasound can discriminate patients at high risk for stroke and TIA from those at low risk of these events.[23] Recently, a greater association

between ultrasonographic plaque features and its pathological correlates has been well described.

The main morphological ultrasonographic plaque parameters are:

- plaque ulceration
- plaque echogenicity.

Determinations of such morphological ultrasonographic plaque features are not always possible in clinical practice. There are many methodological differences between various studies that have reported on ultrasonographic morphological characteristics of plaque.

Plaque ulceration

Ultrasonographic criteria most commonly employed in the determination of plaque ulceration include the following (Figures 8.5 and 8.6):

- plaque recess at least 2 mm long and 2 mm deep
- well-defined wall at its base
- reversed flow at the crater, not representing aliasing.

Detection of ulcerated plaques by duplex ultrasound is limited by the ultrasound technique (e.g. resolution of ultrasound) and irregular characteristics of plaques. Irregular heterogeneous plaques may be ulcerated, but sensitivity and specificity of duplex ultrasound to detect ulceration in these plaques are low. The mechanisms

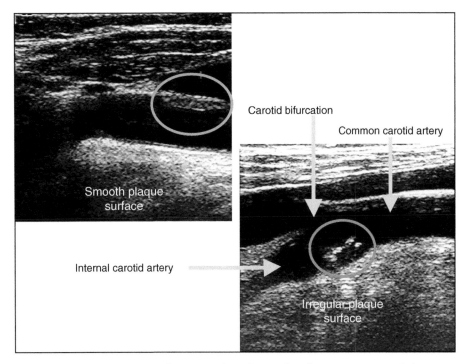

Figure 8.5 Carotid plaque surface: smooth and irregular plaque. Existence of plaque ulceration in irregular plaque cannot be completely ruled out.

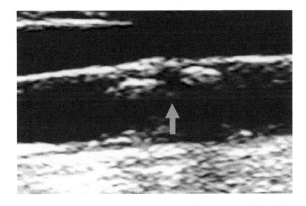

Figure 8.6 An ulcerated plaque (red arrow) with well-defined arterial wall at its base and a recess over 2 mm in the length and depth. (See color plate section.)

through which plaque ulceration may predispose to a higher stroke risk include denudation of the endothelium, exposure of thrombogenic structures, and the formation of in-situ thrombosis with subsequent distal embolization and/or further lumen reduction.

Ultrasound studies of carotid plaque ulceration in asymptomatic patients are sparse. One study reported that ulcerated carotid plaque was more common in symptomatic than asymptomatic patients (77% vs 41%).[24]

However, despite frequently postulated association between plaque ulceration and cerebral symptomatology from carotid stenosis, a definite causal confirmation from the ultrasonographic studies is lacking.[25] The evidence regarding plaque ulceration and increased risk of stroke mainly comes from the angiographic studies primarily in symptomatic patients.[26,27]

Why are ultrasonographic studies of ulcerated plaques in asymptomatic carotid disease sparse?

There are several reasons why ultrasonographic studies of plaque ulceration are sparse, including technical limitations of ultrasound methods and a low prevalence of plaque ulceration in the general population. One of the important reasons, however, may be a consequence of plaque 'instability'. Unstable plaques are dynamic lesions. They most likely become ulcerated at the time of symptom onset, they 'heal' quickly, and it is therefore difficult to capture them in the asymptomatic phase. Methodological problems in determining the presence of plaque ulceration were reported in angiographic as well as ultrasound studies. Data from NASCET showed a less than optimal correlation between angiographic features and the presence of plaque ulceration from surgical specimens.[27] Similar findings were observed from an ultrasonographic study,[24] where the sensitivity of detecting an ulcerated carotid plaque in lesions >50% of stenosis was low (41%).

In order to improve the yield of detection of plaque ulceration, novel non-invasive methods such as high-definition and 3D ultrasound, MRA, and computed tomographic angiography (CTA) are emerging. Color Doppler flow imaging (CDFI) and power Doppler imaging (PDI) are better ultrasound techniques in defining the contours of an ulcerated plaque than duplex ultrasound.[28] Recently, 3D ultrasound has been employed for better definition of plaque characteristics. This appears to be a promising technology, since not only detection of plaque and its characteristics but also the rate of progression and regression can be determined more precisely.[29] All newer ultrasound systems are already equipped with CDFI and PDI. These techniques are already available for better assessment of carotid plaque ulcerations in clinical practice. However, 3D ultrasound is still at the research and development phase and is not yet a validated technology for assessment of plaque morphology.

Plaque echogenicity

Plaque echogenicity is defined as hyperechoic (bright on ultrasound) and hypoechoic (dark on ultrasound) in comparison to the echodensity of surrounding media as the reference, such as blood (dark on ultrasound, lowest reflection of the ultrasound beam), vessel wall (lighter than blood), soft tissue (lighter than blood), and bone (the brightest on ultrasound, the highest reflection of the ultrasound beam).[30]

Classification of plaques by echogenicity

1. Hypoechoic or echolucent: dark on ultrasound (lipid-rich content, blood).
2. Hyperechoic or echodense: Bright on ultrasound (calcified).

Plaques can be further divided into heterogeneous, when a non-uniform pattern with mixed echo intensities is detected, and homogeneous, when a uniform or predominant echo intensity is present. Homogeneous plaques usually show a regular, smooth surface, whereas heterogeneous plaques usually show an irregular surface.[31]

Classification of plaques by uniformity of echo intensities

- Heterogeneous: non-uniform pattern with mixed echo intensities.
- Homogeneous: uniform echo intensity.

Echolucent plaque

Plaque echolucency (low ultrasound reflective properties) is a marker of unstable plaque (Figure 8.7) and is associated with an increased risk of future stroke.[32,33] In the large population-based Cardiovascular Health Study among asymptomatic individuals who were followed up for a mean of 3 years, echolucent carotid plaques were associated with a 2-fold increased risk for stroke, and with a 2.3-fold increased risk of stroke among those who had echolucent plaques in combination with carotid stenosis >50%.[32] In the Tromso study among asymptomatic CAS patients, echolucent plaques were associated with a 5 times greater risk of stroke. This increased risk was independent of the degree of stenosis and other cardiovascular risk factors.[33] Conversely, several studies have reported that only symptomatic patients with echolucent plaques have increased risk of subsequent stroke.[34]

An echolucent plaque has a high content of lipid in its core as well as intraplaque hemorrhage, both conditions predisposing to denudation of the endothelial wall and triggering of the thrombotic cascade.[35] Lipid-rich plaques are associated with elevated serum lipoproteins and triglycerides and this correlation appears stronger in women than in men.[36–38] Lipid-rich plaques are also surrounded by the inflammation process. This may help to explain unstable plaque characteristics through continuing inflammation and may suggest that the effect of various classes of antiplatelet, lipid-lowering, and blood pressure-lowering medications in reducing the risk is beyond their presumed primary mechanism. These medications may play a role in plaque stabilization. Similarly, higher serum levels of interleukin-6 (IL-6), C-reactive protein, and white blood cell count were observed in patients with hypoechoic plaques[39] or larger plaques,[40] providing more evidence for a role of active inflammation in hypoechoic plaques. (A detailed discussion on the role of inflammation in plaque formation is provided in Chapter 11.)

Echolucent plaques may have a higher emboligenic potential and therefore increased risk of future

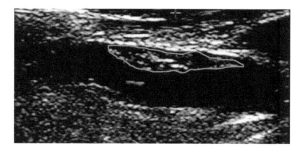

Figure 8.7 Echolucent heterogeneous plaque (outlined in red). (See color plate section.)

TIA or stroke. Furthermore, they may carry a greater risk of embolization during endovascular procedures increasing peri- and postprocedural risk of stroke.[41,42]

Echodense (calcified) plaque

The higher degree of calcium deposition in symptomatic and asymptomatic carotid plaques was associated with plaque stability. The mechanism by which the 'protective' effects of plaque calcification may explain plaque stability is that such calcification, often seen in long-standing plaques, is the last 'healing' event in the process of plaque activity. These plaques become less 'active' by being less prone to rupture, subintimal dissection, and hemorrhage, and therefore become stabile. Supportive evidence for a stable course and lower risk of stroke for patients with carotid plaques with higher calcium content came from a computed tomographic (CT) study.[43] Although B-mode ultrasound may be less technically accurate and greater operator-dependent for detection of plaque calcification, there is a histopathological evidence that echodense plaques represent a higher calcium to lipid ratio content, with the highest calcium content in homogeneously echodense plaques (Figure 8.8). These homogeneously calcified plaques are considered in several studies as a good prognostic feature based on the lower rates of stroke.[31,35,44,45] However, some recent studies have shown quite the opposite results. Echodense carotid plaques have been associated with an increased risk of stroke.[46,47] A similar observation was reported for coronary calcium score, which was significantly associated with an increased risk of vascular events.[48]

The logical conclusion from such opposite results is that both protective and deleterious effects of carotid plaque calcification are possible. Echodense, calcified carotid plaque may be a marker of carotid plaque inactivity and stability and therefore associated with reduced risk of stroke. At the same time, calcified plaque may be a marker of an active and unstable plaque present in other cerebral arteries or other vascular beds

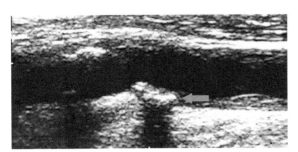

Figure 8.8 Echodense (calcified, bright) homogeneous plaque with acoustic shadowing (red arrow). (See color plate section.)

and may be associated with an increased risk of stroke and vascular events. Therefore, a patient with an evidence of echodense or calcified 'non-vulnerable' carotid plaque may still be considered a 'vulnerable patient'.

Plaque echodensity and echolucency are descriptive and subjective ultrasonographic morphological plaque characteristics. The ultrasound examiner subjectivity represents the main limitation of the ultrasound morphological assessments of plaque features. Several studies have reported that ultrasonographic plaque morphology evaluation has a low interobserver reliability.[49] Novel, computerized, and standardized ultrasound technologies such as the gray-scale median (GSM) analyses of plaque echogenicity are more objective methods and their evaluation is currently underway.[50]

The gray-scale median: a computer-assisted index of plaque echogenicity

In order to obtain the GSM index, images from a standard B-mode ultrasound of the vessel walls are captured and further analyzed on a computerized platform using a specific algorithm. GSM is generated after the color Doppler effect has been subtracted and echo frequencies analyzed in individual pixels determining differences in echogenicity. Although employing slightly different cut-off GSM values, several studies have consistently correlated low GSM numbers (hypoechoic plaques) with lipid-rich and necrotic material as well as intraplaque hemorrhage.[50–55] Moreover, selected areas of the plaque can be further scrutinized by normalized image analysis to increase the precision of the plaque echogenicity index.[56]

It seems that the GSM analysis of the plaque echolucency is a useful tool in assessment of carotid plaque embolic potential. However, this methodology is not ready yet for a prime-time use in clinical practice. Despite the relatively large number of studies reporting reliability of ultrasound evaluation of plaque echogenicity and a relatively high correlation with pathological specimens, criticism remains as to whether results have been consistent and whether some basic technical guidelines can be followed. A recent critical review of major studies on the correlation between ultrasonographic plaque features and histological characteristics has emphasized a poor consistency among different studies.[57]

SUMMARY

There is clear evidence that some but not all ultrasonographic features of atherosclerotic carotid plaque have a significant prognostic value for increased risk of cerebral ischemia. Sufficient data to support their predictive role for increased risk of stroke and other vascular events exist for the ultrasonographically determined degree of carotid stenosis, progression of carotid stenosis, and plaque size. Evidence regarding the predictive value of plaque echogenicity (echolucency or echodensity) for future vascular events is accumulating, but full confirmation in asymptomatic CAS patients is still awaited. The role of duplex ultrasound in assessing the degree of carotid stenosis, its progression, plaque size, and morphology is, however, indispensable in routine clinical practice.

REFERENCES

1. Tegos TJ, Sabetai MM, Nicolaides AN et al. Correlates of embolic events detected by means of transcranial Doppler in patients with carotid atheroma. J Vasc Surg 2001; 33: 131–8.
2. Siebler M, Kleinschmidt A, Sitzer M et al. Cerebral microembolism in symptomatic and asymptomatic high-grade internal carotid artery stenosis. Neurology 1994; 44: 615–18.
3. Molloy J, Markus HS. Asymptomatic embolization predicts stroke and TIA risk in patients with carotid artery stenosis. Stroke 1999; 30: 1440–3.
4. Spence JD, Tamayo A, Lownie SP, Ng WP, Ferguson GG. Absence of microemboli on transcranial Doppler identifies low-risk patients with asymptomatic carotid stenosis. Stroke 2005; 36: 2373–8.
5. Abbott AL, Chambers BR, Stork JL et al. Embolic signals and prediction of ipsilateral stroke or transient ischemic attack in asymptomatic carotid stenosis: a multicenter prospective cohort study. Stroke 2005; 36: 1128–33.
6. Johnston DC, Goldstein LB. Clinical carotid endarterectomy decision making: noninvasive vascular imaging versus angiography. Neurology 2001; 56: 1009–15.
7. North American Symptomatic Carotid Endarterectomy Trial Collaborators. Beneficial effect of carotid endarterectomy in symptomatic patients with high grade stenosis. N Engl J Med 1991; 325: 445–53.
8. European Carotid Surgery Triallists Collaborative Group. MRC European Carotid Surgery Trial: interim results for symptomatic patients with severe (70–99%) or mild (0–29%) carotid stenosis. Lancet 1991; 337: 1235–43.
9. Carra G, Visona A, Bonanome A et al. Carotid plaque morphology and cerebrovascular events. Int Angiol 2003; 22: 284–9.
10. Rothwell PM. Risk modeling to identify patients with symptomatic carotid stenosis most at risk of stroke. Neurol Res 2005; 27 (Suppl 1): S18–S28.
11. Chambers BR, Norris JW. Outcome in patients with asymptomatic neck bruits. N Engl J Med 1986; 315: 860–5.
12. Mackey AE, Abrahamowicz M, Langlois Y et al. Outcome of asymptomatic patients with carotid disease. Neurology 1997; 48: 896–903.
13. Bock RW, Gray-Weale AC, Mock PA et al. The natural history of asymptomatic carotid artery disease. J Vasc Surg 1993; 17(1): 160–9.
14. Halliday A, Mansfield A, Marro J et al; MRC Asymptomatic Carotid Surgery Trial (ACST) Collaborative Group. Prevention of disabling and fatal strokes by successful carotid endarterectomy in patients without recent neurological symptoms: randomised controlled trial. Lancet 2004; 363 (9420): 1491–502.
15. Nicolaides AN, Kakkos SK, Griffin M et al; Asymptomatic Carotid Stenosis and Risk of Stroke (ACSRS) Study Group. Severity of asymptomatic carotid stenosis and risk of ipsilateral hemispheric ischaemic events: results from the ACSRS study. Eur J Vasc Endovasc Surg 2005; 30: 275–84.
16. Lewis RF, Abrahamowicz M, Cote R, Battista RN. Predictive power of duplex ultrasonography in asymptomatic carotid disease. Ann Intern Med 1997; 127: 13–20.
17. Roederer GO, Langlois YE, Jager KA et al. The natural history of carotid arterial disease in asymptomatic patients with cervical bruits. Stroke 1984; 15: 605–13.
18. Sabeti S, Exner M, Mlekusch W et al. Prognostic impact of fibrinogen in carotid atherosclerosis: nonspecific indicator of inflammation or independent predictor of disease progression? Stroke 2005; 36(7): 1400–4.
19. Klop RB, Eikelboom BC, Taks AC. Screening of the internal carotid arteries in patients with peripheral vascular disease by colour-flow duplex scanning. Eur J Vasc Surg 1991; 5: 41–5.
20. Spence JD, Eliasziw M, DiCicco M. Carotid plaque area. A tool for targeting and evaluating vascular preventive therapy. Stroke 2002; 33: 2916–22.
21. Manolio TA, Burke GL, O'Leary DH et al. Relationships of cerebral MRI findings to ultrasonographic carotid atherosclerosis in older adults: the Cardiovascular Health Study. CHS Collaborative Research Group. Arterioscler Thromb Vasc Biol 1999; 19: 356–65.
22. Iemolo F, Martiniuk A, Steinman DA, Spence D. Sex differences in carotid plaque and stenosis. Stroke 2004; 35: 477–81.
23. Liapis CD, Kakisis JD, Kostakis AG. Carotid stenosis: factors affecting symptomatology. Stroke 2001; 32: 2782–6.
24. Steinke W, Hennerici M, Rautenberg W, Mohr JP. Symptomatic and asymptomatic high-grade stenoses in Doppler color-flow imaging. Neurology 1992; 42: 131–8.
25. Sitzer M, Müller W, Siebler M et al. Plaque ulceration and lumen thrombus are the main sources of cerebral microemboli in high-grade internal carotid artery stenosis. Stroke 1995; 26: 1231–3.
26. Eliasziw M, Streifler JY, Fox AJ et al. Significance of plaque ulceration in symptomatic patients with high-grade carotid stenosis. Stroke 1994; 25: 304–8.
27. Streifler JY, Eliasziw M, Fox AJ et al. Angiographic detection of carotid plaque ulceration. Comparison with surgical observations in a multicenter study. North American Symptomatic Carotid Endarterectomy Trial. Stroke 1994; 25(6): 1130–2.
28. Sztajzel R. Ultrasonographic assessment of the morphological characteristics of the carotid plaque. Swiss Med Wkly 2005; 135: 635–43.
29. Schminke U, Motsch L, Hilker L, Kessler C. Three-dimensional ultrasound observation of carotid artery plaque ulceration. Stroke 2000; 31: 1651–5.
30. De Bray JM, Baud JM, Dauzat M. Consensus concerning the morphology and the risk of carotid plaques. Cerebrovasc Dis 1996; 7: 289–96.
31. Reilly LM, Lusby RJ, Hugues L et al. Carotid plaque histology using real-time ultrasonography: clinical and therapeutic implications. Am J Surg 1997; 113: 1352–8.
32. Polak JF, Shemanski L, O'Leary DH et al. Hypoechoic plaque at US of the carotid artery: an independent risk factor for incident stroke in adults aged 65 years or older. Radiology 1998; 208: 649–54.
33. Mathiesen EB, Bonaa KH, Joakimsen O. Echolucent plaques are associated with high risk of ischemic cerebrovascular events in carotid stenosis: the Tromso study. Circulation 2001; 103: 2171–5.
34. Gronholdt ML, Nordestgaard BG, Schroeder TV et al. Ultrasonic echolucent carotid plaques predict future strokes. Circulation 2001; 104: 68–73.
35. European Carotid Plaque Study Group. Carotid artery plaque composition and relationship to clinical presentation and ultrasound B-mode imaging. Eur J Vasc Endovasc Surg 1995; 10: 23–30.
36. Grønholdt ML, Nordestgaard BG, Wiebe BM, Wilhjelm JE, Sillesen H. Echo-lucency of computerized ultrasound images of

carotid atherosclerotic plaques are associated with increased levels of triglyceride-rich lipoproteins as well as increased plaque lipid content. Circulation 1998; 97: 34–40.

37. Kofoed SC, Grønholdt ML, Bismuth J et al. Echolucent, rupture-prone carotid plaques associated with elevated triglyceride-rich lipoproteins, particularly in women. J Vasc Surg 2002; 36: 783–92.

38. Grønholdt ML, Nordestgaard BG, Bentzon J et al. Macrophages are associated with lipid-rich carotid artery plaques, echolucency on B-mode imaging, and elevated plasma lipid levels. J Vasc Surg 2002; 35: 137–45.

39. Yamagami H, Kitagawa K, Nagai Y et al. Higher levels of interleukin-6 are associated with lower echogenicity of carotid artery plaques. Stroke 2004; 35: 677–81.

40. Elkind MS, Cheng J, Boden-Albala B et al. Elevated white blood cell count and carotid plaque thickness: the Northern Manhattan Stroke Study. Stroke 2001; 32: 842–9.

41. Biasi GM, Froio A, Dietrich EB et al. Carotid plaque echolucency increases the risk of stroke in carotid stenting. The Imaging in Carotid Angioplasty and Risk of Stroke (ICAROS) Study. Circulation 2004; 110: 756–62.

42. Ohki T, Marin ML, Lyon RT et al. Ex vivo human carotid artery bifurcation stenting: correlation of lesion characteristics with embolic potential. J Vasc Surg 1998; 27: 463–71.

43. Shaalan WE, Cheng H, Gewertz B et al. Degree of carotid plaque calcification in relation to symptomatic outcome and plaque inflammation. J Vasc Surg 2004; 40: 262–9.

44. Johnson JM, Kennelly MM, Decesare D, Morgan S, Sparrow A. Natural history of asymptomatic carotid plaque. Arch Surg 1985; 120: 1010–12.

45. Gray-Weale AC, Graham JC, Burnett JR, Byrne K, Lusby RJ. Carotid artery atheroma: comparison of preoperative B-mode ultrasound appearance with carotid endarterectomy specimen pathology. J Cardiovasc Surg 1988; 29: 676–81.

46. Fanning NF, Walters TD, Fox AJ, Symons SP. Association between calcification of the cervical carotid artery bifurcation and white matter ischemia. AJNR Am J Neuroradiol 2006; 27(2): 378–83.

47. Nandalur KR, Baskurt E, Hagspiel KD et al. Carotid artery calcification on CT may independently predict stroke risk. AJR Am J Roentgenol 2006; 186(2): 547–52.

48. Greenland P, LaBree L, Azen SP, Doherty TM, Detrano RC. Coronary artery calcium score combined with Framingham score for risk prediction in asymptomatic individuals. JAMA 2004; 291: 210–15.

49. Hartmann A, Mohr JP, Thompson JL, Ramos O, Mast H. Interrater reliability of plaque morphology classification in patients with severe carotid artery stenosis. Acta Neurol Scand 1999; 99: 61–4.

50. Biasi GM, Sampaolo A, Mingazzini P et al. Computer analysis of ultrasonic plaque echolucency in identifying high risk carotid bifurcation lesions. Eur J Vasc Endovasc Surg 1999; 17: 476–9.

51. Gronholdt MLM. Ultrasound and lipoproteins as predictors of lipid-rich, rupture-prone plaques in the carotid artery. Arterioscler Thromb Vasc Biol 1999; 19: 2–13.

52. Matsagas MI, Vasdekis SN, Gugulakis AG et al. Computer-assisted ultrasonographic analysis of carotid plaques in relation to cerebrovascular symptoms, cerebral infarction, and histology. Ann Vasc Surg 2000; 14: 130–7.

53. El-Barghouty NM, Levine T, Ladva S et al. Histological verification of computerized carotid plaque characterization. Eur J Vasc Endovasc Surg 1996; 11: 414–16.

54. Tegos TJ, Sohail M, Sabetai MM et al. Echomorphologic and histopathologic characteristics of unstable carotid plaques. AJNR Am J Neuroradiol 2000; 21: 1937–44.

55. Sztajzel R, Momjian S, Momjian-Mayor I et al. Stratified grey-scale median analysis and color mapping of the carotid plaque: correlation with endarterectomy specimen histology of 28 patients. Stroke 2005; 36: 741–5.

56. Denzel C, Balzer K, Muller KM et al. Relative value of normalized sonographic in vitro analysis of arteriosclerotic plaques of internal carotid artery. Stroke 2003; 34: 1901–6.

57. Lovett JK, Redgrave JN, Rothwell PM. A critical appraisal of the performance, reporting, and interpretation of studies comparing carotid plaque imaging with histology. Stroke 2005; 36: 1091–7.

9

Risk stratification of patients with asymptomatic carotid artery stenosis: transcranial Doppler-based evaluation of asymptomatic cerebral microemboli

Lee Birnbaum, Tatjana Rundek and Andrei V Alexandrov

Take-Home Messages

1. Cerebral embolism accounts for up to 70% of all ischemic strokes. These emboli originate from carotid occlusive disease, diseases of the heart, aortic arch atheroma, and plaques in vertebral and intracranial arteries.
2. Cerebral microembolic signals (MES) detected by Transcranial Doppler (TCD) are defined as HITS of duration <300 ms, exceeding the background signal by at least 3 dB, and are unidirectional within the Doppler velocity spectrum.
3. The detection of cerebral MES by TCD relies on subjective operator analysis. Automated computer-assisted MES detection systems are in development, and further studies are needed to confirm their reliability before their widespread use in clinical practice.
4. In patients with asymptomatic carotid artery stenosis (CAS) the prevalence of MES varies between 1 and 23%, whereas in patients with symptomatic CAS that prevalence varies between 27 and 82%.
5. The variability in prevalence of cerebral MES in patients with asymptomatic CAS depends on the severity of the carotid stenosis and morphology of the carotid plaque, and the frequency and duration of TCD monitoring.
6. The presence of cerebral MES in patients with asymptomatic CAS is associated with a 4–5-fold increased risk of stroke. However, the clinical utility of this technique to discriminate among patients who will benefit from carotid revascularization vs patients who would not awaits confirmation in prospective trials.

INTRODUCTION

Transcranial Doppler (TCD) is a non-invasive ultrasonic technique that monitors blood flow velocity and blood flow direction in large intracranial arteries.[1] In 1982 Aaslid and colleagues introduced TCD to clinical practice by monitoring blood flow in the basal cerebral arteries.[2] Since then, TCD has been utilized to detect microemboli during carotid endarterectomy (CEA),[3,4] cardiac surgery,[5] stroke associated with atrial fibrillation (AF),[6] and in patients with prosthetic heart valves (PHVs).[7] Recent reports suggest that these microemboli

may indicate an increased risk of stroke or have clinical sequelae.[8–13] Nonetheless, studies have yet to clearly show that the reduction of cerebral emboli detected by TCD results in improved outcomes.[14]

BACKGROUND

Cerebral embolism from any source is thought to account for the majority of stroke cases. It has been reported as the underlying pathology in anywhere from 15% to 70% of all ischemic strokes.[15–20] These emboli may originate from the heart, aortic arch, carotid, vertebral, and intracranial arteries, or the venous system. Although determining the exact source of embolism remains a challenge, cardiogenic embolism is believed to be the major category of embolic stroke, followed by artery-to-artery embolism.

The pathophysiology behind embolism involves a particle of variable constitution that travels through the cerebral bloodstream until it wedges into an artery whose diameter is smaller than that of the particle. The embolic material is most commonly mural thrombi and platelet aggregates.[21] These short-lived aggregates often disorganize and allow for recanalization in the occluded vessel. Within the first 48 hours of stroke, TCD serial studies have shown recanalization of middle cerebral artery (MCA) mainstem or branch occlusions in up to 52% of cases.[22–24] One of these studies suggests that cardiogenic emboli are more likely to disorganize and allow for recanalization than arterial emboli.[23] Although TCD provides useful information, it is not able to determine which emboli will dissolve nor from where they originated.

As use becomes more widespread, TCD is being criticized for its variability by center, protocol, and diagnostic criteria. To improve reliability and promote standardization, certified ultrasound laboratories have been established and a Neurosonology proficiency examination by the American Society of Neuroimaging (www.asnweb.org). This is the only test that comprehensively assesses the physician's knowledge of TCD. In addition, the Therapeutics and Technology Assessment Subcommittee of the American Academy of Neurology published a report on TCD applications for clinical use.[14] They assigned type B, class II–IV evidence for TCD use in the detection of cerebral MES. This report states that 'TCD is probably useful to detect cerebral microembolic signals in a wide variety of cardiovascular and cerebrovascular disorders and procedures'.

TCD has established itself as a relatively easy, non-invasive, and safe tool in the diagnosis of stroke. In the hands of a proficient operator, TCD appears to be a sensitive test for the detection of intracranial emboli.[3–5] Because TCD has become an important tool in the armamentarium against stroke, clinicians should better understand its basic concepts and applications.

CEREBRAL MICROEMBOLIC SIGNALS

TCD detects microemboli in real time by measuring an increase in the returned Doppler-shifted ultrasonic power.[25] A range-gated, pulsed-Doppler ultrasonic beam of 1–2 MHz is transmitted through a skull window.[2] The temporal, orbital, and foramen magnum windows are exploited to insonate intracranial arteries. The transmitted

ultrasonic beam interfaces with a moving erythrocyte or microemboli, and is reflected back to the device recorder. This reflected ultrasonic power is called backscatter, and the difference between the transmitted signal and the received signal is called the Doppler shift.[26]

Because erythrocytes move at different speeds, returned Doppler signals from an artery fluctuate.[27,28] This intrinsic fluctuation of frequency creates a standard scatter. A passing microembolus can only be detected by TCD when its backscatter is greater than the standard scatter by a certain chosen threshold in decibels (dB). Thus, some emboli may pass the recorder undetected. The backscatter from solid emboli is typically higher than the standard scatter, and that from gaseous emboli of similar size is even higher. Thus far, however, reliable conclusions regarding the composition and size of a microembolus cannot be made due to the limitation of technical parameters.[29,30] Such parameters include size of the sample volume, recording time, and instrument settings. These parameters are set by the various manufacturers and operators of the equipment.

MES are also called transient high-intensity signals (HITS). These two acronyms are used interchangeably in clinical practice and in the literature (Figure 9.1).

Definition of cerebral microemboli or high-intensity hit signals

Cerebral microemboli are defined by the following criteria:

1. Duration of HITS less than 300 ms.
2. HITS exceed the background by at least 3 dB.
3. HITS are unidirectional within the Doppler velocity spectrum.[30]

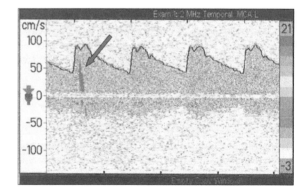

Figure 9.1 Cerebral microembolic signals (MES) or high-intensity transient signals (HITS) detected in the middle cerebral artery (red arrow) in the Doppler spectrum obtained by TCD monitoring. (See color plate section.)

However, these criteria are not uniform. Depending on the reference, a baseline excess of anywhere from 3 to 9 dB above standard scatter defines a true HITS.[30–32] Although criteria are helpful, differentiation between artifact and solid emboli still remains a technical challenge.

The reliability of TCD-HITS monitoring has been criticized because most studies have relied on subjective operator analysis to distinguish between true HITS and artifact. Although high interobserver agreement of HITS detection has been shown in several studies, high cost and reliability issues remain the driving force for development of an automated computer-assisted HITS detection system.[33–36] Automatic recognition of HITS is necessary for widespread use of detection of microemboli by TCD in clinical practice. Such a system needs to reliably discriminate between artifact and microemboli as well as to classify microemboli.

Multifrequency TCD has been clinically shown to differentiate between solid and gaseous microemboli,[37] but this observation was not confirmed in most recent studies. The distinction of emboli composition may be achieved by insonating microemboli simultaneously with two different ultrasound frequencies. Solid and gaseous emboli reflect more ultrasound power at a higher and lower frequency, respectively. Reflection of ultrasound power depends on both the size and composition of the embolus. By exploiting this principle, automated differentiation is possible.[38,39] Nonetheless, some sources of error with multifrequency TCD include microembolus size limits, resonance effects of tiny gaseous emboli,

and a problem of detection when multiple emboli are passing through the sample volume at the same time.[37]

Although the development of multifrequency TCD systems shows promise, an automated system has yet to completely satisfy the requirements of reliably discriminating between artifact and microemboli and classifying microemboli by their composition. These systems are not yet ready for routine clinical use. Further studies to address these limitations are pivotal to ensure validity of automated HITS detection by multifrequency TCD.

CEREBRAL MICROEMBOLI IN STROKE

Cerebral microemboli can be detected in a wide variety of pathological conditions as well as in association with various cerebrovascular procedures (Figure 9.2). HITS detection may be helpful in determining the pathogenesis of stroke. HITS are most commonly found in patients with persistent neurological deficits from large-artery strokes.[40] Such strokes are probably a result of carotid or cardiogenic emboli. HITS are also commonly detected in elderly patients with large aortic arch atheromas (Figure 9.3).[41] This finding supports the role of aortic arch plaque emboli in the pathogenesis of stroke. Patients with small-vessel strokes, on the other hand, infrequently exhibit HITS on TCD monitoring.[40]

In addition to determining pathogenesis of stroke, the detection of recurrent HITS by TCD may also be helpful in clinical trials and stroke prevention strategies.[42]

Cerebral microemboli can be detected:

- during procedures including angiography, carotid angioplasty and stenting, open heart surgery, carotid endarterectomy
- in patients with transient ischemic attacks or stroke
- asymptomatic carotid stenosis
- heart valve prosthesis
- intracranial arterial disease
- large aortic arch atheromas

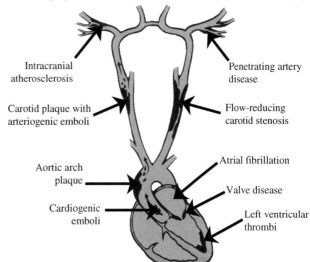

Figure 9.2 Sources of cerebral microemboli.

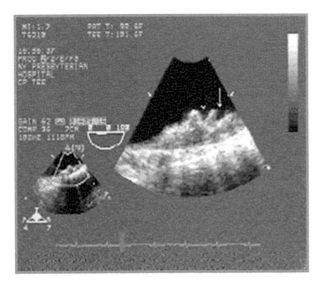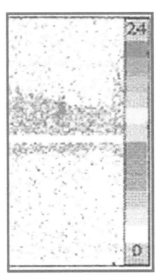

Figure 9.3 Cerebral microembolic signals (MES) detected by TCD in a stroke patient with aortic arch atheroma visualized by transesophageal echocardiography (TEE). TEE courtesy of Marco R Di Tullio MD. (See color plate section.)

Detection of HITS by TCD may be a useful predictor of sequential stroke risk and a surrogate endpoint of stroke in clinical trials.

TCD, unfortunately, only suffices two of the three necessary criteria to serve as a valid surrogate measure.[43] First, TCD-detected emboli can serve as a clinical marker for stroke. Secondly, TCD-detected emboli can reliably predict stroke. Cerebral microemboli on TCD have been correlated with ischemic events in both CEA and carotid stenosis.[44] The third criteria involves demonstration that a therapy which reduces the number of TCD-detected emboli translates into a reduction of stroke incidence. Adequate fulfillment of this last criterion has been questioned based on various study results. Two pharmacological agents that are known to reduce platelet aggregation have been clinically shown to significantly reduce the number of TCD-detected emboli in patients immediately post-CEA.[45] Nonetheless, 5 of the 42 (12%) patients treated with these agents still experienced post-CEA neurological events even though they did not have HITS demonstrated on TCD after the treatment. Future studies are needed to validate the correlation between reduced HITS on TCD and risk reduction of stroke.

CEREBRAL MICROEMBOLI IN PATIENTS WITH CAROTID ARTERY DISEASE

TCD is a helpful tool in detecting and understanding the significance of microembolic material from the

carotid artery atheroma. In 1990, TCD detection of solid, rather than gaseous, emboli in the MCA was reported in patients undergoing CEA.[4] TCD signals similar to that detected from air emboli were recorded prior to opening the carotid artery. These signals were explained as a result of solid emboli that had dislodged from the carotid plaque while the surgeon was dissecting the carotid artery. This was confirmed later by both in-vivo and in-vitro models.[43] After MES were reported during CEA, similar spontaneous signals were identified in patients with symptomatic and asymptomatic carotid stenosis.[46–50]

MES prevalence in patients with carotid stenosis appears to be highest among symptomatic patients and increases as the length of recording time increases. Studies have shown MES detection in 29%[49] and 27%[50] of patients recorded for 30 minutes, 57%[51] of those recorded for 1 hour, and one study[31] detected MES in all 14 patients studied with a mean recording time of 3.2 hours. Although universal recording protocols have yet to be established, a 1-hour recording time on at least one occasion is a minimum standard for patients with carotid artery disease.[30]

The potential applications of this technique in patients with carotid disease include identifying at-risk patients, appropriate assignment to pharmacological and revascularization therapies, monitoring pharmacological effectiveness, and monitoring during interventional procedures such as CEA, carotid angioplasty and stenting, and cerebral angiography. In this section, we focus on the prevalence and prognostic significance of

MES in patients with symptomatic vs asymptomatic carotid disease as well as the effect of carotid lesion severity and morphology on the prevalence of MES in these patients.

Prevalence and prognostic value of cerebral microembolic signals in patients with symptomatic carotid artery stenosis

The prevalence of MES and its prognostic value in predicting recurrent neurological events in patients with symptomatic CAS have been extensively reported.[51–55] In the study by Markus and MacKinnon among 200 symptomatic CAS (>50%) patients, the presence of MES was associated with 4–5 times increased risk of recurrent stroke or transient ischemic attack (TIA) (27% recurrent strokes or TIA; adjusted hazard ratio (HR) = 4.67; 95% CI 1.99–11.01) during 90 days of follow-up.[52] The absence of MES identified a group at low risk for stroke alone and stroke and TIA during follow-up: 0% and 7.5%, respectively, vs 3.5% and 15.5%. Also, in patients with symptomatic stenosis, MES is most frequently detected in the ensuing days or weeks after a TIA or stroke.[31,32,56–58] This finding is in agreement with data from the North American Symptomatic Carotid Endarterectomy Trial (NASCET)[59] and the European Carotid Surgery Trial (ECST)[60] where the risk of recurrent stroke was greatest within the first few months following the last neurological event.

The prevalence of MES in these patients appears to increase when TCD monitoring is performed closer to the acute event. In the largest published series of an unselected group of stroke patients, HITS were detected in 10% of patients who were monitored by TCD within a month of their stroke onset.[50] In comparison to another unselected group, ipsilateral MES were detected in 25% of stroke patients who were monitored by TCD within 2 days of admission.[40] These observations suggest that atherosclerotic plaque or thrombus may have increased 'emboligenicity' or 'vulnerability' at the time of stroke and that repeated TCD examinations may be an important predictor of sequential stroke.

Confirming the relationship between MES and the carotid plaque, MES detection, alongside the ipsilateral stroke risk, significantly decreases after successful CEA.[31,32] The frequency of MES has also been shown to decrease with anticoagulant or antiplatelet therapy[32,61] and TCD monitoring for HITS may predict medical therapy failure prior to another TIA or stroke.

Prevalence and prognostic significance of cerebral microembolic signals in patients with asymptomatic carotid artery stenosis

The prevalence of cerebral MES in patients with asymptomatic CAS (Figure 9.4) varies widely but is significantly less than in patients with symptomatic CAS (see Table 9.1).

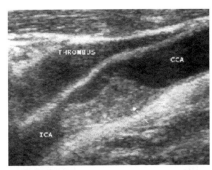

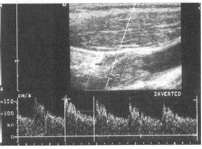

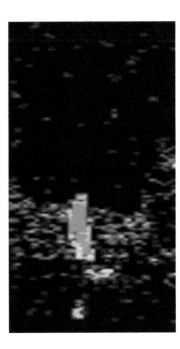

Figure 9.4 Cerebral microembolic signals (MES) detected in the middle cerebral artery (MCA) in an asymptomatic patient with a large irregular atherosclerotic plaque in the carotid artery (60–80% stenosis of the internal carotid artery at the carotid bifurcation) on duplex ultrasound. (See color plate section.)

Table 9.1 Prevalence of cerebral MES in the middle cerebral artery ipsilateral to asymptomatic and symptomatic CAS in the first reported studies to determine the frequency of MES

Study	Degree of CAS (%)	TCD monitoring time (min)	Asymptomatic CAS prevalence of MES N (%)	Symptomatic CAS prevalence of MES N (%)
Siebler et al, 1994[54]	>70	150	9 (16.1)	27 (81.8)
Markus et al, 1995[32]	>70	20	1 (0.6)	8 (34.7)
Orlandi et al, 1997[68]	>70	60	5 (23.3)	17 (56.7)
Georgiadis et al, 1997[72]	>70	30	3 (7.5)	10 (27.0)
Molloy et al, 1998[46]	>70	60	4 (20.0)	10 (50.0)
Droste et al, 1999[17]	>70	60	4 (10.0)	21 (33.0)

CAS, carotid artery stenosis; TCD, transcranial Doppler; MES, microembolic signals.

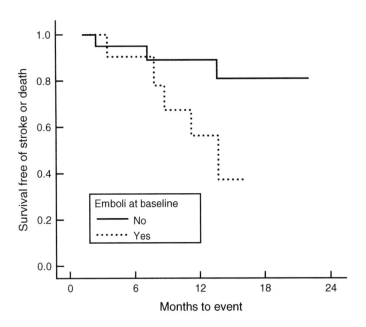

Figure 9.5 Survival free of stroke or death by microembolic status at baseline. A Kaplan–Meier plot shows that patients with microemboli at baseline were more likely to experience a stroke or death during 2 years of follow-up; most of the events occurred soon after the microemboli were detected. Log rank $p < 0.0001$. (Adapted from Spence et al.[65])

Several studies have indicated that TCD-detected MES may be useful in identifying patients with asymptomatic CAS at high risk of ipsilateral stroke or TIA.[62–65] The Asymptomatic Stenosis Embolus Detection (ASED) Study[64] reported on 202 patients with asymptomatic CAS (60–99%), without other apparent cerebroembolic sources, who underwent several 60-minute MES monitoring and intermediate-term follow-up (mean follow-up = 34 months). Patients who had MES-positive arteries had more ipsilateral carotid ischemic events (10%) than those who had MES-negative arteries (7%), but the difference was not statistically significant. The findings of this study were limited by the low rates of MES

detection (7.7% of studies) and the low rate of ipsilateral carotid stroke (annual rate of 1%).

Spence and colleagues[65] demonstrated a clear relationship between cerebral MES positivity and incidence of future stroke in patients with asymptomatic CAS. In this prospective observational study, 319 patients with asymptomatic CAS were monitored for MES prospectively with TCD imaging 2 times for up to 1 hour, 1 week apart. At 1 year, the stroke risk among the 32 (10%) patients with MES was 15% vs 1% in the group without MES ($p < 0.0001$) (Figure 9.5). In this study, the confidence limits of the event rate in patients with negative MES were very small, indicating a high statistical certainty of the very low stroke rate (~1%/year) and that carotid revascularization can be delayed. On the other hand, although patients with positive MES had a 15.6-fold increase in the risk of stroke, the number of strokes were small and the confidence limits were wider, indicating lower statistical certainty of the results. Therefore, the authors concluded that these findings should be tested in clinical trials.

It has been estimated, based on the ASED study,[64] that the required sample size to test the hypothesis that the detection of MES can be used to identify subjects with asymptomatic CAS at high risk of ipsilateral carotid stroke/TIA is ~500–2000 subjects, depending on the projected outcome event rates.

What are the predictors of cerebral microembolic signals in patients with asymptomatic carotid artery stenosis?

In patients with asymptomatic CAS, the prevalence of distal embolization increases with increasing lesion severity until a stenosis of approximately 90%, but then decreases with very tight stenoses.[63] Molloy and Markus[63] found no cerebral MES at all in asymptomatic patients with >90% stenosis. A tight stenosis can be accompanied by reduced flow and distal internal carotid artery collapse, and this might be expected pathophysiologically to confer reduced risk. This is consistent with data from the NASCET trial,[66] demonstrating a reduced risk of stroke above stenoses with distal internal carotid artery (ICA) collapse compared with 90% stenoses without distal collapse.

In addition to lesion severity, there are preliminary data suggesting that cerebral MES is related to carotid plaque morphology. Sitzer and colleagues[67] found a correlation between preoperative MES and intraluminal thrombus and plaque ulceration of CEA specimens of asymptomatic and symptomatic patients with CAS. There were no correlations between MES and plaque fissuring or intraplaque hemorrhage.[67] Other studies have demonstrated a positive association between MES and plaque ulceration based on conventional angiogram.[68]

CEREBRAL MICROEMBOLI FROM THE HEART

TCD has been a useful tool in predicting neurological outcome in cardiopulmonary bypass surgery. Intraoperative MES detected by TCD not only provide an indirect index of cerebral blood flow but also positively correlate with poor neurological and neuropsychological outcomes.[4,5,69,70]

The general use of TCD has most frequently detected MES in patients with mitral valve strands, PHVs, and patent foramen ovale (PFO).[48] Along with its intraoperative use, TCD monitoring to identify MES from cardiac sources may be helpful to determine the cause of stroke and appropriate treatment strategies.

MES are also detected in patients with cardioembolic stroke but without evidence of valvular disease. One prospective study evaluated acute stroke patients with echocardiography-confirmed potential cardiac emboli.[71] Forty of the acute stroke patients (51%) showed MES during at least one of three serial TCD examinations. TCD monitoring time was for 30 minutes at admission, after 24 hours, and again after 48 hours. MES were most commonly detected in those patients with AF, coronary artery disease, low ejection fraction of <30%, and infectious endocarditis. The influence of anticoagulation therapy on the occurrence of MES in these patients remains unclear. Although patients receiving anticoagulation treatment tended to show less MES, this difference was not statistically significant. In a study of 300 patients, bilateral TCD monitoring detected MES in 45% of patients with infective endocarditis, 34% with left ventricular aneurysm, 26% with intracardiac thrombus, 26% with dilative cardiomyopathy, 21% with non-valvular AF and in 15% of patients with valvular disease.[72]

In patients with stroke of unclear etiology, a PFO has been detected in as many as 50% of patients.[73] TCD monitoring of intracranial vessels during intravenous injection of agitated saline may be used to detect intracardiac right-to-left shunts (Figure 9.6). An intracardiac shunt is deemed positive when HITS, in this case representing microbubbles that reach the brain, are detected by TCD.[74–76] When a standardized protocol with Valsalva maneuver is used, TCD monitoring is as effective as transesophageal echocardiography (TEE) for detecting an intracardiac shunt.[77] In addition, TCD not only provides evidence that a cardiac shunt exists but also demonstrates real-time feasibility for paradoxical, embolic flow. TCD can detect HITS from intravenous injection of agitated saline with a sensitivity and specificity that approaches 100%.[78] Factors that influence the detection of PFO include the timing of the Valsalva, the amount of contrast media used, and the patient's positioning during the test.[79,80] However, false-positive results may arise when a patient without a PFO has an intrapulmonary shunt. The use of TCD and echocardiography together greatly reduces this likelihood and approaches 100% specificity.

HITS detected by TCD have been demonstrated in patients with AF.[81] TCD studies examining HITS and anticoagulation in patients with AF have given conflicting results. No clear evidence exists that the frequency of

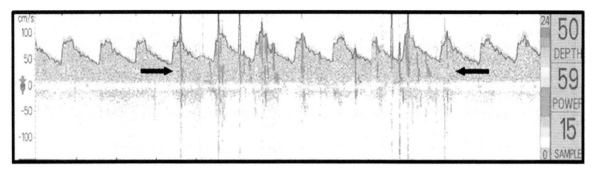

Figure 9.6 Transcranial Doppler (TCD) detection of right-to-left cardiac shunt (PFO; patent foramen ovale). Single-gate spectral TCD waveform display of the middle cerebral artery (MCA) at a depth of 50 mm. Over 15 microemboli of high signal intensity appeared after the intravenous injection of agitated saline (9 ml normal saline mixed with 1 ml air) and rapidly disappeared (between the two arrows). Monitoring started 10 seconds prior to agitated saline injection and continued for 2 minutes after the bolus. (See color plate section.)

HITS decreases after a patient with AF is anticoagulated. In addition, anticoagulation has not been shown to change the frequency of HITS in patients with biomechanical heart valves.[82]

The presence of MES has been noted in a variety of heart valves.[82] Certain PHVs have a higher prevalence of MES than others.[83] Also, the prevalence of MES was higher in patients with mechanical valves (58%) than in patients with porcine (43%) or homograft valves (20%).[83] Adequately anticoagulated, asymptomatic patients with PHV have been shown to have greater than 40 000 MES/day.[21] Fortunately, such MES associated with PHV are predominately benign. For PHV patients already taking coumadin, the addition of aspirin does not influence the rate of MES.[84] Monitoring of PHV patients placed in a hyperbaric chamber demonstrates reduction in the number of HITS.[85] These findings indicate that cavitational gaseous microbubbles can form at prosthetic valves and most likely represent a significant proportion of HITS detected in these patients. These HITS may be less dangerous for future strokes, as gaseous bubbles resorb promptly in cerebral circulation.

SUMMARY

TCD detection of MES is an established and routinely used diagnostic test that will continue to evolve in the future to advance our abilities to diagnose and treat stroke patients as well as asymptomatic patients with carotid stenosis. TCD-detected microemboli can serve as a clinical marker for stroke and can reliably predict stroke in high-risk populations. Clinical trials of various medical therapies and interventional procedures aimed to demonstrate

a reduction of stroke incidence after a reduction of the number of TCD-detected microemboli are currently underway. To ensure better reliability of the MES detection, the International Consensus Group on Microembolus Detection has published MES definitions for spectral Doppler,[36] and subsequent detailed recommendations for reporting MES studies.[86] In addition, the establishment of certified Doppler laboratories ensures appropriate implementation of these guidelines by proficient technicians and physicians alike (www.icavl.org). The future development of automated systems to obtain and process Doppler data and determine HITS will best facilitate standardization and routine use in clinical practice. Until that time, data obtained from certified Doppler laboratories remain the gold standard.

REFERENCES

1. Babikian VL, Feldmann E, Wechsler LR et al. Transcranial Doppler ultrasonography: year 2000 update. J Neuroimaging 2000; 10(2): 101–15.
2. Aaslid R, Markwalder TM, Nornes H. Noninvasive transcranial Doppler ultrasound recording of flow velocity in basal cerebral arteries. J Neurosurg 1982; 57(6): 769–74.
3. Padayachee TS, Gosling RG, Bishop CC et al. Monitoring middle cerebral artery blood velocity during carotid endarterectomy. Br J Surg 1986; 73(2): 98–100.
4. Spencer MP, Thomas GI, Nicholls SC, Sauvage LR. Detection of middle cerebral artery emboli during carotid endarterectomy using transcranial Doppler ultrasonography. Stroke 1990; 21(3): 415–23.
5. Pugsley W. The use of Doppler ultrasound in the assessment of microemboli during cardiac surgery. Perfusion 1986; 4: 115–22.
6. Tegeler CH, Hitchings LP, Eicke M. Microemboli detection in stroke associated with atrial fibrillation. J Cardiovasc Technol 1990; 9: 283–4.
7. Berger M, Davis D, Colley D et al. Detection of sub-clinical microemboli in patients with prosthetic aortic valves. J Cardiovasc Technol 1990; 9: 282–3.

8. Jansen C, Ramos LM, van Heesewijk JP et al. Impact of microembolism and hemodynamic changes in the brain during carotid endarterectomy. Stroke 1994; 25(5): 992–7.

9. Gaunt ME, Martin PJ, Smith JL et al. Clinical relevance of intraoperative embolization detected by transcranial Doppler ultrasonography during carotid endarterectomy: a prospective study of 100 patients. Br J Surg 1994; 81(10): 1435–9.

10. Pugsley W, Klinger L, Paschalis C et al. The impact of microemboli during cardiopulmonary bypass on neuropsychological functioning. Stroke 1994; 25(7): 1393–9.

11. Ackerstaff RG, Jansen C, Moll FL et al. The significance of microemboli detection by means of transcranial Doppler ultrasonography monitoring in carotid endarterectomy. J Vasc Surg 1995; 21(6): 963–9.

12. Spencer MP. Transcranial Doppler monitoring and causes of stroke from carotid endarterectomy. Stroke 1997; 28(4): 685–91.

13. Levi CR, O'Malley HM, Fell G et al. Transcranial Doppler detected cerebral microembolism following carotid endarterectomy. High microembolic signal loads predict postoperative cerebral ischaemia. Brain 1997; 120(Pt 4): 621–9.

14. Sloan MA, Alexandrov AV, Tegeler CH et al. Therapeutics and Technology Assessment Subcommittee of the American Academy of Neurology. Assessment: transcranial Doppler ultrasonography: report of the Therapeutics and Technology Assessment Subcommittee of the American Academy of Neurology. Neurology 2004; 62(9): 1468–81.

15. Foulkes MA, Wolf PA, Price TR et al. The Stroke Data Bank: design, methods, and baseline characteristics. Stroke 1988; 19(5): 547–54.

16. Fieschi C, Argentino C, Lenzi GL et al. Clinical and instrumental evaluation of patients with ischemic stroke within the first six hours. J Neurol Sci 1989; 91(3): 311–21.

17. Droste DW, Dittrich R, Kemeny V et al. Prevalence and frequency of microembolic signals in 105 patients with extracranial carotid artery occlusive disease. J Neurol Neurosurg Psychiatry 1999; 67(4): 525–8.

18. Kunitz SC, Gross CR, Heyman A et al. The pilot Stroke Data Bank: definition, design, and data. Stroke 1984; 15(4): 740–6.

19. Mohr JP, Caplan LR, Melski JW et al. The Harvard Cooperative Stroke Registry: a prospective registry. Neurology 1978; 28(8): 754–62.

20. Kolominsky-Rabas PL, Weber M, Gefeller O et al. Epidemiology of ischemic stroke subtypes according to TOAST criteria: incidence, recurrence, and long-term survival in ischemic stroke subtypes: a population-based study. Stroke 2001; 32(12): 2735–40.

21. Mohr JP, Choi DW, Grotta JC et al. Stroke: Pathophysiology, Diagnosis, and Management, 3rd edn. New York: Churchill Livingstone, 1998.

22. Kase CS, White RL, Vinson TL, Eichelberger RP. Shotgun pellet embolus to the middle cerebral artery. Neurology 1981; 31(4): 458–61.

23. Zanette EM, Roberti C, Mancini G et al. Spontaneous middle cerebral artery reperfusion in ischemic stroke. A follow-up study with transcranial Doppler. Stroke 1995; 26(3): 430–3.

24. Toni D, Fiorelli M, Zanette EM et al. Early spontaneous improvement and deterioration of ischemic stroke patients. A serial study with transcranial Doppler ultrasonography. Stroke 1998; 29(6): 1144–8.

25. Babikian VL, Wechsler LR, eds. Transcranial Doppler Ultrasonography. 2nd edn. Boston: Butterworth-Heinemann, 1999.

26. Aaslid R. The Doppler principle applied to measurement of blood flow velocities in cerebral arteries. In: Aaslid R, ed. Transcranial Doppler Sonography. Vienna: Springer-Verlag, 1986: 22–38.

27. Angelsen BA. A theoretical study of the scattering of ultrasound from blood. IEEE Trans Biomed Eng 1980; 27(2): 61–7.

28. Mo LY, Cobbold RS. A stochastic model of the backscattered Doppler ultrasound from blood. IEEE Trans Biomed Eng 1986; 33(1): 20–7.

29. Russell D. The detection of cerebral emboli using Doppler ultrasound. In: Newell DW, Aaslid R, eds. Transcranial Doppler. New York: Raven, 1992; 52–8.

30. Ackerstaff RG, Babikian VL, Georgiadis D et al. Basic identification criteria of Doppler microemboli signals: Consensus Committee of the Ninth International Cerebral Hemodynamics Symposium. Stroke 1995; 26: 1123.

31. Siebler M, Sitzer M, Rose G et al. Silent cerebral embolism caused by neurologically symptomatic high-grade carotid stenosis. Event rates before and after carotid endarterectomy. Brain 1993; 16(Pt 5): 1005–15.

32. Markus HS, Thomson ND, Brown MM. Asymptomatic cerebral embolic signals in symptomatic and asymptomatic carotid artery disease. Brain 1995; 118(Pt 4): 1005–11.

33. Georgiadis D, Kaps M, Siebler M et al. Variability of Doppler microembolic signal counts in patients with prosthetic cardiac valves. Stroke 1995; 26(3): 439–43.

34. Markus H, Bland JM, Rose G et al. How good is intercenter agreement in the identification of embolic signals in carotid artery disease? Stroke 1996; 27(7): 1249–52.

35. Van Zuilen EV, Mess WH, Jansen C et al. Automatic embolus detection compared with human experts. A Doppler ultrasound study. Stroke 1996; 27(10): 1840–3.

36. The International Cerebral Hemodynamics Society Consensus Statement. Stroke 1995; 26: 1123.

37. Russell D, Brucher R. Online automatic discrimination between solid and gaseous cerebral microemboli with the first multifrequency transcranial Doppler. Stroke 2002; 33(8): 1975–80.

38. Lubbers J, van der Berg JW. An ultrasonic detector for microgas emboli in a blood flow line. Ultrasound Med Biol 1976; 2: 301–10.

39. Moehring MA, Klepper JR. Pulse Doppler ultrasound detection, characterization and size estimation of emboli in flowing blood. IEEE Trans Biomed Eng 1994; 41(1): 35–44.

40. Daffertshofer M, Ries S, Schminke U, Hennerici M. High-intensity transient signals in patients with cerebral ischemia. Stroke 1996; 27(10): 1844–9.

41. Rundek T, Di Tullio MR, Sciacca RR et al. Association between large aortic arch atheromas and high-intensity transient signals in elderly stroke patients. Stroke 1999; 30(12): 2683–6.

42. Dittrich R, Ritter MA, Kaps M et al. The use of embolic signal detection in multicenter trials to evaluate antiplatelet efficacy: signal analysis and quality control mechanisms in the CARESS (Clopidogrel and Aspirin for Reduction of Emboli in Symptomatic carotid Stenosis) trial. Stroke 2006; 37(4): 1065–9

43. Grotta JC, Alexandrov AV. Preventing stroke: is preventing microemboli enough? Circulation 2001; 103(19): 2321–2.

44. Barnett HJ, Eliasziw M, Meldrum HE. Drugs and surgery in the prevention of ischemic stroke. N Engl J Med 1995; 332(4): 238–48.

45. Kaposzta Z, Baskerville PA, Madge D et al. L-arginine and S-nitrosoglutathione reduce embolization in humans. Circulation 2001; 103(19): 2371–5.

46. Molloy J, Khan N, Markus HS. Temporal variability of asymptomatic embolization in carotid artery stenosis and optimal recording protocol. Stroke 1998; 29: 1129–32.

47. Siebler M, Sitzer M, Steinmetz H. Detection of intracranial emboli in patients with symptomatic extracranial carotid artery disease. Stroke 1992; 23(11): 1652–4.

48. Grosset DG, Georgiadis D, Abdullah I et al. Doppler emboli signals vary according to stroke subtype. Stroke 1994; 25(2): 382–4.

49. Markus HS, Droste DW, Brown MM. Detection of asymptomatic cerebral embolic signals with Doppler ultrasound. Lancet 1994; 343(8904): 1011–12.

50. Daffertshofer M, Ries S, Schminke U, Hennerici M. High-intensity transient signals in patients with cerebral ischemia. Stroke 1996; 27(10): 1844–9.

51. Eicke BM, von Lorentz J, Paulus W. Embolus detection in different degrees of carotid disease. Neurol Res 1995; 17(3): 181–4.

52. Markus HS, MacKinnon A. Asymptomatic embolization detected by Doppler ultrasound predicts stroke risk in symptomatic carotid artery stenosis. Stroke 2005; 36: 971–5.

53. Wijman CA, Babikian VL, Matjucha IC et al. Cerebral microembolism in patients with retinal ischemia. Stroke 1998; 29(6): 1139–43.

54. Siebler M, Kleinschmidt A, Sitzer M et al. Cerebral microembolism in symptomatic and asymptomatic high-grade internal carotid artery stenosis. Neurology 1994; 44(4): 615–18.

55. Babikian VL, Hyde C, Pochay V, Winter MR. Clinical correlates of high-intensity transient signals detected on transcranial Doppler sonography in patients with cerebrovascular disease. Stroke 1994; 25(8): 1570–3.

56. Forteza AM, Babikian VL, Hyde C et al. Effect of time and cerebrovascular symptoms of the prevalence of microembolic signals in patients with cervical carotid stenosis. Stroke 1996; 27(4): 687–90.

57. Valton L, Larrue V, le Traon AP et al. Microembolic signals and risk of early recurrence in patients with stroke or transient ischemic attack. Stroke 1998; 29(10): 2125–8.

58. Babikian VL, Wijman CA, Hyde C et al. Cerebral microembolism and early recurrent cerebral or retinal ischemic events. Stroke 1997; 28(7): 1314–18.

59. Beneficial effect of carotid endarterectomy in symptomatic patients with high-grade carotid stenosis. North American Symptomatic Carotid Endarterectomy Trial Collaborators. N Engl J Med 1991; 325(7): 445–53.

60. MRC European Carotid Surgery Trial. Interim results for symptomatic patients with severe (70–99%) or with mild (0–29%) carotid stenosis. European Carotid Surgery Trialists' Collaborative Group. Lancet 1991; 337(8752): 1235–43.

61. Markus HS, Droste D, Brown MM. Ultrasonic detection of cerebral emboli in carotid stenosis. Lancet 1993; 341(8860): 1606.

62. Siebler M, Nachtmann A, Sitzer M et al. Cerebral microembolism and the risk of ischemia in asymptomatic high-grade internal carotid artery stenosis. Stroke. 1995; 26: 2184–6.

63. Molloy J, Markus HS. Asymptomatic embolization predicts stroke and TIA risk in patients with carotid artery stenosis. Stroke 1999; 30: 1440–3.

64. Abbott AL, Chambers BR, Stork JL et al. Embolic signals and prediction of ipsilateral stroke or transient ischemic attack in asymptomatic carotid stenosis: a multicenter prospective cohort study. Stroke 2005; 36: 1128–33.

65. Spence JD, Tamayo A, Lownie SP, Ng WP, Ferguson GG. Absence of microemboli on transcranial Doppler identifies low-risk patients with asymptomatic carotid stenosis. Stroke. 2005; 36: 2373–8.

66. Morgenstern LB, Fox AJ, Sharpe BL et al. The risks and benefits of carotid endarterectomy in patients with near occlusion of the carotid artery: North American Symptomatic Carotid Endarterectomy Trial (NASCET) Group. Neurology 1997; 48: 911–5.

67. Sitzer M, Muller W, Siebler M et al. Plaque ulceration and lumen thrombus are the main sources of cerebral microemboli in high-grade internal carotid artery stenosis. Stroke 1995; 26(7): 1231–3.

68. Orlandi G, Parenti G, Bertolucci A et al. Carotid plaque features on angiography and asymptomatic cerebral microembolism. Acta Neurol Scand 1997; 96(3): 183–6.

69. Harrison MJ, Pugsley W, Newman S et al. Detection of middle cerebral emboli during coronary artery bypass surgery using transcranial Doppler sonography. Stroke 1990; 21(10): 1512.

70. Clark RE, Brillman J, Davis DA et al. Microemboli during coronary artery bypass grafting. Genesis and effect on outcome. J Thorac Cardiovasc Surg 1995; 109(2): 249–58.

71. Sliwka U, Lingnau A, Stohlmann WD et al. Prevalence and time course of microembolic signals in patients with acute stroke. A prospective study. Stroke 1997; 28(2): 358–63.

72. Georgiadis D, Lindner A, Manz M et al. Intracranial microembolic signals in 500 patients with potential cardiac or carotid embolic source and in normal controls. Stroke 1997; 28(6): 1203–7.

73. Lechat P, Mas JL, Lascault G et al. Prevalence of patent foramen ovale in patients with stroke. N Engl J Med 1988; 318(18): 1148–52.

74. Chimowitz MI, Nemec JJ, Marwick TH et al. Transcranial Doppler ultrasound identifies patients with right-to-left cardiac or pulmonary shunts. Neurology 1991; 41(12): 1902–4.

75. Di Tullio M, Sacco RL, Venketasubramanian N et al. Comparison of diagnostic techniques for the detection of a patent foramen ovale in stroke patients. Stroke 1993; 24(7): 1020–4.

76. Itoh T, Matsumoto M, Handa N et al. Paradoxical embolism as a cause of ischemic stroke of uncertain etiology. A transcranial Doppler sonographic study. Stroke 1994; 25(4): 771–5.

77. Jauss M, Kaps M, Keberle M et al. A comparison of transesophageal echocardiography and transcranial Doppler sonography with contrast medium for detection of patent foramen ovale. Stroke 1994; 25(6): 1265–7.

78. Nemec JJ, Marwick TH, Lorig RJ et al. Comparison of transcranial Doppler ultrasound and transesophageal contrast echocardiography in the detection of interatrial right-to-left shunts. Am J Cardiol 1991; 68(15): 1498–502.

79. Schwarze JJ, Sander D, Kukla C et al. Methodological parameters influence the detection of right-to-left shunts by contrast transcranial Doppler ultrasonography. Stroke 1999; 30(6): 1234–9.

80. Droste DW, Jekentaite R, Stypmann J et al. Contrast transcranial Doppler ultrasound in the detection of right-to-left shunts: comparison of Echovist-200 and Echovist-300, timing of the Valsalva maneuver, and general recommendations for the performance of the test. Cerebrovasc Dis 2002; 13(4): 235–41.

81. Tegeler CH, Hitchings LP, Eicke M et al. Microemboli detection in stroke associated with atrial fibrillation. J Cardiovasc Technol 1990; 9: 283–4.

82. Rams JJ, Davis DA, Lolley DM et al. Detection of microemboli in patients with artificial heart valves using transcranial Doppler: preliminary observations. J Heart Valve Dis 1993; 2(1): 37–41.

83. Georgiadis D, Grosset DG, Kelman A et al. Prevalence and characteristics of intracranial microemboli signals in patients with different types of prosthetic cardiac valves. Stroke 1994; 25(3): 587–92.

84. Sturzenegger M, Beer JH, Rihs F. Monitoring combined antithrombotic treatments in patients with prosthetic heart valves using transcranial Doppler and coagulation markers. Stroke 1995; 26(1): 63–9.

85. Kaps M, Hansen J, Weiher M et al. Clinically silent microemboli in patients with artificial prosthetic aortic valves are predominantly gaseous and not solid. Stroke 1997; 28: 322–5.

86. Ringelstein EB, Droste DW, Babikian VL et al. Consensus on microembolus detection by TCD. International Consensus Group on Microembolus Detection. Stroke 1998; 29: 725–9.

10

Risk stratification of patients with asymptomatic carotid artery stenosis: evaluation of cerebrovascular reserve

Jennifer A Frontera and Randolph Marshall

Take-Home Messages

1. Cerebrovascular reserve (CVR) is the brain capacity to maintain a constant cerebral blood volume (CBF) during a wide range of changes of mean arterial blood pressure (MAP).
2. CVR is altered by several disease states, including hypertension, diabetes, carotid occlusive disease, and stroke/transient ischemic attack (TIA).
3. CVR can be tested by increasing pCO_2 or altering MAP, which can be accomplished by breath-holding (passive CO_2 accumulation), acetazolamide challenge, inhaled CO_2, Valsalva maneuver, rapid leg cuff deflation, or transient carotid artery occlusion.
4. Changes in CBF during the CVR testing may be measured by transcranial Doppler (TCD), positive emission tomography (PET), magnetic resonance imaging (MRI) based techniques, single-photon emission computed tomography (SPECT), and xenon computed tomography (CT).
5. Brain imaging modalities such as PET, MRI, SPECT, and CT offer very precise assessment of CVR and more direct measurements of CBF than TCD. However, these imaging modalities are time-consuming and expensive.
6. TCD vasomotor reactivity testing in both symptomatic and asymptomatic patients with >70% stenosis or occlusion is a useful tool for risk stratification.
7. Patients with asymptomatic CAS and impaired cerebral vasoreactivity are at higher risk of ischemic neurological events. These patients should be strongly considered for carotid revascularization.

DEFINITION AND MECHANISMS OF CEREBROVASCULAR RESERVE

Definition of cerebrovascular reserve

CVR refers to the capacity of the brain to increase cerebral blood volume (CBV) to maintain a constant CBF in the face of low cerebral perfusion pressure (CPP). Regional cerebral blood flow is determined by the ratio of CPP to cerebrovascular resistance by the formula:

$$CBF = CPP/vascular\ resistance$$

Cerebral perfusion pressure is related to systemic MAP and intracranial pressure (ICP) by the equation:

$$CPP = MAP - ICP$$

In healthy individuals, a constant CBF is maintained over a wide range of CPP, with mean CBF values approximately 50 ml/100 g/min (Figure 10.1). When CBF values fall below 20 ml/100 g/min, ischemia ensues. Infarction occurs at CBF levels <10–15 ml/100 g/min.

Cerebral hemodynamic insufficiency can be described by the following three stages:[1]

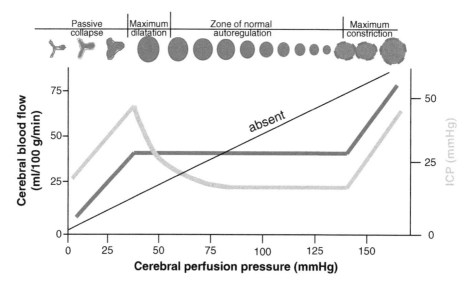

Figure 10.1 Relationship of cerebral perfusion pressure (CPP), cerebral blood flow (CBF), and intracranial pressure (ICP). (Courtesy of Stephan A Mayer MD.) (See color plate section.)

- *Stage 0:* CPP is normal. CBF and metabolic demand are closely matched. With moderate reductions in CPP, the maintenance of CBF in normal brain is largely dependent on changes in cerebrovascular resistance at the arteriolar level. Vasodilatation of the arterioles allows for maintenance of CBF when CPP falls.
- *Stage I hemodynamic failure:* at extremely low perfusion pressures, the vasodilatory capacity of the arterioles becomes exhausted and further reduction of perfusion pressure results in a fall in CBF. Similarly, in conditions of high CPP, arterioles, which normally constrict to prevent excessive rises in CBF, passively allow for an increase in CBF. Thus, at extremes of CPP small arterioles are unable to regulate changes in CBF.[2,3] A secondary consequence of loss of arteriolar reactivity is change in ICP. When cerebral arterioles are maximally dilated, CBV and CBF increase and, hence, ICP increases. In states of prolonged hypertension, the autoregulatory curve is shifted to the right, such that autoregulation is maintained at higher perfusion pressures. In disease states, the autoregulatory curve may be lost altogether (see Figure 10.1).
- *Stage II hemodynamic failure:* when CPP falls below a certain level, changes in arteriolar resistance are no longer able to maintain CBF. At that point the brain's oxygen extraction fraction (OEF) will increase to maintain constant cerebral oxygen metabolism (Figure 10.2). This hemodynamic state is often

referred to as misery perfusion.[4,5] Normally, OEF is about one-third of the total oxygen content, whereas glucose extraction fraction is approximately one-tenth.[6,7] If CPP continues to fall, increased OEF can no longer meet the brain's energy requirements and ischemia will occur.

Mechanism of cerebrovascular reserve

The basis of CVR is mechanistically complex. Neuronal, metabolic, mechanical, and chemical stimuli can effect changes in arteriolar tone. Cerebral blood vessels receive both autonomic and general sensory innervation. Sympathetic stimuli constrict large arteries, but dilate smaller downstream vessels. Under normotensive conditions sympathetic stimulation has little effect on CBF, but during acute hypertension increases in CBF are attenuated by sympathetic outflow.[8] In contrast, parasympathetic innervation may increase CBF.[9,10] General sensory innervation from the trigeminal ganglion produces vasodilatory effects via calcitonin gene-related peptide (CGRP).[11] Increases in CGRP lead to the production of cAMP, which activates K_{ATP} channels, diminishing calcium entry into cells and causing vasodilation.[11] Under normal conditions, CBF and metabolism are coupled such that more active neural tissue preferentially receives more blood flow. This process is referred to as neurovascular coupling (Figure 10.3). Gray matter receives 2–3 times the amount of CBF as white matter, and regional CBF can fluctuate by 10–20%, depending on neuronal activity.

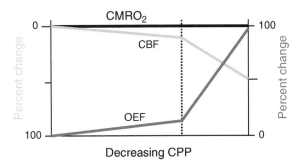

Figure 10.2 Relationship of cerebral blood flow (CBF) and metabolism (oxygen extraction fraction – OEF, cerebral metabolic rate of oxygen – $CMRO_2$) to decreasing cerebral perfusion pressure (CPP). (See color plate section.)

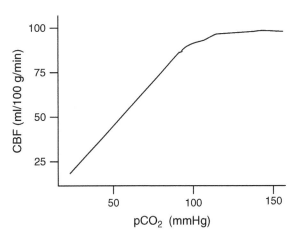

Figure 10.4 Relationship of partial pressure of CO_2 (pCO_2) and cerebral blood flow (CBF).

Vasoactive mediators

Whether exogenously administered or produced as a consequence of metabolic or neuronal activity, several vasoactive mediators are implicated in the maintenance of arteriolar tone.

pCO_2

Changes in pCO_2 cause changes in intracellular and extracellular pH, which, in turn, exert effects on vascular smooth muscle via second messenger systems and by directly altering smooth muscle calcium concentrations.[16] At a range of 20–80 mmHg pCO_2, CBF changes by 1–2 ml/100 g/min/mmHg CO_2 (Figure 10.4).[16] Sustained hypocapnia leads to a compensatory decrease in CSF bicarbonate concentration over a period of hours, allowing CBF to recover to baseline with correction of extracellular pH.[17]

Nitric oxide

Nitric oxide (NO), which is tonically produced by the brain, provides constant vasodilatory tone. Nitric oxide synthesis is responsive to metabolic stimuli such as CO_2 production.[18] Inhibition of nitric oxide synthase removes baseline vasodilation and may alter the response to other vasoactive signals, thus impairing cerebrovascular reactivity.[19] Downstream from NO is cGMP, which activates voltage-gated K_{ATP} channels to diminish calcium entry into cells, thereby relaxing smooth muscle.[16] NO mechanisms may be more closely related to the chemoregulation response of arterioles than to the mechanoregulatory changes of vascular tone in response to changes in blood pressure. After exposure to exogenous nitric oxide, in the form of sodium nitroprusside, healthy volunteers had preserved CBF in response to changes

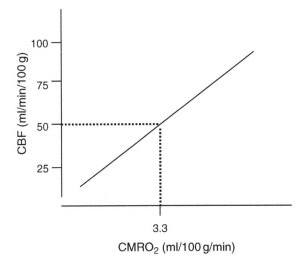

Figure 10.3 Coupling of cerebral blood flow (CBF) and metabolism (cerebral metabolic rate for oxygen – $CMRO_2$).

In states of extreme metabolic variation, such as seizure or coma, CBF can change by up to 40%.[12,13] Neuronal dysfunction associated with CBF abnormalities is exemplified by the spreading depression model of uncoupling in the posterior cerebral artery territory that occurs in migraine with aura.[14] Dynamic cerebral autoregulation (see below) is significantly different in migraineurs compared with controls.[15] In coma, cerebral oxygen metabolism is greatly reduced due to decreased synaptic activity, yet CBF is not always correspondingly low, indicating neurovascular uncoupling. Myogenic responses to changes in systemic blood pressure provide a mechanical basis for autoregulation. Hypoxia and hypercapnia are potent chemical cerebral vasodilators.

in blood pressure but had blunted cerebrovascular reactivity after hypo- or hyperventilation.[20]

Adenosine

Adenosine is another key factor in the autoregulatory cascade. Adenosine levels increase in the brain with hypotension, and modulate vasodilation via adenosine A_{2A} receptors.[21] Adenosine also activates K_{ATP} channels to relax arteries.

Endothelium-derived factors

Endothelium-derived hyperpolarizing, contracting, and relaxing factors are among many other postulated substances that contribute to vascular tone.[18]

METHODS OF ESTIMATING CEREBROVASCULAR RESERVE

Transcranial Doppler in estimation of cerebrovascular reserve

Transcranial Doppler (TCD) measures blood flow velocities in the circle of Willis. Provided that the caliber of the insonated vessel remains constant during measurement, mean flow velocities (MFV) will estimate cerebral blood flow. This is a reasonable assumption in normal brain,[3,22] although caution must be applied in states of acute brain injury when vessel diameter may fluctuate in response to changes in ICP or due to vasospasm.[23,24]

Provocative stimuli given during MFV measurement can assess the reactivity of the arterioles that are responsible for maintaining CVR. Stimuli are aimed at either increasing pCO_2 or altering MAP. Breath-holding (passive CO_2 accumulation), acetazolamide challenge, inhaled CO_2, Valsalva, rapid leg cuff deflation, or transient carotid artery occlusion may be used.[25–32]

TCD–CO_2 vasoreactivity testing

TCD–CO_2 vasoreactivity testing is performed by administering a 5–8% CO_2–air mixture for 2 minutes while bilaterally insonating the middle cerebral arteries.[29,33] CO_2 reactivity is calculated according to the equation:

$$\text{Percent change in MFV/change in end-tidal } pCO_2 \text{ during 2 min of } CO_2 \text{ inhalation}$$

A normal reactivity is considered to be 2% change in MFV/mmHg of CO_2 based on age-matched normative data.[33] CO_2 reactivity has been compared with xenon blood flow and found to be comparable.[34]

TCD–acetazolamide vasoreactivity testing

An acetazolamide (Diamox) challenge is performed by assessing baseline TCD followed by an intravenous injection of 1 g of acetazolamide. Middle cerebral artery flow velocities are then assessed at regular time intervals.[35–37]

TCD–breath-holding and hyperventilation vasoreactivity testing

Breath-holding and hyperventilation have also been employed to test arteriolar reactivity.[38,39] A breath-holding index is the quotient of the percent change in MFV and the time of breath-holding.[40]

TCD–dynamic cerebral autoregulation

Dynamic cerebral autoregulation (DCA) monitoring has emerged as a new TCD-based technique for estimating CVR. It relies on correlations between continuous measures of blood pressure MFV. Provocative blood pressure challenges such as rapid thigh pressure cuff deflation has been utilized;[41] however, natural fluctuations in blood pressure during a 10-minute monitoring period with spontaneous respiration has also proven adequate to perform DCA calculations.[42] Changes in MFV in response to small changes in MAP give an estimation of autoregulation.

Direct correlation of MFV and MAP suggest a loss of autoregulation

Cerebral blood flow has been noted to vary around a steady state. This may represent cyclical perturbations in CPP, intrinsic variation in vasomotor tone, or be due to central control mechanisms.[43–46] Because cerebral autoregulation responds to changes in MAP within several seconds,[41,47–49] variation in CBF due to changes in MAP will be dampened in the low-frequency (<0.15 Hz) range for blood pressure variation, indicating intact autoregulation. Autoregulation is less effective in the high-frequency range (>0.15 Hz).[41,50] At these ranges, MAP may transfer directly to changes in MFV, indicating a loss of autoregulation.

Mathematical techniques for estimating dynamic cerebral autoregulation

Many different mathematical techniques for estimating DCA have been used. Moving correlation coefficients, which are overlapping, averaged Pearson's correlation coefficients can be used to compare MAP and MFV. Increasing correlation coefficients imply a direct dependency of MFV on MAP and, hence, a loss of autoregulation.[51,52] Transfer function analysis involves fast-Fourier transformation of MAP and MFV time-locked waveforms, followed by smoothing and calculation of phase shift, gain, and coherence. The phase and transfer magnitude (gain) represent the time relationship and relative amplitude, respectively, between arterial blood pressure and cerebral blood flow over a specified frequency range. The shift in degrees required to align the input (MAP) and output signal (MFV) at a specific frequency is termed the phase.[53] As the phase shift approaches 0, the relationship between arterial pressure and CBF becomes direct, indicating a loss of autoregulation. Conversely, as the coherence between the two waveforms approaches unity, a direct relationship is present. When the coherence approaches 0, there is a non-linear or no relationship between signals, implying intact autoregulation.[41] The gain is a rough indicator of the magnitude of change of the MFV in response to changes in MAP. Smaller gains represent more intact autoregulation.[53]

Comparison between DCA and CO2 vasoreactivity techniques

DCA and CO_2 reactivity have been compared in individuals with carotid stenosis. Some investigators have found that DCA was impaired while CO_2 reactivity remained in the normal range.[54] Others have found that the correlation between phase shift and CO_2 reactivity is relatively high ($r = 0.55$) and therefore acceptable.[51,54,55] It is likely that the two methods of estimating autoregulation are complementary. CO_2 reactivity represents the response to a chemical challenge (chemoregulation) and assesses the vasodilatory capacity of the arterioles, whereas DCA represents the response of arterioles to physiological fluctuations in blood pressure (mechanoregulation) and takes into account both the vasodilatory and vasoconstrictive capability of the vessels. In settings where low CPP is the pathological state of interest, such as in carotid artery stenosis, the pertinent assessment is of vasodilatory capacity. Therefore, in patients with carotid stenosis, TCD–CO_2 vasoreactivity may be the most useful test of cerebral vasoreactive capacity in order to estimate the risk of cerebral ischemia.

Advantages and disadvantages of TCD estimation of cerebral autoregulation

The major advantages of TCD-based estimations of autoregulation, such as CO_2 reactivity and DCA, are that they are non-invasive, portable, reliable, can be performed at the bedside, and are non-expensive. Furthermore, results can be quickly assessed without excessive off-line calculations, and repeated evaluations are feasible since studies are not time-consuming. A limited penetration of ultrasound through the thick skull bones ('poor ultrasound windows' found in the elderly) is the only disadvantage of TCD reactivity testing.

Brain imaging modalities in estimation of cerebrovascular reserve

Positive emission tomography

Positive emission tomography (PET) has been considered the gold standard for estimating CVR. Using oxygen-15 (O-15) labeled radiotracers, PET is able to give estimates of CBV, CBF, cerebral metabolic rate of oxygen ($CMRO_2$), and OEF (Figures 10.5 and 10.6).

CBF is related to CBV by the equation:

$$CBF = CBV/MTT \text{ (mean transit time)}$$

CBV is maximal during states of oligemia when arteriolar dilatation and collateral flow are able to compensate to maintain CBF. In progressive states of ischemia, vascular collapse, and metabolic depression, CBV declines. It has been assumed, based on the three-stage hemodynamic failure model, that CBV will increase prior to increases in OEF. In some patients, however, stroke may occur with increased OEF but normal or reduced CBV, although patients, with elevated CBV and OEF have higher stroke rates than patients with elevated OEF and normal or reduced CBV.[5]

PET hemodynamic scan technique

PET hemodynamic scans depend on the fact that oxygen rapidly diffuses into tissue at the capillary level and the rate of diffusion and clearance of oxygen is related to CBF. To estimate OEF, the patient inhales O-15 labeled oxygen, which is then bound to hemoglobin and used for oxidative metabolism. The O-15 degrades over approximately 15 minutes by emitting a positron. This positron travels a few millimeters, encounters an electron, and annihilates. In this process, two photons of energy are produced and can be quantitatively detected. This method requires arterial sampling and quantitative measures of CBF and CBV provided from separate PET examinations.[56] A count-based method for estimating OEF has been developed which relies on the comparison of PET counts in an O-15 labeled oxygen scan with the PET counts in an O-15 labeled water scan. The ratio of these two counts is linearly proportional to quantitative regional OEF.[57] Acetazolamide challenges can be given to assess the vasodilatory capacity of the arterioles, where CBF is estimated by PET at 5-minute intervals after the vasodilator injection.

Magnetic resonance imaging based techniques

Dynamic contrast-enhanced perfusion magnetic resonance imaging

Dynamic contrast-enhanced perfusion magnetic resonance imaging (MRI) provides relative estimates of CBV derived

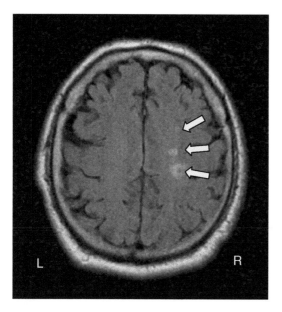

Figure 10.5 Brain MRI of a patient with symptomatic right internal carotid artery (RICA) occlusion (indicated by arrows).

from perfusion images by tracking a bolus of paramagnetic contrast agent. However, it cannot provide absolute CBV measurements and may be inaccurate when there is breakdown of the blood–brain barrier.[58] As with PET, an acetazolamide challenge can be administered with this technique to estimate vasodilatory capacity.[59]

Blood oxygen level-dependent magnetic resonance imaging

Focal increases in CBF in response to a vasodilatory challenge, or a focal increase in metabolism during a functional task (e.g. repetitive hand movement), results in a change of the oxy- to deoxyhemoglobin ratio and a consequent signal change on MRI because deoxyhemoglobin is a paramagnetic molecule.[60,61] When arterioles are maximally dilated to maintain flow in conditions such as carotid stenosis, a decreased or absent blood oxygen-level dependent (BOLD) signal is seen.[62]

Quantitative magnetic resonance angiography

Quantitative magnetic resonance angiography (MRA) can estimate the relative contribution of arteries to blood

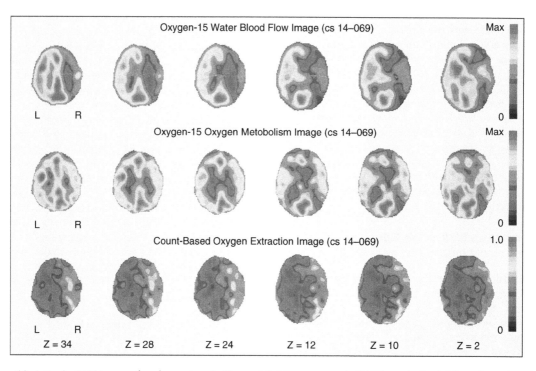

Figure 10.6 Brain PET images for the patient in Figure 10.5 (symptomatic RICA occlusion). Note the reduced blood flow and increased oxygen extraction in the right hemisphere. (Study acquired for the Carotid Occlusion Surgery Study (COSS); Courtesy of William J Powers, Principal Investigator of COSS.) (See color plate section.)

flow in different regions of the brain and, thus, assess collateral circulation. Arterial spin labeling MRA estimates CBF by tracking the transit of a volume of arterial blood intracranially that has been 'tagged' with a radiofrequency magnetic pulse in the neck. Quantitative measures of CBF are possible because the input function is known.[63] Arterial spin labeling MRA allows for frequent and repeated measures of CBF.

Single-photon emission computed tomography and xenon computed tomography

Technetium single-photon emission computed tomography (SPECT) and xenon computed tomography (CT) have also been used to estimate CBF. Xenon CT provides quantitative CBF values, whereas SPECT values are relative values of CBF change.

Advantages and disadvantages of brain imaging modalities in estimation of cerebral autoregulation

Brain imaging modalities offer precise assessment of CVR by providing more direct measurements of CBF than TCD. Brain imaging modalities also provide additional information on the brain structure and can simultaneously delineate ischemia, infarction, and edema or give a variety of quantitative metabolic measures. The limitations of brain imaging modalities for estimating CVR are that such studies are time-consuming, expensive, require technically skilled support staff, are difficult in critically ill patients, and require an extensive post-processing.

CAROTID ARTERY STENOSIS AND CEREBROVASCULAR RESERVE

Symptomatic carotid stenosis or occlusion

High-grade carotid stenosis or occlusion that is associated with poor hemodynamic reserve carries a high risk of subsequent stroke.[27,33,55,64] When compared with control groups, patients with symptomatic high-grade stenosis or occlusion have significantly lower CO_2 reactivity values and are more likely to have ischemic events at 6 months.[33] Patients with recent stroke ($<$3 months) and patients with carotid occlusion and contralateral stenosis also have significantly impaired CO_2 reactivity.[39] Correlation coefficients and transfer function parameters have been shown to be abnormal ipsilateral to carotid stenosis.[51,55] The absence of sufficient collateral circulation further contributes to poor hemodynamic

reserve.[55] Increased OEF, indicating stage II hemodynamic failure, is a powerful independent predictor of stroke risk in patients with symptomatic stenosis or occlusion.[64–66] In a prospective series of 81 patients with symptomatic carotid occlusion and increased OEF on PET scanning, the age-adjusted relative risk of ipsilateral stroke was 7.0.[64]

For complete carotid occlusion, extracranial–intracranial (EC/IC) bypass has also been shown to improve CO_2 reactivity, decrease OEF, and improve CBF in small cohorts of patients.[67,68] The first EC/IC Bypass Study failed to show a surgical benefit for patients with symptomatic carotid artery occlusion.[69] There has been a revival of interest in EC/IC bypass since surgical techniques have improved and more specific patient selection criteria have developed. A large, prospective, blinded, longitudinal cohort study showed that patients with ipsilateral stage II hemodynamic failure (increased OEF on PET) had a 27% stroke rate over 2 years compared with a 5% stroke rate in patients with normal OEF.[64] Patients who had hemispheric symptoms within 120 days had the worst prognosis, with a 2-year ipsilateral stroke rate of 12% in patients with normal OEF and 50% in patients with increased OEF.[70] These data spurred the Carotid Occlusion Surgery Study (COSS), a large prospective multicenter trial aimed at randomizing patients with carotid occlusion and stage II hemodynamic failure to superficial temporal artery–MCA bypass surgery plus best medical therapy vs medical therapy alone. A Markov model to estimate the cost-effectiveness demonstrated that PET screening prior to EC/IC bypass conferred 23.2 additional quality-adjusted life-years (QALYs) at a cost of $20 000 per QALY compared with medical therapy alone, suggesting that EC/IC bypass may be cost-effective in selecting patients with impaired autoregulation.[71]

Asymptomatic carotid stenosis or occlusion

The need for and timing of carotid revascularization in asymptomatic patients remain the subject of ongoing debate.[72–77] Overall, patients with asymptomatic carotid occlusion are less likely to have abnormal OEF than symptomatic patients (42% vs 16%) even when other baseline risk factors are similar.[78] Although both the Asymptomatic Carotid Atherosclerosis Study (ACAS) and the Asymptomatic Carotid Surgery Trail (ACST) showed superiority of carotid endarterectomy (CEA) over medical therapy alone,[79,80] about 40 asymptomatic patients need to be treated to prevent 1 disabling or fatal stroke after 5 years.[81] Risk stratification, therefore, may be helpful to identify patients who are appropriate for either medical therapy or an interventional

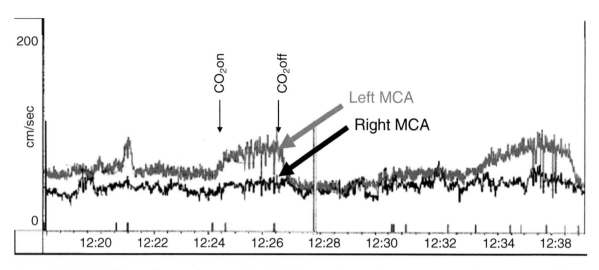

Figure 10.7 TCD-CO_2 cerebrovascular reactivity (CVR) in a patient with asymptomatic right internal carotid artery stenosis. Bilateral recording of mean blood flow velocities (MBFV) in both middle cerebral arteries (MCA) during breath-hold, after CO_2 inhalation, and at rest. Note that MBFV were increased in the left MCA (normal CVR, green arrow) and diminished in the right MCA (black arrow), indicating impaired CVR on the right. (See color plate section.)

Table 10.1 Annual risk of stroke in patients with asymptomatic carotid artery stenosis and impaired cerebrovascular reserve

Study	Degree of ICA stenosis	Method	Sample size N	Annual stroke risk (%)
Yamauchi et al, 1992[65]	>70%	PET (oxygen extraction fraction)	40	57
Gur et al, 1996[82]	>70%	TCD with acetazolamide	44	10.5
Vernieri et al, 1999[27]	Occlusion	TCD with breath-holding index	42	11.9
Silvestrini et al, 2000[26]	>70%	TCD with breath-holding index	94	13.9
Markus et al, 2001[29]	>70%	TCD with CO_2 challenge	59	3.8
Marshall et al, 2003[33]	>80% or occlusion	TCD with CO_2 challenge	35	20

ICA, internal carotid artery; PET, position emission tomography; TCD, transcranial Doppler.

approach. Asymptomatic carotid stenosis can be associated with poor cerebral vasoreactivity (Figure 10.7), which is an independent predictor of stroke and TIA (Table 10.1).[26–36,82] A breath-holding index of 0.69 in asymptomatic patients reliably identified patients at high risk for TIA or stroke.[27] In a prospective cohort of 94 patients with asymptomatic carotid stenosis ≥70%, the annual ischemic event rate was 4% in patients with normal CVR and 14% in patients with an abnormal

breath-holding index.[26] Furthermore, it has been suggested that abnormal CVR is a more robust predictor of future stroke than the degree of carotid stenosis. This is probably because adequacy of collateral circulation varies among patients with similar degrees of stenosis and may compensate for the flow failure in some patients. Most patients with poor collateral circulation will have impaired CVR. Identifying asymptomatic patients with poor CVR may be a useful tool in selecting patients for carotid surgery or angioplasty. According to the American Academy of Neurology consensus panel, TCD vasomotor reactivity testing in both symptomatic and asymptomatic patients with >70% stenosis or occlusion is considered useful (type B, class II–III evidence).[83]

Carotid revascularization and cerebrovascular reserve

Carotid revascularization procedures can improve intracerebral hemodynamics. CEA has been shown to improve ipsilateral CO_2 reactivity in patients with abnormal reactivity at baseline and may improve hemodynamics in the contralateral hemisphere.[84,85] Percutaneous transluminal angioplasty has been reported to improve CO_2 reactivity to a degree equal or greater than that of CEA.[42,86]

Although improvement of CO_2 reactivity can be noticed as soon as 2 days after carotid angioplasty, a marked improvement has been observed at 1 month after a procedure, suggesting a delay in return to maximal cerebral microvasculature reactivity.[86]

Diminished autoregulatory capacity has been postulated to be responsible for the hyperperfusion syndrome that can occur within the first several days following a revascularization procedure.[87–92] The hyperperfusion syndrome has been reported to occur in 1.4–9% of patients following carotid revascularization.[93–96] Several studies have demonstrated that in the acute period following CEA, patients with symptoms or signs of cerebral hyperperfusion (headache, hemorrhage, seizure, or focal deficits) had markedly elevated ipsilateral MCA mean flow velocities compared with baseline values.[89,90,97] Reductions in arterial blood pressure can reduce MFV and alleviate symptoms.[90] The response to antihypertensive treatment implies a passive dependence of CBF on MAP, i.e. impaired autoregulation. MRI perfusion weighted imaging may be used in detecting relative increases in CBF in patients who develop hyperperfusion syndrome.[98]

SUMMARY

The ability of the brain to regulate its blood flow to meet metabolic demands and to compensate for acute and chronic changes in CPP is a crucial physiological brain property to mediate against cerebral ischemia. Although autoregulation is mechanistically complex and dependent on neuronal, endothelial, and metabolic factors, it can readily be assessed using either TCD or brain imaging-based modalities. Each of these techniques has its advantages and disadvantages. Selection of a specific method for CVR testing will depend on availability, required precision, and cost.

Autoregulation is abnormal in a variety of disease states. Patients with carotid stenosis or occlusion may have impaired cerebral autoregulation and therefore may have a greater risk of stroke or TIA than patients with intact cerebral autoregulation. Assessment of CVR can help to stratify patients by their risk for stroke or TIA. In particular, in asymptomatic carotid disease, estimation of CVR can help in selecting the patients who may benefit the most from revascularization therapy. Also, cerebral vasoreactivity testing may be useful to monitor cerebral autoregulation after revascularization procedures as a surrogate endpoint of vascular events.

REFERENCES

1. Powers WJ, Press GA, Grubb RL Jr, Gado M, Raichle ME. The effect of hemodynamically significant carotid artery disease on the hemodynamic status of the cerebral circulation. Ann Intern Med 1987; 106(1): 27–34.
2. Powers WJ. Cerebral hemodynamics in ischemic cerebrovascular disease. Ann Neurol 1991; 29(3): 231–40.
3. Aaslid R, Lindegaard KF, Sorteberg W, Nornes H. Cerebral autoregulation dynamics in humans. Stroke 1989; 20(1): 45–52.
4. Baron JC, Bousser MG, Rey A et al. Reversal of focal "misery-perfusion syndrome" by extra-intracranial arterial bypass in hemodynamic cerebral ischemia. A case study with 15O positron emission tomography. Stroke 1981; 12(4): 454–9.
5. Derdeyn CP, Videen TO, Yundt KD et al. Variability of cerebral blood volume and oxygen extraction: stages of cerebral haemodynamic impairment revisited. Brain 2002; 125(Pt 3): 595–607.
6. Lebrun-Grandie P, Baron JC, Soussaline F et al. Coupling between regional blood flow and oxygen utilization in the normal human brain. A study with positron tomography and oxygen 15. Arch Neurol 1983; 40(4): 230–6.
7. Rhodes CG, Wise RJ, Gibbs JM et al. In vivo disturbance of the oxidative metabolism of glucose in human cerebral gliomas. Ann Neurol 1983; 14(6): 614–26.
8. Heistad DD, Marcus ML. Effect of sympathetic stimulation on permeability of the blood–brain barrier to albumin during acute hypertension in cats. Circ Res 1979; 45(3): 331–8.
9. Morita-Tsuzuki Y, Hardebo JE, Bouskela E. Inhibition of nitric oxide synthase attenuates the cerebral blood flow response to stimulation of postganglionic parasympathetic nerves in the rat. J Cereb Blood Flow Metab 1993; 13(6): 993–7.
10. Moskowitz MA, Wei EP, Saito K, Kontos HA. Trigeminalectomy modifies pial arteriolar responses to hypertension or norepinephrine. Am J Physiol 1988; 255(1 Pt 2): H1–6.
11. Shin HK, Hong KW. Importance of calcitonin gene-related peptide, adenosine and reactive oxygen species in cerebral autoregulation under normal and diseased conditions. Clin Exp Pharmacol Physiol 2004; 31(1–2): 1–7.
12. Lassen NA. Cerebral blood flow and oxygen consumption in man. Physiol Rev 1959; 39(2): 183–238.
13. Reivich M. Blood flow metabolism couple in brain. Res Publ Assoc Res Nerv Ment Dis 1974; 53: 125–40.
14. Daffertshofer M, Hennerici M. Cerebrovascular regulation and vasoneuronal coupling. J Clin Ultrasound 1995; 23(2): 125–38.

15. Muller M, Marziniak M. The linear behavior of the system middle cerebral artery flow velocity and blood pressure in patients with migraine: lack of autonomic control? Stroke 2005; 36(9): 1886–90.

16. Brian JE Jr. Carbon dioxide and the cerebral circulation. Anesthesiology 1998; 88(5): 1365–86.

17. Muizelaar JP, van der Poel HG, Li ZC, Kontos HA, Levasseur JE. Pial arteriolar vessel diameter and CO_2 reactivity during prolonged hyperventilation in the rabbit. J Neurosurg 1988; 69(6): 923–7.

18. Faraci FM, Heistad DD. Regulation of the cerebral circulation: role of endothelium and potassium channels. Physiol Rev 1998; 78(1): 53–97.

19. Faraci FM, Brian JE Jr. Nitric oxide and the cerebral circulation. Stroke 1994; 25(3): 692–703.

20. Lavi S, Egbarya R, Lavi R, Jacob G. Role of nitric oxide in the regulation of cerebral blood flow in humans: chemoregulation versus mechanoregulation. Circulation 2003; 107(14): 1901–5.

21. Shin HK, Park SN, Hong KW. Implication of adenosine A2A receptors in hypotension-induced vasodilation and cerebral blood flow autoregulation in rat pial arteries. Life Sci 2000; 67(12): 1435–45.

22. Dahl A, Russell D, Nyberg-Hansen R, Rootwelt K. Effect of nitroglycerin on cerebral circulation measured by transcranial Doppler and SPECT. Stroke 1989; 20(12): 1733–6.

23. Kontos HA. Validity of cerebral arterial blood flow calculations from velocity measurements. Stroke 1989; 20(1): 1–3.

24. Kontos HA, Wei EP, Navari RM et al. Responses of cerebral arteries and arterioles to acute hypotension and hypertension. Am J Physiol 1978; 234(4): H371–383.

25. Settakis G, Lengyel A, Molnar C et al. Transcranial Doppler study of the cerebral hemodynamic changes during breath-holding and hyperventilation tests. J Neuroimaging 2002; 12(3): 252–8.

26. Silvestrini M, Vernieri F, Pasqualetti P et al. Impaired cerebral vasoreactivity and risk of stroke in patients with asymptomatic carotid artery stenosis. JAMA 2000; 283(16): 2122–7.

27. Vernieri F, Pasqualetti P, Passarelli F, Rossini PM, Silvestrini M. Outcome of carotid artery occlusion is predicted by cerebrovascular reactivity. Stroke 1999; 30(3): 593–8.

28. Vernieri F, Pasqualetti P, Matteis M et al. Effect of collateral blood flow and cerebral vasomotor reactivity on the outcome of carotid artery occlusion. Stroke 2001; 32(7): 1552–8.

29. Markus H, Cullinane M. Severely impaired cerebrovascular reactivity predicts stroke and TIA risk in patients with carotid artery stenosis and occlusion. Brain 2001; 124(Pt 3): 457–67.

30. Ringelstein EB, Van Eyck S, Mertens I. Evaluation of cerebral vasomotor reactivity by various vasodilating stimuli: comparison of CO_2 to acetazolamide. J Cereb Blood Flow Metab 1992; 12(1): 162–8.

31. Russell D, Dybevold S, Kjartansson O et al. Cerebral vasoreactivity and blood flow before and 3 months after carotid endarterectomy. Stroke 1990; 21(7): 1029–32.

32. Muller M, Schimrigk K. Vasomotor reactivity and pattern of collateral blood flow in severe occlusive carotid artery disease. Stroke 1996; 27(2): 296–9.

33. Marshall RS, Rundek T, Sproule DM et al. Monitoring of cerebral vasodilatory capacity with transcranial Doppler carbon dioxide inhalation in patients with severe carotid artery disease. Stroke 2003; 34(4): 945–9.

34. Ng SC, Poon WS, Chan MT et al. Transcranial Doppler ultrasonography (TCD) in ventilated head injured patients: correlation with stable xenon-enhanced CT. Acta Neurochir Suppl 2000; 76: 479–82.

35. Kleinschmidt A, Steinmetz H, Sitzer M, Merboldt KD, Frahm J. Magnetic resonance imaging of regional cerebral blood oxygenation changes under acetazolamide in carotid occlusive disease. Stroke 1995; 26(1): 106–10.

36. Ficzere A, Valikovics A, Fulesdi B et al. Cerebrovascular reactivity in hypertensive patients: a transcranial Doppler study. J Clin Ultrasound 1997; 25(7): 383–9.

37. Piepgras A, Schmiedek P, Leinsinger G et al. A simple test to assess cerebrovascular reserve capacity using transcranial Doppler sonography and acetazolamide. Stroke 1990; 21(9): 1306–11.

38. Widder B. Use of breath holding for evaluating cerebrovascular reserve capacity. Stroke 1992; 23(11): 1680–1.

39. Widder B, Kleiser B, Krapf H. Course of cerebrovascular reactivity in patients with carotid artery occlusions. Stroke 1994; 25(10): 1963–7.

40. Markus HS, Harrison MJ. Estimation of cerebrovascular reactivity using transcranial Doppler, including the use of breath-holding as the vasodilatory stimulus. Stroke 1992; 23(5): 668–73.

41. Zhang R, Zuckerman JH, Giller CA, Levine BD. Transfer function analysis of dynamic cerebral autoregulation in humans. Am J Physiol 1998; 274(1 Pt 2): H233–41.

42. Reinhard M, Roth M, Muller T et al. Effect of carotid endarterectomy or stenting on impairment of dynamic cerebral autoregulation. Stroke 2004; 35(6): 1381–7.

43. Zernikow B, Michel E, Kohlmann G et al. Cerebral autoregulation of preterm neonates – a non-linear control system? Arch Dis Child Fetal Neonatal Ed 1994; 70(3): F166–73.

44. Fujii K, Heistad DD, Faraci FM. Vasomotion of basilar arteries in vivo. Am J Physiol 1990; 258(6 Pt 2): H1829–34.

45. Hudetz AG, Roman RJ, Harder DR. Spontaneous flow oscillations in the cerebral cortex during acute changes in mean arterial pressure. J Cereb Blood Flow Metab 1992; 12(3): 491–9.

46. Newell DW, Aaslid R, Stooss R, Reulen HJ. The relationship of blood flow velocity fluctuations to intracranial pressure B waves. J Neurosurg 1992; 76(3): 415–21.

47. Paulson OB, Strandgaard S, Edvinsson L. Cerebral autoregulation. Cerebrovasc Brain Metab Rev 1990; 2(2): 161–92.

48. Florence G, Seylaz J. Rapid autoregulation of cerebral blood flow: a laser-Doppler flowmetry study. J Cereb Blood Flow Metab 1992; 12(4): 674–80.

49. Aaslid R, Newell DW, Stooss R, Sorteberg W, Lindegaard KF. Assessment of cerebral autoregulation dynamics from simultaneous arterial and venous transcranial Doppler recordings in humans. Stroke 1991; 22(9): 1148–54.

50. Diehl RR, Linden D, Lucke D, Berlit P. Phase relationship between cerebral blood flow velocity and blood pressure. A clinical test of autoregulation. Stroke 1995; 26(10): 1801–4.

51. Reinhard M, Roth M, Muller T et al. Cerebral autoregulation in carotid artery occlusive disease assessed from spontaneous blood pressure fluctuations by the correlation coefficient index. Stroke 2003; 34(9): 2138–44.

52. Soehle M, Czosnyka M, Pickard JD, Kirkpatrick PJ. Continuous assessment of cerebral autoregulation in subarachnoid hemorrhage. Anesth Analg 2004; 98(4): 1133–9, table of contents.

53. Blaber AP, Bondar RL, Stein F et al. Transfer function analysis of cerebral autoregulation dynamics in autonomic failure patients. Stroke 1997; 28(9): 1686–92.

54. White RP, Markus HS. Impaired dynamic cerebral autoregulation in carotid artery stenosis. Stroke 1997; 28(7): 1340–4.

55. Reinhard M, Muller T, Roth M et al. Bilateral severe carotid artery stenosis or occlusion – cerebral autoregulation dynamics and collateral flow patterns. Acta Neurochir (Wien) 2003; 145(12): 1053–9; discussion 1059–60.

56. Mintun MA, Raichle ME, Martin WR, Herscovitch P. Brain oxygen utilization measured with O-15 radiotracers and positron emission tomography. J Nucl Med 1984; 25(2): 177–87.

57. Derdeyn CP, Videen TO, Simmons NR et al. Count-based PET method for predicting ischemic stroke in patients with symptomatic carotid arterial occlusion. Radiology 1999; 212(2): 499–506.

58. Cha S. Perfusion MR imaging: basic principles and clinical applications. Magn Reson Imaging Clin N Am 2003; 11(3): 403–13.

59. Ohnishi T, Nakano S, Yano T et al. Susceptibility-weighted MR for evaluation of vasodilatory capacity with acetazolamide challenge. AJNR Am J Neuroradiol 1996; 17(4): 631–7.

60. Ogawa S, Menon RS, Tank DW et al. Functional brain mapping by blood oxygenation level-dependent contrast magnetic resonance imaging. A comparison of signal characteristics with a biophysical model. Biophys J 1993; 64(3): 803–12.

61. Ogawa S, Menon RS, Kim SG, Ugurbil K. On the characteristics of functional magnetic resonance imaging of the brain. Annu Rev Biophys Biomol Struct 1998; 27: 447–74.

62. Carusone LM, Srinivasan J, Gitelman DR, Mesulam MM, Parrish TB. Hemodynamic response changes in cerebrovascular disease: implications for functional MR imaging. AJNR Am J Neuroradiol 2002; 23(7): 1222–8.

63 Golay X, Hendrikse J, Lim TC. Perfusion imaging using arterial spin labeling. Top Magn Reson Imaging 2004; 15(1): 10–27.

64. Grubb RL Jr, Derdeyn CP, Fritsch SM et al. Importance of hemodynamic factors in the prognosis of symptomatic carotid occlusion. JAMA 1998; 280(12): 1055–60.

65. Yamauchi H, Fukuyama H, Fujimoto N, Nabatame H, Kimura J. Significance of low perfusion with increased oxygen extraction fraction in a case of internal carotid artery stenosis. Stroke 1992; 23(3): 431–2.

66. Yamauchi H, Fukuyama H, Nagahama Y et al. Evidence of misery perfusion and risk for recurrent stroke in major cerebral arterial occlusive diseases from PET. J Neurol Neurosurg Psychiatry 1996; 61(1): 18–25.

67. Takagi Y, Hashimoto N, Iwama T, Hayashida K. Improvement of oxygen metabolic reserve after extracranial–intracranial bypass surgery in patients with severe haemodynamic insufficiency. Acta Neurochir (Wien) 1997; 139(1): 52–6, discussion 56–7.

68. Miller JD, Smith RR, Holaday HR. Carbon dioxide reactivity in the evaluation of cerebral ischemia. Neurosurgery 1992; 30(4): 518–21.

69. Failure of extracranial–intracranial arterial bypass to reduce the risk of ischemic stroke. Results of an international randomized trial. The EC/IC Bypass Study Group. N Engl J Med 1985; 313(19): 1191–200.

70. Grubb RL Jr, Powers WJ, Derdeyn CP, Adams HP Jr, Clarke WR. The carotid occlusion surgery study. Neurosurg Focus 2003; 14(3): e9.

71. Derdeyn CP, Gage BF, Grubb RL, Powers WJ. Cost-effectiveness of PET screening prior to EC/IC bypass in patients with carotid occlusion. Clin Positron Imaging 1999; 2(6): 341.

72. North American Symptomatic Carotid Endarterectomy Trial. Methods, patient characteristics, and progress. Stroke 1991; 22(6): 711–20.

73. MRC European Carotid Surgery Trial: interim results for symptomatic patients with severe (70–99%) or with mild (0–29%) carotid stenosis. European Carotid Surgery Trialists' Collaborative Group. Lancet 1991; 337(8752): 1235–43.

74. Endovascular versus surgical treatment in patients with carotid stenosis in the Carotid and Vertebral Artery Transluminal Angioplasty Study (CAVATAS): a randomised trial. Lancet 2001; 357(9270): 1729–37.

75. Halliday AW, Thomas DJ, Mansfield AO. The asymptomatic carotid surgery trial (ACST). Int Angiol 1995; 14(1): 18–20.

76. Yadav JS, Wholey MH, Kuntz RE et al. Protected carotid-artery stenting versus endarterectomy in high-risk patients. N Engl J Med 2004; 351(15): 1493–501.

77. Halliday A, Mansfield A, Marro J et al. Prevention of disabling and fatal strokes by successful carotid endarterectomy in patients without recent neurological symptoms: randomised controlled trial. Lancet 2004; 363(9420): 1491–502.

78. Derdeyn CP, Yundt KD, Videen TO et al. Increased oxygen extraction fraction is associated with prior ischemic events in patients with carotid occlusion. Stroke 1998; 29(4): 754–8.

79. Endarterectomy for asymptomatic carotid artery stenosis. Executive Committee for the Asymptomatic Carotid Atherosclerosis Study. JAMA 1995; 273(18): 1421–8.

80. Halliday A, Mansfield A, Marro J et al. Prevention of disabling and fatal strokes by successful carotid endarterectomy in patients without recent neurological symptoms: randomised controlled trial. Lancet 2004; 363: 1491–502.

81. Rothwell PM, Goldstein LB. Carotid endarterectomy for asymptomatic carotid stenosis: asymptomatic carotid surgery trial. Stroke 2004; 35: 2425–7.

82. Gur AY, Bova I, Bornstein NM. Is impaired cerebral vasomotor reactivity a predictive factor for stroke in asymptomatic patients. Stroke 1996; 27: 2188–90.

83. Sloan MA, Alexandrov AV, Tegeler CH et al. Assessment: transcranial Doppler ultrasonography: report of the Therapeutics and Technology Assessment Subcommittee of the American Academy of Neurology. Neurology 2004; 62(9): 1468–81.

84. Visser GH, van Huffelen AC, Wieneke GH, Eikelboom BC. Bilateral increase in CO_2 reactivity after unilateral carotid endarterectomy. Stroke 1997; 28(5): 899–905.

85. Hartl WH, Janssen I, Furst H. Effect of carotid endarterectomy on patterns of cerebrovascular reactivity in patients with unilateral carotid artery stenosis. Stroke 1994; 25(10): 1952–7.

86. Markus HS, Clifton A, Buckenham T, Taylor R, Brown MM. Improvement in cerebral hemodynamics after carotid angioplasty. Stroke 1996; 27(4): 612–16.

87. Phatouros CC, Meyers PM, Higashida RT et al. Intracranial hemorrhage and cerebral hyperperfusion syndrome after extracranial carotid artery angioplasty and stent placement. AJNR Am J Neuroradiol 2002; 23(3): 503–4.

88. Sbarigia E, Speziale F, Giannoni MF et al. Post-carotid endarterectomy hyperperfusion syndrome: preliminary observations for identifying at risk patients by transcranial Doppler sonography and the acetazolamide test. Eur J Vasc Surg 1993; 7(3): 252–6.

89. Ascher E, Markevich N, Schutzer RW et al. Cerebral hyperperfusion syndrome after carotid endarterectomy: predictive factors and hemodynamic changes. J Vasc Surg 2003; 37(4): 769–77.

90. Jorgensen LG, Schroeder TV. Defective cerebrovascular autoregulation after carotid endarterectomy. Eur J Vasc Surg 1993; 7(4): 370–9.

91. Gonzalez A, Mayol A, Gil-Peralta A et al. Hyperperfusion syndrome as a complication of percutaneous transluminal angioplasty of the internal carotid artery. Rev Neurol 1999; 29(10): 923–5.

92. Penn AA, Schomer DF, Steinberg GK. Imaging studies of cerebral hyperperfusion after carotid endarterectomy. Case report. J Neurosurg 1995; 83(1): 133–7.

93. Dalman JE, Beenakkers IC, Moll FL, Leusink JA, Ackerstaff RG. Transcranial Doppler monitoring during carotid endarterectomy helps to identify patients at risk of postoperative hyperperfusion. Eur J Vasc Endovasc Surg 1999; 18(3): 222–7.

94. Gossetti B, Martinelli O, Guerricchio R, Irace L, Benedetti-Valentini F. Transcranial Doppler in 178 patients before, during, and after carotid endarterectomy. J Neuroimaging 1997; 7(4): 213–16.

95. Meyers PM, Higashida RT, Phatouros CC et al. Cerebral hyperperfusion syndrome after percutaneous transluminal stenting of the craniocervical arteries. Neurosurgery 2000; 47(2): 335–43, discussion 343–5.

96. Morrish W, Grahovac S, Douen A et al. Intracranial hemorrhage after stenting and angioplasty of extracranial carotid stenosis. AJNR Am J Neuroradiol 2000; 21(10): 1911–16.

97. Fujimoto S, Toyoda K, Inoue T et al. Diagnostic impact of transcranial color-coded real-time sonography with echo contrast agents for hyperperfusion syndrome after carotid endarterectomy. Stroke 2004; 35(8): 1852–6.

98. Karapanayiotides T, Meuli R, Devuyst G et al. Postcarotid endarterectomy hyperperfusion or reperfusion syndrome. Stroke 2005; 36(1): 21–6.

11

Risk stratification of patients with asymptomatic carotid artery stenosis: role of inflammatory biomarkers for atherosclerosis

Mitchell SV Elkind and Marie C Eugene

Take-Home Messages

1. Inflammatory processes play an important role in atherosclerosis, including carotid artery disease.
2. Limited evidence suggests that inflammation is found more commonly in plaques from patients with symptomatic than asymptomatic disease, indicating that inflammation may be a marker of plaque instability.
3. Serum biomarkers of inflammation, including high-sensitivity C-reactive protein (hsCRP) and lipoprotein-associated phospholipase A_2 (Lp-PLA$_2$), predict risk of first ischemic stroke and may predict prognosis after ischemic stroke, including mortality and recurrence.
4. Limited evidence suggests an association between serum levels of inflammatory biomarkers and carotid atherosclerosis, including the risk of stroke in patients with asymptomatic stenosis.
5. Serum levels of inflammatory biomarkers may allow risk stratification in patients with asymptomatic stenosis. Patients with higher levels of these markers, for example, may be particularly appropriate for revascularization procedures to reduce incidence of stroke.
6. Several behavioral and medical interventions, particularly statins, reduce levels of inflammatory biomarkers. These interventions may thus reduce risk of stroke in the setting of asymptomatic carotid stenosis.
7. Further well-designed studies will be needed to confirm these hypotheses and to determine the role of markers of inflammation in the management of patients with asymptomatic carotid stenosis.

INTRODUCTION

The importance of inflammation in atherosclerosis, including carotid artery disease, has been increasingly appreciated in recent years. According to the current theory developed by Sir Russell Ross[1] and others,[2] atherosclerosis is predominantly an inflammatory condition produced by a 'response to injury.' Many different toxic stimuli can cause endothelial injury, with the final result being a cascade of immunologically mediated events: adhesion of monocytes and lymphocytes to the endothelial surface, migration of these leukocytes beneath the endothelial surface, and subsequent subendothelial localization. Macrophages then take up lipid, forming foam cells, these and other macrophages are activated, and cytokines and growth factors are released. This leads to smooth muscle cell proliferation and plaque formation. The potential causes of the underlying endothelial injury include oxidized low-density lipoprotein (LDL), high shear force as is present in hypertension, homocysteine, toxic constituents of cigarette smoke, and possibly even infections. Inflammation also plays a role in plaque rupture, potentially precipitating a clinical event.[2]

The basic science relevant to the role of inflammation in atherosclerosis has been reviewed elsewhere.[1,2] The current chapter reviews:

- the epidemiological and clinical literature regarding the value of several inflammatory markers, including hsCRP, in predicting ischemic stroke and prognosis after stroke
- studies on the relationship of these markers to carotid artery disease and associated clinical events
- potential therapeutic implications

Because the available data on the role of these markers in treating patients with carotid stenosis are limited, the chapter will conclude with several suggestions for future research.

INFLAMMATORY MARKERS AND RISK OF ISCHEMIC STROKE

Leukocytes

Relative increases in levels of certain inflammatory markers, even within the normal range, appear to be associated with markers of subclinical atherosclerosis and risk of stroke (Table 11.1). Leukocyte count, for example, is independently associated with carotid plaque thickness cross-sectionally[3] and progression of carotid intima-media thickness (IMT) over time.[4] Leukocyte counts are also associated with aortic arch atherosclerotic disease, and with aortic arch plaque ≥4 mm, the degree of thickening conventionally considered to be associated with increased risk of stroke.[5] Leukocyte levels are also inversely associated with endothelial reactivity.[6] Levels of leukocytes may also serve as predictors of future risk of ischemic cardiac and cerebrovascular events, even after adjustment for smoking.[7–13] In the Northern Manhattan Study (NOMAS), leukocyte count measured on average approximately 3 years before the occurrence of stroke in essentially healthy, elderly individuals was predictive of first ischemic stroke, even after adjusting for several vascular risk factors, including the metabolic syndrome[14] (Figure 11.1).

High-sensitivity C-reactive protein

Among inflammatory markers, acute phase proteins, and hsCRP in particular, have been most extensively studied.[15] Part of the innate immune response, C-reactive protein (CRP) is produced by the liver in response to stimulation by interleukin-6 (IL-6). It is a stable protein, its measurement is not affected greatly by freezing and

Table 11.1 Inflammatory markers associated with atherosclerosis and risk of stroke

Acute phase reactants
C-reactive protein (CRP)
High-sensitivity C-reactive protein (hsCRP)
Serum amyloid A
Fibrinogen

Cytokines
Interleukin-1β
Interleukin-2
Interleukin-6
Interleukin-8
Interleukin-10
Tumor necrosis factor-α
Tumor necrosis factor receptor 1
Tumor necrosis factor receptor 2

Soluble adhesion molecules
E-selectin
P-selectin
Intercellular adhesion molecule-1
Vascular cell adhesion molecule-1
CD40 ligand

Others
Leukocytes
Myeloperoxidase
Monocyte chemoattractant protein-1
Lipoprotein-associated phospholipase A_2 (Lp-PLA$_2$)

thawing cycles in large, epidemiological studies, it has little diurnal variation, and is minimally affected by eating. All of these characteristics make it a good, reproducible assay, and there is currently a widely available, standardized, Food and Drug Administration (FDA)-approved immunonephelometric assay. Disadvantages to the use of hsCRP are that it is very non-specific and so acute increases in levels of hsCRP may occur in the setting of acute infection or other illness. The mechanisms by which hsCRP is associated with cardiac disease or stroke, moreover, remain uncertain. HsCRP may be an 'epiphenomenon,' or marker of the inflammation that is present in atherosclerosis but not directly responsible for it. Alternatively, growing evidence suggests that CRP may play a direct or causative role, or serve as another risk factor, for atherosclerosis.[15]

HsCRP is also associated with a number of other factors (Table 11.2), many of which are themselver associated with ischemic events, including age,[16–18]

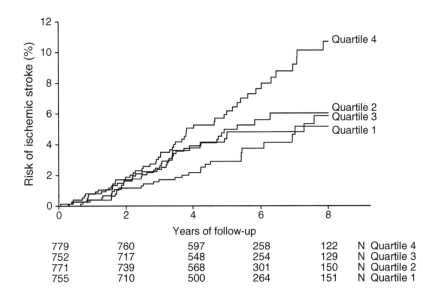

Figure 11.1 Kaplan–Meier estimate of risk of ischemic stroke according to quartile of baseline leukocyte count, from the Northern Manhattan Study. Quartile 1: $\leq 4.8 \times 10^3$ cells/L. Quartile 2: $4.9–6.2 \times 10^3$ cells/L. Quartile 3: $6.3–7.2 \times 10^3$ cells/L. Quartile 4: $\geq 7.3 \times 10^3$ cells/L. (Adapted from Elkind MS, Sciacca R, Boden-Albala B et al. Relative elevation in leukocyte count predicts first cerebral infarction. Neurology 2005; 64: 2121–5, with permission from Lippincott, Williams & Wilkins.)

779	760	597	258	122	N Quartile 4
752	717	548	254	129	N Quartile 3
771	739	568	301	150	N Quartile 2
755	710	500	264	151	N Quartile 1

Table 11.2 Patient factors associated with high-sensitivity C-reactive protein (hsCRP) level

Increased hsCRP
Hypertension
Body mass index
Obesity
Diabetes mellitus
Metabolic syndrome
Smoking
Hormone use

Decreased hsCRP
Moderate alcohol consumption
Physical activity
Weight loss
Medications:
- Statins
- Angiotensin-converting enzyme inhibitors
- Others

---

smoking,[18–20] blood pressure,[18] obesity,[21,22] dietary glucose load,[23] glucose tolerance and metabolic syndrome,[24–27] cocaine exposure,[28] physical activity,[29–32] alcohol consumption,[33] infection with *Helicobacter pylori*[21] and *Chlamydia pneumoniae*,[21] and periodontitis.[34] In most attempts to account for these other risk factors in statistical analyses, however, hsCRP has remained a statistically significant independent predictor

of risk of cardiac disease.[35] Nonetheless, because hsCRP is strongly associated with obesity and diabetes mellitus, it remains unsettled whether increased levels are simply due to presence of these risk factors.[36] Furthermore, even in populations in which hsCRP is independently predictive of events, it remains unclear that the addition of hsCRP to existing risk-prediction models improves their predictive power in a clinically meaningful way.[37]

HsCRP has been shown to predict incident cardiovascular events in several populations.[15,38] Its relationship to stroke has not been as thoroughly investigated, but there is growing evidence to support this association. In the Women's Health Study (WHS), hsCRP, IL-6, soluble intercellular adhesion molecule-1 (SICAM-1), and serum amyloid A (SAA) all predicted incident cardiovascular events, including stroke.[39,40] Of note, in multivariate models, hsCRP was the only inflammatory marker that independently predicted risk, and the inclusion of hsCRP improved the predictive ability of the models over those containing lipid values and other risk factors alone.[39,41,42] An important limitation of these studies is that they focused on predominantly healthy middle-aged individuals without a significant burden of risk factors. In at least one elderly population (the Cardiovascular Health Study),[43] however, hsCRP predicted stroke modestly (adjusted hazard ratio for the highest quartile 1.60, 95% CI 1.23–2.08).

The relationship of hsCRP to incident stroke risk appears to depend on the study design and population studied. HsCRP levels measured prior to onset of clinical disease were an independent predictor of first ischemic stroke (relative risk 1.9 for those in the highest quartile [hsCRP ≥ 2.1] vs those in the lowest quartile) in the Physicians' Health Study.[38] In a cross-sectional analysis, hsCRP ≥ 0.55 mg/dl was significantly associated with a self-reported past history of stroke.[44] In a study among very elderly subjects (≥85 years) in Europe, hsCRP was associated with an increased risk of fatal stroke, but also with a risk of death from all causes.[45] In the Framingham Study, during >10 years of follow-up, men in the highest quartile of hsCRP had twice the risk of stroke of those in the lowest and women had three times the risk.[46] For men, the increased risk was not statistically significant after adjusting for confounders. Ischemic stroke subtypes were incompletely characterized in these studies, as well. In healthy Japanese-American men in the Honolulu Heart Program, using a nested case–control study design, investigators found a 3.8 times increased risk in the population overall among those in the highest compared with lowest quartile of hsCRP after 10–15 years of follow-up.[47] The associations were strongest among those aged 55, and without a history of hypertension or diabetes. This result provides evidence that the greatest predictive value of hsCRP may be found among those with the lowest baseline risk of an event. This may explain why the association between hsCRP and ischemic stroke is attenuated in certain older populations and those with more risk factors.[43] The determination of an association is also limited by the fact that there are many different subtypes of stroke, and not all stroke is secondary to atherosclerosis.

Other inflammatory markers

Recently, in large epidemiological studies,[48,49] investigators have described an increased risk of incident coronary events associated with elevated serum levels of lipoprotein-associated phospholipase A_2 (Lp-PLA$_2$), a macrophage-derived enzyme involved in the metabolism of LDL in arterial walls that is responsible for the release of inflammatory mediators. Further evidence has suggested that this marker also predicts stroke.[50,51] Recent analyses from the NOMAS also provide evidence that this marker may be less susceptible to changes after stroke, and may be a better marker of the risk of recurrence after a first stroke than hsCRP.[52]

CD40 ligand (CD40L) is a proinflammatory molecule produced by endothelial cells, macrophages, lymphocytes, platelets, and smooth muscle cells. It is involved in leukocyte interactions with one another and with endothelium, as well as platelet–platelet interactions, and promotes a cascade of events associated with atherosclerosis and acute coronary syndromes and potentially stroke, including increasing production of metalloproteinases, tissue factor, cytokines, and adhesion molecules.[53] Soluble CD40L (sCD40L) is shed from stimulated lymphocytes as well as activated platelets, and is biologically active. CD40L plays an important role in experimental models of atherosclerosis. Blockage of CD40L, as well as other immunomodulatory molecules expressed by macrophages, T cells, endothelium, and smooth cells in atherosclerotic plaques, can reduce lesion formation.[54–57]

In clinical studies, sCD40L predicted a first myocardial infarction (MI), stroke, or vascular event among participants in the WHS, with a relative risk of approximately 2.8 after adjusting for other risk factors.[58] There was no correlation between CD40L and hsCRP. There is also evidence that sCD40L predicts prognosis in cardiac patients independently of aspirin therapy and troponin levels.[53,59,60] Soluble CD40L has also been demonstrated to be up-regulated in patients with acute ischemic stroke, and this up-regulation continues for at least 3 months after the infarction.[61] Soluble CD40L may thus be an appropriate and useful marker of future risk of recurrent cardiovascular events in stroke patients, and potentially for response to antiplatelet or other therapy. It may also serve as a marker of risk among those patients with carotid artery disease.

RELATIONSHIP OF INFLAMMATION AND INFLAMMATORY MARKERS TO CAROTID ARTERY DISEASE

Several studies have assessed the role of inflammation and associated inflammatory markers in patients with carotid atherosclerosis specifically. There is evidence that plaques from symptomatic patients have a more inflammatory profile than plaques from asymptomatic patients. There is also limited evidence that serum levels of markers are higher in those patients with symptoms, and perhaps most importantly, those patients most likely to develop symptoms or stroke later. Whether these levels could be used to predict who will have events remains unsettled, but if proven, could have a significant clinical impact.

Carotid plaque characteristics

Plaques from symptomatic patients undergoing carotid endarterectomy (CEA) have significantly more inflammatory cells on immunohistochemical analysis than plaques from asymptomatic patients.[62] Macrophages and T lymphocytes are prominent in the cellular infiltrate and there is increased expression of endothelial adhesion molecules.[63] In one study, concentrations of the interleukins IL-6, IL-8, and IL-18 were significantly higher in 40 unstable plaques than in 24 stable plaques.[64]

IL-18 was found to be >3 times higher in symptomatic vs asymptomatic plaques.[65]

Adhesion molecules, including sICAM-1 and vascular cell adhesion molecule-1 (VCAM-1), are expressed on endothelial cells and allow leukocytes to attach to the endothelium. In one study, increased expression of ICAM-1 was found in the high-grade regions of plaques obtained from symptomatic patients compared with plaques removed from asymptomatic patients,[66] although other studies have not confirmed this finding.[67]

Serum inflammatory markers and carotid disease

In the offspring cohort of the Framingham Heart Study, participants in the highest quartile of hsCRP had a significantly higher prevalence of carotid stenosis compared with those in the lowest quartile.[68] However, this remained significant only in women after adjustment was made for various factors such as menopausal status and estrogen replacement therapy. In another recent study among clinic patients undergoing duplex Doppler ultrasound, fibrinogen, hsCRP, and antibodies to cytotoxic *H. pylori*, *C. pneumoniae*, and cytomegalovirus were associated with increasing levels of IMT.[69] In multivariable analyses, elevated fibrinogen, hsCRP, infectious serologies, and the presence of increased IMT (IMT ≥ 0.9 mm) or carotid plaque predicted clinical outcome events. In the Inflammation and Carotid Artery – Risk for Atherosclerosis Study (ICARAS), hsCRP and SAA were measured in 1268 asymptomatic participants followed with carotid ultrasound.[70] Progression of atherosclerosis was significantly associated with hsCRP and SAA levels. In a community-based study among 1111 participants, however, monocyte count was a better independent predictor of carotid plaque formation than IL-6, hs-CRP, fibrinogen, or total white cell count.[71]

Carotid plaques with lower echogenicity (echolucent plaques) have higher lipid content and are more prone to rupture, whereas plaques with higher echogenicity (echorich) have more fibrous tissue and tend to be more stable. In one study of 246 patients, higher levels of IL-6 and hsCRP were significantly correlated with plaques of lower echogenicity.[72] This finding remained significant for IL-6 after adjusting for plaque thickness and medication, but was of borderline significance for hsCRP.

In a cross-sectional study of the difference in level of hsCRP between symptomatic and asymptomatic carotid stenosis, hsCRP concentration was higher in 125 symptomatic patients compared with 12 asymptomatic patients.[73] Among 62 patients admitted for endarterectomy, there was a significant association between increased serum hsCRP and plaque instability (defined by ulceration or recent intraplaque hemorrhage consisting of diffuse blood in the subendothelial space).[74] HsCRP levels in serum were also correlated with the number of macrophages and T lymphocytes in the plaques.

In another preliminary analysis among 668 selected patients undergoing carotid ultrasound, inflammatory markers, including hsCRP, and infectious markers, including antibodies to *H. pylori*, *C. pneumoniae*, and cytomegalovirus, were all associated with degree of atherosclerosis.[75] HsCRP and infectious serologies also appeared to predict stroke and transient ischemic attack (TIA) after accounting for degree of carotid atherosclerosis. Further studies will be needed to confirm these findings.

There is also evidence that hsCRP predicts which patients develop neointimal hyperplasia after carotid artery stenting, a complication that is associated with increased risk of restenosis and adverse clinical events. In one study of 68 asymptomatic and 32 symptomatic patients undergoing carotid angioplasty and stenting, 14% had neointimal hyperplasia, and this was significantly associated with preprocedural hsCRP ($p = 0.024$).[76]

Tumor necrosis factor-α (TNF-α) is a cytokine secreted by many cells, including activated macrophages or monocytes, fibroblasts, smooth muscle cells, and neurons. It is a proinflammatory cytokine capable of stimulating an acute phase response through its actions on the liver. TNF receptor 1 and TNF receptor 2 are released as soluble receptors by many of the cells with which TNF-α interacts. In 279 stroke-free NOMAS participants, levels of TNF receptors 1 and 2, but not TNF-α, were associated with increased maximal carotid plaque thickness, but only in patients <70 years of age.[77] After adjusting for numerous factors, this association remained significant for TNF receptor 1 and was of marginal significance for TNF receptor 2.

Studies of serum levels of adhesion molecules, while involving a small number of patients, have also provided conflicting evidence of an association with the symptomatic state. In a study of 29 symptomatic and 25 asymptomatic patients undergoing CEA for greater than 60% stenosis, serum levels of soluble forms of soluble ICAM-1 were significantly elevated in symptomatic vs asymptomatic patients.[78] Furthermore, sICAM-1 levels were significantly higher in patients with carotid artery stenosis than in five control patients who did not have stenosis.

Recent studies have also provided evidence that high-resolution carotid magnetic resonance imaging (MRI) provides an alternative technique to assess the stability of carotid plaque,[79] and that visualized abnormalities are associated with relatively elevated levels of serum inflammatory markers.[80] Treatment to lower levels of LDL has also been associated with MRI-visualized carotid plaque regression.[81]

Whereas inflammation is likely to play a crucial role in the activation and progression of carotid artery disease, the cross-sectional design of many of the studies presented may limit their application to clinical practice. Prospective randomized controlled trials that focus on particular markers are necessary to determine more specifically the implications of inflammatory markers for management of asymptomatic carotid artery stenosis.

POTENTIAL THERAPEUTIC IMPLICATIONS

Recognition of the importance of inflammatory measures in atherosclerosis could have important therapeutic implications in at least two major ways (Table 11.3). First, inflammatory biomarkers may permit risk-stratification of patients with carotid stenosis, thereby permitting more informed decisions regarding the appropriateness of invasive therapy. Secondly, inflammatory markers may themselves be targets of specific therapies, including statins.

The importance of risk stratification

The role of procedural revascularization in many asymptomatic patients remains unsettled. Improved ability to predict risk among these patients could help choose the best candidates for more aggressive medical therapy or procedures. Contemporary studies have provided evidence, for example, that several measures of cerebral hemodynamics may provide prognostic information in patients with severe carotid stenosis or occlusion.[82–84] While unproven, use of hemodynamic parameters may thus be of use in selecting patients for interventions, as those at highest risk are likely to derive most benefit from a procedure.

Measures of inflammatory status could have similar prognostic and therapeutic implications in patients with carotid disease (see Table 11.3). Elevations in inflammatory marker levels could be used to identify patients with asymptomatic carotid disease who are at high absolute risk of stroke, or to identify patients with symptomatic but moderate stenosis (50–69%) who might benefit from surgery. For example, in one small study, levels of sCD40L were found to predict risk of a cardiovascular event among patients with asymptomatic carotid stenosis, independently of hsCRP and other risk factors.[85] In addition to targeting these patients for traditional secondary prevention medications – including antiplatelet drugs, statins, and antihypertensive agents – these patients could be considered candidates for CEA or angioplasty and stenting. Such an approach would be consistent with the emerging paradigm used in primary prevention and secondary prevention after cardiac disease, according to which the overall baseline level of risk, rather than a specific risk factor, should be treated with all therapies efficacious in reducing risk of vascular events.[86,87]

Levels of these markers, moreover, may identify patients likely to respond to specific therapies. For example, the benefit from aspirin was seen primarily in those in the highest quartile of hsCRP in the Physicians' Health Study.[38] Baseline levels of hsCRP also predicted response to clopidogrel among patients treated with percutaneous coronary procedures in a small, single-center study.[88] In a trial of abciximab, a glycoprotein IIb/IIIa inhibitor, in unstable cardiac patients undergoing angioplasty, the effect of abciximab on lowering the risk of a recurrent event was seen only in those patients with elevated levels of CD40L, indicating that CD40L could be used as a marker of likelihood of response to therapy.[59] Whether these findings also apply to patients undergoing carotid procedures remains unknown.

Finally, it remains possible, although untested, that levels of hsCRP or other biomarkers would help determine whether patients should undergo CEA as opposed to angioplasty and stenting.

Behavioral approaches to reduce inflammation

Potential anti-inflammatory therapies include both behavioral changes and medications (Table 11.4). Behavioral changes include exercise, weight loss, and smoking cessation. In a group of 31 men, half of whom had the metabolic syndrome, a 3-week course of monitored aerobic exercise led to significant reductions in hsCRP, adhesion molecule levels, and many other markers of systemic inflammation.[89] Controlled studies have similarly shown reductions in levels of

---

Table 11.3 Potential future use of inflammatory marker data in management of patients with asymptomatic carotid disease

Determine patients at increased risk

Determine frequency of follow-up evaluations in conservative management

Determine patients who may benefit from intervention

Determine the type of intervention (carotid endarterectomy vs angioplasty and stenting)

Prognosis after intervention

Determine risk of neointimal hyperplasia and restenosis

Encourage behavioral modifications

Choice of medical therapy

Table 11.4 Potential strategies to reduce levels of inflammation
Behavioral
Exercise
Physical activity
Weight loss
Smoking cessation
Medications
Statins
Antiplatelet therapy
Angiotensin-converting enzyme (ACE) inhibitors
Angiotensin receptor blockers
Peroxisome proliferator-activated receptor (PPAR)-γ agonists

hsCRP after exercise regimens in different patient populations.[90,91] Other studies, however, have not confirmed these findings, and have found that the reductions in insulin sensitivity in obese, non-diabetic subjects after moderate to intense physical activity programs do not correlate with changes in inflammatory markers.[92]

There is similar evidence that weight loss can reduce levels of inflammatory markers, including hsCRP, although whether these changes are sustained or correlate with measures of subclinical atherosclerosis, such as endothelial dysfunction, remains uncertain.[93] In one study, weight loss associated with 6 months of treatment with orlistat in obese subjects was correlated with reductions in hsCRP and IL-6.[94] In the Diabetes Prevention Program (DPP) clinical trial comparing intensive lifestyle intervention, metformin, and placebo in 3234 adults with impaired glucose tolerance, reductions in the median hsCRP from baseline to 1 year were approximately 30% in the lifestyle group and 10% in the metformin group. Levels remained the same or increased slightly in the placebo group. Weight loss rather than exercise appeared to account for most of the change in hsCRP.[95] Caloric intake, rather than relative protein or carbohydrate intake, appears to be most important in determining CRP levels.[96,97]

Among smokers, smoking cessation appears to result in reductions in levels of CRP after about 5 years.[98,99]

Medical therapies to reduce inflammation

Statins

3-Hydroxy-3-methylglutaryl coenzyme A (HMG-CoA) reductase inhibitors, or statins, are the best studied medications shown to reduce levels of inflammation. Several studies have shown that statins lower inflammatory

marker levels, even over a relatively short time. In one trial,[100] 24 weeks of pravastatin 40 mg daily ($n = 865$ active treatment patients) led to a 17% reduction in hsCRP levels compared with placebo ($p < 0.001$). The effect was seen as early as 12 weeks. There was no correlation between reductions in lipid levels and changes in hsCRP, indicating that the effects of the statin treatment on lipid and inflammatory parameters were independent. Cerivastatin reduced hsCRP levels by 25% over 8 weeks among 785 patients with hypercholesterolemia, also without a reduction in lipid levels.[101] There was no dose–response relationship at the doses (0.4 and 0.8 mg) tested. In a small study of patients undergoing CEA, those patients randomized to intensive treatment with atorvastatin for 1 month prior to surgery had a reduction in inflammatory parameters of plaque composition as well as reduced levels of peripheral leukocyte activation.[102]

A pre-specified secondary analysis of the PRavastatin Or AtorVastatin Evaluation and Infection – Thrombolysis in Myocardial Infarction 22 (PROVE IT-TIMI 22) study provided confirmation of the hypothesis that treatment to lower target levels of hsCRP may have important clinical consequences in reducing cardiac ischemic events.[103] In this trial, 3745 patients with acute coronary syndromes were randomized to receive atorvastatin 80 mg daily or pravastatin 40 mg daily. HsCRP and LDL levels were measured at baseline, 30 days, and intervals during the study. Correlation of LDL and hsCRP levels was very low, suggesting measurement of independent phenomena. Event rates were lower in those treated to LDL levels <70 mg/dl (2.7 vs 4.0 events per 100 person-years). Lower event rates were also present, with a similar magnitude of benefit, in those patients in whom hsCRP levels were lowered to <2 mg/L, independent of lowering of LDL level (2.8 vs 3.9 events per 100 person-years follow-up). The lowest event rates were seen in those with LDL <70 mg/dl and hsCRP <1 mg/L (1.9 events per 100 person-years), suggesting an additive benefit of lowering lipid and inflammatory measures. Of note, the benefit of lowering these markers was independent of the specific agent (atorvastatin or pravastatin) used, and depended on the degree of success in lowering these parameters. Similar results were seen in a simultaneously published study on the effect of these two statins on slowing progression of coronary atheroma using intravascular ultrasound.[104] More recent data from PROVE-IT also provide evidence that measurement of Lp-PLA$_2$ activity 30 days, but not immediately, after coronary syndromes has prognostic significance, and that more intensive statin therapy lowers Lp-PLA$_2$ levels more than less intense therapy.[105]

Further studies focused solely on hsCRP or other inflammatory biomarker modification as a strategy to reduce risk will be needed before targeting such markers is incorporated into future guidelines regarding the use of statin agents in cardiac prevention. The measurement of hsCRP and other inflammatory marker levels in the Heart Protection Study (HPS)[106] is ongoing and should provide further insight into these questions. The role of these measures in stroke prevention and treatment of carotid disease will remain unsettled until similar studies in these patient populations are also performed.

Antiplatelet agents

There is little evidence that aspirin alone, particularly at doses typically used in vascular prophylaxis, significantly lowers levels of hsCRP or other inflammatory markers.[107,108] One small study ($n = 40$) among patients with chronic angina showed an effect of aspirin 300 mg daily on inflammatory markers.[109] There are no data to indicate that aspirin reduces levels of these markers in patients with stroke. There may be a disassociation between the anti-inflammatory and anti-aggregatory effects of aspirin. Aspirin 300 mg daily, for example, did not decrease levels of P-selectin, CD11b/CD18 (leukocyte adhesion molecule), or the formation of platelet–leukocyte aggregates, despite an effect on platelet aggregation.[110–112]

There is some evidence that the addition of a second antiplatelet agent, even against a background of aspirin and statin use, may have an additional effect on reduction of inflammation. For example, the addition of ticlopidine to aspirin during coronary procedures led to a reduction in levels of monocyte expression of CD11b/CD18 while aspirin alone did not.[113] There may also be different anti-inflammatory effects among antiplatelet agents. Clopidogrel reduced P-selectin expression on platelets and formation of platelet–leukocyte aggregates in healthy volunteers, whereas abciximab, an antibody to the platelet glycoprotein IIb/IIIa receptor, did not.[114] In a small, randomized trial, the addition of clopidogrel to aspirin in patients with acute ischemic stroke led to a statistically significant reduction over 7 days in hsCRP levels and platelet P-selectin expression compared with patients receiving aspirin and heparin.[115]

Anti-hypertensive agents

There is emerging evidence of an association between hsCRP levels and hypertension in cross-sectional studies,[116,117] and hsCRP was an independent risk factor for the development of hypertension among 20 525 women in a prospective cohort study.[118] Studies in other populations have not found associations of inflammatory markers with hypertension,[119] particularly after adjusting for other risk factors.[120] Some

antihypertensive agents may lower levels of hsCRP and other inflammatory markers. There is evidence that agents that interfere with the renin–angiotensin system (RAS) have a greater effect on reducing inflammation than other antihypertensive agents,[121] although whether this translates into a greater reduction in risk than what would be predicted by their blood pressure-lowering effects alone remains undetermined. Angiotensin-converting enzyme (ACE) inhibitors, for example, have been associated with lower hsCRP levels at the time of ischemic stroke and better long-term outcomes, even after adjusting for blood pressure levels.[122] Angiotensin type 2 receptor blockers (ARBs) may be even more effective in lowering levels of inflammatory markers than traditional ACE inhibitors.[123]

PPAR-γ agonists

The thiazolidinedione oral hypoglycemic agents (or peroxisome proliferator-activated receptor [PPAR]-γ agonists) also have an anti-inflammatory effect.[124] These selective ligands of the nuclear transcription factor PPAR-γ include rosiglitazone and pioglitazone, and are used extensively in the treatment of type 2 diabetes mellitus. By their effects on PPAR-γ, they are capable of regulating gene transcription and affecting several protein pathways, including reducing TNF-α production by monocytes and reducing macrophage activation.[125] Animal models have also shown decreases in cytokine production and inflammation.[125] In non-diabetic obese patients, troglitazone (which has since been removed from the market due to risk of hepatotoxicity) also reduces proinflammatory nuclear factor-κB in monocytes.[126] In diabetic patients, these agents reduce hsCRP by 20% over several months,[127] and they may also reduce matrix metalloproteinase-9, leukocyte count, sICAM-1, monocyte chemoattractant protein-1, plasminogen activator inhibitor-1, and sCD40L.[125,127]

FUTURE RESEARCH

Further research is needed to more fully explore the role for measurement of inflammatory biomarkers in the management of patients with stroke in general, and in those patients with asymptomatic carotid artery disease in particular. Measurement of levels of hsCRP and other markers in a population of patients with asymptomatic carotid disease, with follow-up for outcomes, would be a useful study design. Ideally such a study would involve many centers nationally or internationally. Repeated measurements, moreover, would allow determination of whether changes over time lead to increased risk. Such natural history studies may be difficult to conduct in the present era, however, in which interventions are increasingly offered to patients on the basis of clinical trial results demonstrating a general benefit in stroke risk reduction. It may be increasingly important, however, to evaluate these markers in asymptomatic carotid stenosis patients considered at high risk of procedures, who are being followed conservatively. Patients who elect to be followed with only medical treatment would be another group of patients to be studied. Careful assessment of medical therapy will be needed in such studies, however, as the medical therapy may itself influence levels of these markers. Correlation of levels of inflammatory markers with short-term and long-term outcomes after endarterectomy and stenting procedures may also be useful in determining whether these markers have a role in choice of medical therapy after these procedures.

Clinical trials of anti-inflammatory therapies should also be considered in carotid stenosis patients, including those patients who undergo procedures. Randomized trials of high- vs low-dose statins, dual antiplatelet regimens, and thiazolidinediones should all be considered, with repeated measurements of inflammatory markers. MRI assessment of carotid plaque characteristics, as well as serum biomarkers, could be utilized. Ultimately, correlation with clinical outcomes will be needed to demonstrate efficacy.

REFERENCES

1. Ross R. Atherosclerosis – an inflammatory disease. N Engl J Med 1999; 340: 115–26.
2. Libby P, Theroux P. Pathophysiology of coronary artery disease. Circulation 2005; 111: 3481–8.
3. Elkind MS, Cheng J, Boden-Albala B et al. Elevated white blood cell count and carotid plaque thickness: The Northern Manhattan Stroke Study. Stroke 2001; 32: 842–9.
4. Salonen R, Salonen JT. Progression of carotid atherosclerosis and its determinants: a population-based ultrasonography study. Atherosclerosis 1990; 81(1): 33–40.
5. Elkind MS, Sciacca R, Boden-Albala B et al. Leukocyte count is associated with aortic arch plaque thickness. Stroke 2002; 33: 2587–92.
6. Elkind MS, Sciacca R, Boden-Albala B et al. Leukocyte count is associated with reduced endothelial reactivity. Atherosclerosis 2005; 181: 329–38.
7. Friedman GD, Klatsky AL, Siegelaub AB. The leukocyte count as a predictor of myocardial infarction. N Engl J Med 1974; 290: 1275–8.
8. Zalokar JB, Richard JL, Claude JR. Leukocyte count, smoking, and myocardial infarction. N Engl J Med 1981; 304: 465–8.
9. Prentice RL, Szatrowski TP, Fujikura T et al. Leukocyte counts and coronary heart disease in a Japanese cohort. Am J Epidemiol 1982; 116: 496–509.
10. Grimm RH, Neaton JD, Ludwig W. Prognostic importance of the white blood cell count for coronary, cancer, and all-cause mortality. JAMA 1985; 254: 1932–7.
11. Yarnell JW, Baker IA, Sweetnam PM et al. Fibrinogen, viscosity, and white blood cell count are major risk factors for ischemic heart disease. Circulation 1991; 83: 836–44.
12. Kannel WB, Anderson K, Wilson PW. White blood cell count and cardiovascular disease. Insights from the Framingham Study. JAMA 1992; 267: 1253–6.
13. Grau AJ, Buggle F, Becher H et al. The association of leukocyte count, fibrinogen and C-reactive protein with vascular risk factors and ischemic vascular diseases. Thromb Res 1996; 82(3): 245–55.
14. Elkind MS, Sciacca R, Boden-Albala B et al. Relative elevation in leukocyte count predicts first cerebral infarction. Neurology 2005; 64: 2121–5.
15. Pearson TA, Mensah GA, Alexander RW et al. Markers of inflammation and cardiovascular disease. Application to clinical and public health practice. A statement for healthcare professionals from the Centers for Disease Control and Prevention and the American Heart Association. Circulation 2003; 107: 499–511.
16. Ford ES, Giles WH, Myers GL, Mannino DM. Population distribution of high-sensitivity C-reactive protein among US men: findings from National Health and Nutrition Examination Survey 1999–2000. Clin Chem 2003; 49: 686–90.
17. Imhof A, Fröhlich M, Loewel H et al. Distributions of C-reactive protein measured by high-sensitivity assays in apparently healthy men and women from different populations in Europe. Clin Chem 2003; 49: 669–72.
18. Yamada S, Gotoh T, Nakashima Y et al. Distribution of serum C-reactive protein and its association with atherosclerotic risk factors in a Japanese population. Am J Epidemiol 2001; 153: 1183–90.
19. Bermudez EA, Rifai N, Buring JE et al. Relation between markers of systemic vascular inflammation and smoking in women. Am J Cardiol 2002; 89: 1117–19.
20. Tracy R, Macy E, Bovill EG et al. Lifetime smoking exposure affects the association of C-reactive protein with cardiovascular disease risk factors and subclinical disease in healthy elderly subjects. Arterioscler Thromb Vasc Biol 1997; 17: 2167–76.
21. Mendall MA, Patel P, Ballam L et al. C-reactive protein and its relation to cardiovascular risk factors: a population-based cross sectional study. BMJ 1996; 312: 1061–5.
22. Visser M, Bouter LM, McQuillan GM et al. Elevated C-reactive protein levels in overweight and obese adults. JAMA 1999; 282: 2131–5.
23. Liu S, Manson JE, Buring JE et al. Relation between a diet with high glycemic load and plasma concentrations of high-sensitivity C-reactive protein in middle-aged women. Am J Clin Nutr 2002; 75: 492–8.
24. Wu T, Dorn JP, Donahue RP et al. Associations of serum C-reactive protein with fasting insulin, glucose, and glycosylated hemoglobin: the Third National Health and Nutrition Examination Survey, 1988–94. Am J Epidemiol 2002; 155: 65–71.
25. Ridker PM, Buring JE, Cook NR et al. C-reactive protein, the metabolic syndrome, and risk of incident cardiovascular events: an 8-year follow-up of 14,719 initially healthy American women. Circulation 2003; 107: 391–7.
26. Festa A, D'Agostino RJs, Howard G et al. Chronic subclinical inflammation as part of the insulin resistance syndrome: the Insulin Resistance Atherosclerosis Study (IRAS). Circulation 2000; 102: 42–7.
27. Hak AE, Stehouwer CD, Bots ML et al. Associations of C-reactive protein with measures of obesity, insulin resistance, and subclinical atherosclerosis in healthy, middle-aged women. Arterioscler Thromb Vasc Biol 1999; 19: 1986–91.
28. Siegel AJ, Mendelson JH, Sholar MB et al. Effect of cocaine usage on C-reactive protein, von Willebrand factor, and fibrinogen. Am J Cardiol 2002; 89: 1133–5.

29. Manns PJ, Williams DP, Snow CM, Wander RC. Physical activity, body fat, and serum C-reactive protein in postmenopausal women with and without hormone replacement. Am J Hum Biol 2003; 15: 91–100.

30. Pitsavos C, Chrysohoou C, Panagiotakos DB et al. Association of leisure-time physical activity on inflammation markers (C-reactive protein, white cell blood count, serum amyloid A, and fibrinogen) in healthy subjects (from the ATTICA study). Am J Cardiol 2003; 91: 368–70.

31. Abramson JL, Vaccarino V. Relationship between physical activity and inflammation among apparently healthy middle-aged and older US adults. Arch Intern Med 2001: 162: 1286–92.

32. Rothenbacher D, Hoffmeister A, Brenner H, Koenig W. Physical activity, coronary heart disease, and inflammatory response. Arch Intern Med 2003; 163: 1200–5.

33. Imhof A, Froehlich M, Brenner H et al. Effect of alcohol consumption on systemic markers of inflammation. Lancet 2001; 357: 763–7.

34. Slade GD, Ghezzi EM, Heiss G et al. Relationship between periodontal disease and C-reactive protein among adults in the Atherosclerosis Risk in Communities Study. Arch Intern Med 2003; 163: 1172–9.

35. Ridker PM, Rifai N, Rose L et al. Comparison of C-reactive protein and low-density lipoprotein cholesterol levels in the prediction of first cardiovascular events. N Engl J Med 2002; 347: 1557–65.

36. Miller M, Zhan M, Havas S. High attributable risk of elevated C-reactive protein level to conventional coronary heart disease risk factors. Arch Intern Med 2005; 165: 2063–8.

37. Greenland P, O'Malley PG. When is a new prediction marker useful? Arch Intern Med 2005; 165: 2454–6.

38. Ridker PM, Cushman M, Stampfer MJ et al. Inflammation, aspirin, and the risk of cardiovascular disease in apparently healthy men. N Engl J Med 1997; 336: 973–9.

39. Ridker PM, Buring JE, Shih J et al. Prospective study of C-reactive protein and the risk of future cardiovascular events among apparently healthy women. Circulation 1998; 98(8): 731–3.

40. Ridker PM, Hennekens CH, Buring JE et al. C-reactive protein and other markers of inflammation in the prediction of cardiovascular disease in women. N Engl J Med 2000; 342(12): 836–43.

41. Ridker PM, Rifai N, Rose L et al. Comparison of C-reactive protein and low-density lipoprotein cholesterol levels in the prediction of first cardiovascular events. New Engl J Med 2002; 347: 1557–65.

42. Ridker PM, Glynn RJ, Hennekens CH. C-reactive protein adds to the predictive value of total and HDL cholesterol in determining risk of first myocardial infarction. Circulation 1998; 97(20): 2007–11.

43. Cao JJ, Thach C, Manolio TA et al. C-reactive protein, carotid intima-media thickness, and incidence of ischemic stroke in the elderly: the Cardiovascular Health Study. Circulation 2003; 108: 166–70.

44. Ford ES, Giles WH. Serum C-reactive protein and self-reported stroke: findings from the Third National Health and Nutrition Examination Survey. Arterioscler Thromb Vasc Biol 2000; 20(4): 1052–6.

45. Gussekloo J, Schaap MC, Frolich M et al. C-reactive protein is a strong but nonspecific risk factor of fatal stroke in elderly persons. Arterioscler Thromb Vasc Biol 2000; 20(4): 1047–51.

46. Rost NS, Wolf PA, Kase CS et al. Plasma concentration of C-reactive protein and risk of ischemic stroke and transient ischemic attack. Stroke 2001; 32: 2575–9.

47. Curb JD, Abbott RD, Rodriguez BL et al. C-reactive protein and the future risk of thromboembolic stroke in healthy men. Circulation 2003; 107: 2016–20.

48. Packard CJ, O'Reilly DSJ, Caslake MJ et al. Lipoprotein-associated phospholipase A2 as an independent predictor of coronary heart disease. N Engl J Med 2000; 343: 1148–55.

49. Ballantyne CM, Hoogeveen RC, Bang H et al. Lipoprotein-associated phospholipase A2, high-sensitivity C-reactive protein, and risk for incident coronary heart disease in middle-aged men and women in the Atherosclerosis Risk in Communities (ARIC) Study. Circulation 2004; 109: 837–42.

50. Oei HH, van der Meer IM, Hofman A et al. Lipoprotein-associated phospholipase A2 activity is associated with risk of coronary heart disease and ischemic stroke: the Rotterdam Study. Circulation 2005; 111: 570–5.

51. Ballantyne CM, Hoogeveen RC, Bang H et al. Lipoprotein-associated phospholipase A2, high-sensitivity C-reactive protein, and risk for incident ischemic stroke in middle-aged men and women in the Atherosclerosis Risk in Communities (ARIC) Study. Arch Intern Med 2005; 165: 2479–84.

52. Elkind MS, Tai W, Coates K, Paik MC, Sacco RL. Lipoprotein-associated phospholipase A2, C-reactive protein, and outcome after ischemic stroke. Arch Int Med (in press).

53. Kinlay S, Schwartz GG, Olsson AG et al. Effect of atorvastatin on risk of recurrent cardiovascular events after an acute coronary syndrome associated with high soluble CD40 ligand in the Myocardial Ischemia Reduction with Aggressive Cholesterol Lowering (MIRACL) Study. Circulation 2004; 110: 386–91.

54. Hollenbaugh D, Mischel-Petty N, Edwards CP et al. Expression of functional CD40 by vascular endothelial cells. J Exp Med 1995; 182: 33–40.

55. Mach F, Schonbeck U, Bonnefoy J-Y et al. Activation of monocyte/macrophage functions related to acute atheroma complication by ligation of CD40: induction of collagenase, stromelysin, and tissue factor. Circulation 1997; 96: 396–9.

56. Schönbeck U, Mach F, Bonnefoy J-Y et al. Ligation of CD40 activates interleukin 1(beta)-converting enzyme (caspase-1) activity in vascular smooth muscle and endothelial cells and promotes elaboration of active interleukin 1(beta). J Biol Chem 1997; 272: 19569–74.

57. Mach F, Schönbeck U, Sukhova GK et al. Reduction of atherosclerosis in mice by inhibition of CD40 signalling. Nature 1998; 394: 200–3.

58. Schönbeck U, Varo N, Libby P et al. Soluble CD40L and cardiovascular risk in women. Circulation 2001; 104: 2266–8.

59. Heeschen C, Dimmeler S, Hamm CW et al. Soluble CD40 ligand in acute coronary syndromes. New Engl J Med 2003; 348: 1104–11.

60. Varo N, de Lemos JA, Libby P et al. Soluble CD40L: risk prediction after acute coronary syndromes. Circulation 2003; 108: 1049–52.

61. Garlichs CD, Kozina S, Fateh-Moghadam S et al. Upregulation of CD40-CD40 Ligand (CD154) in patients with acute cerebral ischemia. Stroke 2003; 34: 1412–18.

62. Schumacher H, Kaiser E, Schnabel PA et al. Immunophenotypic characterisation of carotid plaque: increased amount of inflammatory cells as an independent predictor for ischaemic symptoms. Eur J Vasc Endovasc Surg 2001; 21: 494–501.

63. Golledge J, Chir M, Greenhalgh RM et al. The symptomatic carotid plaque. Stroke 2000; 31: 774–81.

64. Formato M, Farina M, Spirito R et al. Evidence for a proinflammatory and proteolytic environment in plaques from endarterectomy segments of human carotid arteries. Arterioscler Thromb Vasc Biol 2004; 24: 129–35.

65. Mallat Z, Corbaz A, Scoazec A et al. Expression of interleukin-18 in human atherosclerotic plaques and relation to plaque instability. Circulation 2001; 104: 1598–603.

66. DeGraba T, Siren AL, Penix L et al. Increased endothelial expression of intercellular adhesion molecule-1 in symptomatic versus

asymptomatic human carotid atherosclerotic plaque. Stroke 1998; 29: 1405–10.

67. Nuotio K, Lindsberg PJ, Carpen O et al. Adhesion molecule expression in symptomatic and symptomatic carotid stenosis. Neurology 2003; 60: 1890–9.

68. Wang TJ, Nam B, Wilson PW et al. Association of C-reactive protein with carotid atherosclerosis in men and women: the Framingham Heart Study. Arterioscler Thromb Vasc Biol 2002; 22: 1662–7.

69. Corrado E, Rizzo M, Tantillo R et al. Markers of inflammation and infection influence the outcome of patients with baseline asymptomatic carotid lesions: a 5-year follow-up study. Stroke 2006; 37: 482–6.

70. Schillinger M, Exner M, Mlekusch W et al. Inflammation and Carotid Artery – Risk for Atherosclerosis Study (ICARAS). Circulation 2005; 111: 2203–9.

71. Chapman CML, Beilby JP, McQuillan BM et al. Monocyte count, but not C-reactive protein or interleukin-6, is an independent risk marker for subclinical carotid atherosclerosis. Stroke 2004; 35: 1619–24.

72. Yamagami H, Kitagawa K, Nagai Y et al. Higher levels of interleukin-6 are associated with lower echogenicity of carotid artery plaques. Stroke 2004; 35: 677–81.

73. Rerkasem K, Shearman CP, Williams JA et al. C-reactive protein is elevated in symptomatic compared with asymptomatic patients with carotid artery disease. Eur J Vasc Endovasc Surg 2002; 23: 505–9.

74. Garcia AB, Ruiz C, Chacon P et al. High-sensitivity C-reactive protein in high-grade carotid stenosis: risk marker for unstable carotid plaque. J Vasc Surg 2003; 38: 1018–24.

75. Corrado E, Rizzo M, Tantillo R et al. Markers of inflammation and infection influence the outcome of patients with baseline asymptomatic carotid lesions: a 5-year follow-up study. Stroke 2006; 37: 482–6.

76. Schillinger M, Exner M, Sabeti S et al. Excessive carotid in-stent neointimal formation predicts late cardiovascular events. J Endovasc Ther 2004; 11: 229–39.

77. Elkind MS, Cheng J, Boden-Albala B et al. Tumor necrosis factor receptor levels are associated with carotid atherosclerosis. Stroke 2002; 33: 31–8.

78. Mocco J, Choudhri TF, Mack WJ et al. Elevation of soluble intercellular adhesion molecule-1 levels in symptomatic and asymptomatic carotid atherosclerosis. Neurosurgery 2001; 48(4): 718–22.

79. Raggi P, Taylor A, Fayad Z et al. Atherosclerotic plaque imaging. Contemporary role in preventive cardiology. Arch Intern Med 2005; 165: 2345–53.

80. Weiss CR, Arai AE, Bui MN et al. Arterial wall MRI characteristics are associated with elevated serum markers of inflammation in humans. J Magn Reson Imaging 2001; 14: 698–704.

81. Corti R, Fuster V, Fayad ZA et al. Effects of aggressive versus conventional lipid-lowering therapy by simvastatin on human atherosclerotic lesions: a prospective, randomized, double-blind trial with high-resolution magnetic resonance imaging. J Am Coll Cardiol 2005; 46: 106–12.

82. Grubb RL Jr, Derdeyn CP, Fritsch SM et al. Importance of hemodynamic factors in the prognosis of symptomatic carotid occlusion. JAMA 1998; 280: 1055–60.

83. Markus H, Cullinane M. Severely impaired cerebrovascular reactivity predicts stroke and TIA risk in patients with carotid artery stenosis and occlusion. Brain 2001; 124: 457–67.

84. Silvestrini M, Vernieri F, Pasqualetti P et al. Impaired cerebral vasoreactivity and risk of stroke in patients with asymptomatic carotid artery stenosis. JAMA 2000; 283: 2122–7.

85. Novo S, Basili S, Tantillo R et al. Soluble CD40L and cardiovascular risk in asymptomatic low-grade carotid stenosis. Stroke 2005; 36: 673–5.

86. Law MR, Wald NJ. Risk factor thresholds: their existence under scrutiny. BMJ 2002; 324: 1570–6.

87. Elkind MSV. Implications of stroke prevention trials: treatment of global risk. Neurology 2005; 65: 17–21.

88. Chew DP, Bhatt DL, Robbins MA et al. Effect of clopidogrel added to aspirin before percutaneous coronary intervention on the risk associated with C-reactive protein. Am J Cardiol 2001; 88: 672–4.

89. Roberts CK, Won D, Pruthi S et al. Effect of a short-term diet and exercise intervention on oxidative stress, inflammation, MMP-9 and monocyte chemotactic activity in men with metabolic syndrome factors. J Appl Physiol 2006; 100: 1657–65.

90. Caulin-Glaser T, Falko J, Hindman L, La Londe M, Snow R. Cardiac rehabilitation is associated with an improvement in C-reactive protein levels in both men and women with cardiovascular disease. J Cardiopulm Rehabil 2005; 25: 332–6.

91. Fairey AS, Courneya KS, Field CJ et al. Effect of exercise training on C-reactive protein in postmenopausal breast cancer survivors: a randomized controlled trial. Brain Behav Immun 2005; 19: 381–8.

92. Marcell TJ, McAuley KA, Traustadottir T et al. Exercise training is not associated with improved levels of C-reactive protein or adiponectin. Metabolism 2005; 54: 533–41.

93. Clifton PM, Keogh JB, Foster PR et al. Effect of weight loss on inflammatory and endothelial markers and FMD using two low-fat diets. Int J Obes (Lond) 2005; 29: 1445–51.

94. Yesilbursa D, Serdar A, Heper Y et al. The effect of orlistat-induced weight loss on interleukin-6 and C-reactive protein levels in obese subjects. Acta Cardiol 2005; 60: 265–9.

95. Haffner S, Temprosa M, Crandall J et al. Intensive lifestyle intervention or metformin on inflammation and coagulation in participants with impaired glucose tolerance. Diabetes 2005; 54: 1566–72.

96. Due A, Toubro S, Stender S, Skov AR, Astrup A. The effect of diets high in protein or carbohydrate on inflammatory markers in overweight subjects. Diabetes Obes Metab 2005; 7: 223–9.

97. O'Brien KD, Brehm BJ, Seeley RJ et al. Diet-induced weight loss is associated with decreases in plasma serum amyloid a and C-reactive protein independent of dietary macronutrient composition in obese subjects. J Clin Endocrinol Metab 2005; 90: 2244–9.

98. Ohsawa M, Okayama A, Nakamura M et al. CRP levels are elevated in smokers but unrelated to the number of cigarettes and are decreased by long-term smoking cessation in male smokers. Prev Med 2005; 41: 651–6.

99. Crook MA, Scott DA, Stapleton JA et al. Circulating concentrations of C-reactive protein and total sialic acid in tobacco smokers remain unchanged following one year of validated smoking cessation. Eur J Clin Invest 2000; 30: 861–5.

100. Albert MA, Danielson E, Rifai N, Ridker PM; PRINCE Investigators. Effect of statin therapy on C-reactive protein levels: the pravastatin inflammation/CRP evaluation (PRINCE): a randomized trial and cohort study. JAMA 2001; 286: 964–70.

101. Ridker PM, Rifai N, Lowenthal SP. Rapid reduction in C-reactive protein with cerivastatin among 785 patients with primary hypercholesterolemia. Circulation 2001; 103: 1191–3.

102. Martin-Ventura JL, Blanco-Colio LM, Gomez-Hernandez A et al. Intensive treatment with atorvastatin reduces inflammation in mononuclear cells and human atherosclerotic lesions in one month. Stroke 2005; 36: 1796–800.

103. Ridker PM, Cannon CP, Morrow D et al. C-reactive protein levels and outcomes after statin therapy. N Engl J Med 2005; 352: 20–8.

104. Nissen SE, Tuzcu EM, Schoenhagen P et al. Statin therapy, LDL cholesterol, C-reactive protein, and coronary artery disease. N Engl J Med 2005; 352: 29–38.

105. O'Donoghue M, Morrow DA, Sabatine MS et al. Lipoprotein-associated phospholipase A2 and its association with cardiovascular outcomes in patients with acute coronary syndromes in the PROVE IT-TIMI 22 (PRavastatin Or atorVastatin Evaluation and Infection Therapy-Thrombolysis In Myocardial Infarction) trial. Circulation 2006; 113: 1745–52.

106. Heart Protection Study Collaborative Group. MRC/BHF Heart Protection Study of cholesterol lowering with simvastatin in 20 536 high-risk individuals: a randomized placebo-controlled trial. Lancet 2002; 360: 7–22.

107. Feng DL, Tracy RP, Lipinska I et al. Effect of short-term aspirin use on C-reactive protein. J Thromb Thrombolysis 2000; 9: 37–41.

108. Feldman M, Jialal I, Devaraj S et al. Effects of low-dose aspirin on serum C-reactive protein and thromboxane B_2 concentrations: a placebo-controlled study using a highly sensitive C-reactive protein assay. J Am Coll Cardiol 2001; 37: 2036–41.

109. Ikonomidis I, Andreotti F, Economou E et al. Increased pro-inflammatory cytokines in patients with chronic stable angina and their reduction by aspirin. Circulation 1999; 100: 793–8.

110. Klinkhardt U, Kirchmaier CM, Westrup D et al. Ex vivo–in vitro interaction between aspirin, clopidogrel, and the glycoprotein IIb/IIIa inhibitors abciximab and SR121566A. Clin Pharmacol Ther 2000; 67: 305–13.

111. Chronos NA, Wilson DJ, Janes SL et al. Aspirin does not affect the flow cytometric detection of fibrinogen binding to, or release of alpha-granules or lysosomes from, human platelets. Clin Sci (Lond) 1994; 87: 575–80.

112. Mickelson JK, Ali MN, Kleiman NS et al. Chimeric 7E3 Fab (ReoPro) decreases detectable CD11b on neutrophils from patients undergoing coronary angioplasty. J Am Coll Cardiol 1999; 33: 97–106.

113. May AE, Neumann FJ, Gawaz M et al. Reduction of monocyte–platelet interaction and monocyte activation in patients receiving antiplatelet therapy after coronary stent implantation. Eur Heart J 1997; 18: 1913–20.

114. Klinkhardt U, Graff J, Harder S. Clopidogrel, but not abciximab, reduces platelet leukocyte conjugates and P-selectin expression in a human ex vivo in vitro model. Clin Pharmacol Ther 2002; 71: 176–85.

115. Cha JK, Jeong MH, Lee KM et al. Changes in platelet P-selectin and in plasma C-reactive protein in acute atherosclerotic ischemic stroke treated with a loading dose of clopidogrel. J Thromb Thrombolysis 2002; 14: 145–50.

116. Schillaci G, Pirro M, Gemelli F et al. Increased C-reactive protein concentrations in never-treated hypertension: the role of systolic and pulse pressures. J Hypertens 2003; 21: 1841–6.

117. Sung KC, Suh JY, Kim BS et al. High sensitivity C-reactive protein as an independent risk factor for essential hypertension. Am J Hypertens 2003; 16: 429–33.

118. Sesso HD, Buring JE, Rifai N et al. C-reactive protein and the risk of developing hypertension. JAMA 2003; 290: 2945–51.

119. Marques-Vidal P, Cambou JP, Bongard V et al. Systolic and diastolic hypertension: no relationship with lipid and inflammatory markers in Haute-Garonne, France. Am J Hypertens 2003; 16: 681–4.

120. Saito M, Ishimitsu T, Minami J et al. Relations of plasma high sensitivity C-reactive protein to traditional cardiovascular risk factors. Atherosclerosis 2003; 167: 73–9.

121. Dohi Y, Ohashi M, Sugiyama M et al. Candesartan reduces oxidative stress and inflammation in patients with essential hypertension. Hypertension Res 2003; 26: 691–7.

122. Di Napoli M, Papa F. Angiotensin-converting enzyme inhibitor use is associated with reduced plasma concentration of C-reactive protein in patients with first-ever ischemic stroke. Stroke 2003; 34: 2922–9.

123. Schieffer B, Bunte C, Witte J et al. Comparative effects of AT-1 antagonism and angiotensin-converting enzyme inhibition on markers of inflammation and platelet aggregation in patients with coronary artery disease. J Am Coll Cardiol 2004; 44: 362–8.

124. Dandona P, Aljada A. A rational approach to pathogenesis and treatment of type 2 diabetes mellitus, insulin resistance, inflammation, and atherosclerosis. Am J Cardiol 2002; 90: 27G–33G.

125. Consoli A, Devangelio E. Thiazolidinediones and inflammation. Lupus 2005; 14: 794–7.

126. Aljada A, Garg R, Ghanim H et al. Nuclear factor-kappaB suppressive and inhibitor-kappaB stimulatory effects of troglitazone in obese patients with type 2 diabetes: evidence of an anti-inflammatory action? J Clin Endocrinol Metab 2001; 86: 3250–6.

127. Haffner SM, Greenberg AS, Weston WM et al. Effect of rosiglitazone treatment on nontraditional markers of cardiovascular disease in patients with type 2 diabetes mellitus. Circulation 2002; 106: 679–84.

12

The role of carotid and cerebral angiography in the management of individuals with asymptomatic carotid artery stenosis

Richard E Temes, H Christian Schumacher, Philip M Meyers and Randall T Higashida

---

Take-Home Messages

1. Among patients with asymptomatic carotid artery stenosis (CAS), angiography of the extracranial and intracranial blood vessels should only be performed when there is discrepancy between duplex ultrasound and magnetic resonance or computed tomography (CT) angiography or prior to carotid revascularization.
2. The objective of angiography is to confirm the severity of stenosis, determine the presence or absence of intracranial tandem lesions, identify the adequacy and source of collateral circulation, and determine the presence or absence of aneurysms and arteriovenous malformations (AVMs).
3. The prevalence of brain AVMs in patients with carotid occlusive disease is low, but if found, they need to be considered in clinical decision-making.
4. If the BAVMs have high-risk hemorrhagic features, it may be preferable to treat them prior to treating the CAS.
5. In patients with symptomatic or asymptomatic CAS, incidental cerebral aneurysms on angiography can be found in 1–9% of patients. In the majority of patients, these aneurysms are small (<10 mm in maximal diameter) and carry a low risk of rupture spontaneously or with carotid revascularization.
6. For patients with larger aneurysms, there is no consensus as to whether they should be treated before carotid revascularization. The treatment plan should follow the current recommendations of the American Heart Association for the treatment of intracranial aneurysms.

INTRODUCTION

Stroke is the leading cause of disability and ranks third in mortality in the USA, Europe, and Asia. Carotid occlusive disease remains a major cause of stroke, accounting for 20–25% of cases in the USA. Population-based studies indicate that the prevalence of carotid artery stenosis (CAS) is 0.5% in the sixth decade of life and increases 20-fold by the age of 80.[1] Intracerebral atherosclerosis accounts for an additional 8–29% of strokes, with a higher reported incidence in Asian, African, and Hispanic ethnicities.[2–4] In the USA alone, an estimated 60 000 to 80 000 strokes per year are due to cerebral atherosclerosis.

Novel techniques such as angioplasty and stent-supported angioplasty have been developed to address the growing burden of disease. Despite these techniques, there remains a mounting debate over the exact role of carotid and cerebral angiography in the management of individuals with asymptomatic carotid and intracerebral occlusive disease. Magnetic resonance imaging (MRI) with and without perfusion, computed tomographic (CT) angiography, Doppler ultrasound, as well as transcranial Doppler ultrasound with and without CO_2 reactivity have all been used to gauge severity of disease. The development of multiple techniques to measure lesion severity, and the role of angiography in the treatment of cerebral pathology such as aneurysms and arteriovenous malformations (AVMs) prior to revascularization add to the dilemma. The focus of this chapter is to provide the clinician with information on the current role of conventional angiography in the detection, grading, and clinical decision-making of asymptomatic carotid and cerebral occlusive disease.

HISTORICAL PERSPECTIVE

The first report on cerebral angiography was presented by Egas Moniz in 1927 where he discussed five patients who underwent successful carotid injections.[5] With the advent of angiography, the first carotid occlusion was discovered by Sjöqvist in 1936.[6] During the 1940s and 1950s, carotid artery disease became a recognized, commonplace entity. In 1955, Millikan et al described the syndrome of 'intermittent insufficiency of the carotid arterial system' and emphasized that these attacks were due to the state of collateral circulation and blood pressure.[7] Carl Fisher[8,9] believed that ulcerative plaques at the carotid bifurcation could cause cerebral embolism and predicted that vascular surgery will bypass the occluded portion of artery.

In 1953, DeBakey performed the first successful carotid endarterectomy (CEA) for the treatment of an occluded extracranial carotid artery.[10] Since then the use of CEA has become widespread throughout the USA and Europe. The NASCET (North American Symptomatic Carotid Endarterectomy Trial),[11] the ECST (European Carotid Surgery Trial),[12] and the ACAS (Asymptomatic Carotid Atherosclerosis Study)[13] all demonstrated the superiority of surgical treatment over medical management for symptomatic CAS.

As revascularization surgery became more and more commonplace, clinicians focused on non-invasive imaging modalities to evaluate carotid and cerebrovascular disease. As discussed elsewhere in this book, carotid and transcranial Doppler ultrasound, MR and CT angiography are all valuable tools to evaluate vascular disease. However, conventional angiography is still regarded by many as being the authoritative method for evaluating the carotid bifurcation as well as small vascular lesions in the cerebral circulation that may be missed by these aforementioned techniques.

With the introduction of endovascular balloon angioplasty in 1980 by Kerber et al,[14] conventional angiography moved from simply a diagnostic technique to one which is therapeutic. Development of carotid stents reduced the rate of recurrent stenosis and appeared to be comparable with endarterectomy in prevention of

ipsilateral stroke. In addition, new methods such as distal protection devices to capture embolic debris during stent angioplasty have been shown to not be inferior to endarterectomy and may provide benefit in those patients who are felt to be high risk for surgery.

ROLE OF CAROTID AND CEREBRAL ANGIOGRAPHY IN THE MANAGEMENT OF PATIENTS WITH CAROTID ARTERY DISEASE

Patients who are referred for angiography are done so to answer specific questions:

1. Is the lesion angiographically significant?
2. What is the etiology of the lesion (e.g. atherosclerotic, dissection, vasculitis)?
3. Is there concomitant cerebral artery disease such as an AVM, aneurysm, or tandem atherosclerotic lesion?
4. What is the status of existing and potential collateral circulation?

The full evaluation of these factors is essential prior to consideration of any revascularization procedure.

Internal carotid artery stenosis

The main goal of cerebral angiography of extracranial atherosclerotic vascular disease is to determine if the vessel is occluded, significantly stenotic, or normal. Because NASCET demonstrated significant benefit of surgery in patients with symptomatic CAS (70–99%), accurate assessment of the maximum stenosis on angiograms is of utmost importance in symptomatic patients. However, the role of angiography in the pre-surgical assessment of asymptomatic patients remains unclear. It has been estimated that the annual risk of ipsilateral stroke in asymptomatic CAS >50% is 2–3%.[13,15,16] It also appears that the annual risk of ipsilateral stroke increases with lesion severity from 1.4% in >50% stenosis to 2.8% in lesions >80%.[16]

Studies to determine the diagnostic accuracy of contrast-enhanced MR angiography and CT angiography in demonstrating internal carotid artery (ICA) stenosis have invariably used conventional digital subtraction angiography (DSA) as the reference standard.[17–21] Conventional DSA, in contrast to rotational conventional angiography, is inherently limited to depicting the carotid bifurcation and carotid arteries in only two or three projections. This limitation, which is inherent to conventional DSA, may, in part, explain the apparent overestimation of ICA stenosis, which is sometimes seen at both unenhanced and contrast-enhanced MR angiography[22] of the carotid artery for which multiple projections are available. Three-dimensional (3D) time-of-flight (TOF) MR angiography, contrast-enhanced MR angiography, DSA, and rotational angiography have been recently compared for depiction of carotid stenosis. Contrast-enhanced MR angiography was shown not to overestimate the degree of stenosis and was highly agreeable with rotational angiography. The authors conclude that, given its safety and ease, contrast-enhanced MR angiography rather than conventional DSA should be the technique of choice.[23]

Although ease and safety are important considerations to make, it is important to note that all of the major clinical trials investigating the indications for carotid endarterectomy (CEA) in both symptomatic and asymptomatic CAS utilized conventional angiography as gold standard for determining the degree of stenosis. In addition, non-invasive imaging modalities (Doppler ultrasound, CT angiography, MR angiography) have their unique pitfalls and vary in accuracy in comparison with conventional angiography.[24,25]

The choice of imaging strategy is perhaps even more important in the case of asymptomatic carotid artery disease. It is important to note that although the perioperative stroke/death rate of 2.3% was seen in ACAS, 1.2% was due to conventional angiography. The high complication rate associated with diagnostic angiography in this trial has been used to justify operating on these patients without angiographic confirmation of stenosis. However, the reported risk of angiography in ACAS is at least twice the currently accepted standard.[26] Relying on duplex ultrasound in clinical practice as the sole imaging modality prior to CEA cannot be justified because of the wide variability in accuracy among various laboratories. Wong and colleagues[27] have shown that the most common cause of inappropriate CEA is stenosis overestimation by duplex ultrasound.

Patients with ultrasound-documented severe carotid stenosis who are being considered for endarterectomy should have confirmative imaging by MR or CT angiography to avoid unnecessary surgery. Non-invasive anatomic imaging removes the potential additional risk of angiography and enables skilled surgeons to reach the 3.0% complication rate of stroke/death suggested by the American Heart Association for CEA to be appropriate for asymptomatic disease.[28]

Measurement of carotid stenosis severity

Several hundred studies have been published over the last few years on imaging and measurement of carotid stenosis. Despite all this research, there is still no consensus about how best to image and measure stenosis. The methods used for determining percent diameter stenosis of the ICA from an angiogram rely on ECST, NASCET, or common carotid[29] criteria. Although

these methods differ in clinically important ways, they all rely for their calculation on measurements of the minimum linear dimension at the level of maximum stenosis as well as the linear dimension of a vessel at a reference location. These two measurements are used to calculate the fractional residual lumen, which can then be converted to percent diameter stenosis.

Historically, the ECST method has been criticized because of vagueness in the definition of the reference diameter, which is chosen as the extrapolated diameter of the carotid bulb at the level of the stenosis, although studies have confirmed that the reproducibility of this method is comparable with that of the NASCET protocol.[30,31] The NASCET method uses the normal distal ICA as a reference point. At very high grades of stenosis, flow reduction can result in a decrease in the size of the distal ICA and therefore reduces the reference diameter in the NASCET measurement. The percent stenosis obtained by the NASCET method is less than (or equal to) the ECST measurement (Figure 12.1) and less than the common carotid value. Conversion factors have been published.[32] When differences in measurement protocols are corrected for, the surgical benefit is comparable between the major studies and, to avoid confusion, most authorities now recommend the use of the NASCET-style measurement for angiography.[33]

Angiographic carotid stenosis morphology

Several angiographic[12,34] and ultrasonographic[35–37] studies have shown, in patients with symptomatic carotid disease, that carotid plaque surface irregularity or ulceration is more commonly associated with recurrent neurological symptoms.

The evidence linking angiographic carotid lesion morphology (ulceration, eccentricity, irregularity) (Figure 12.2) in neurologically asymptomatic individuals with

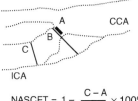

$$NASCET = 1 - \frac{C - A}{C} \times 100\%$$

$$ECST = 1 - \frac{B - A}{B} \times 100\%$$

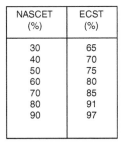

NASCET (%)	ECST (%)
30	65
40	70
50	75
60	80
70	85
80	91
90	97

Figure 12.1 Difference between the NASCET and ECST method of measurement of the degree of internal carotid artery (ICA) stenosis. A = residual lumen diameter, B = lumen diameter at the carotid bulb, C = lumen diameter at the distal ICA.

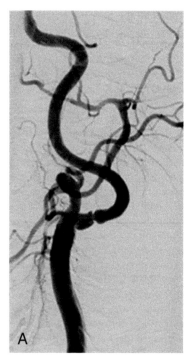 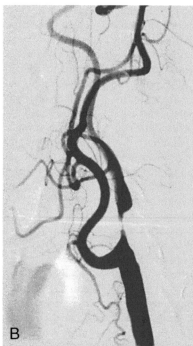 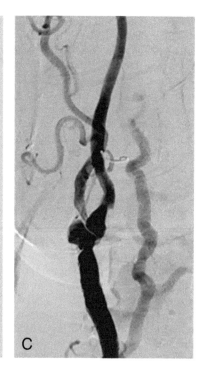

Figure 12.2 Carotid artery stenosis in neurologically asymptomatic individuals. (A) Focal concentric stenosis in left internal carotid artery (ICA). (B) Focal eccentric subtotal stenosis in left ICA. (C) Ulcerated stenosis in right ICA.

the development of future ischemic neurological events is less certain. In an analysis of 5393 carotid bifurcation angiograms from 3007 symptomatic patients in the ECST trial, Rothwell and colleagues[38] demonstrated that patients with angiographic plaque surface irregularity in a symptomatic carotid artery are more likely to have irregular plaques in the asymptomatic carotid artery. It has also been shown that patients with an asymptomatic CAS who had a history of symptomatic contralateral carotid stenosis are more likely to develop ischemic cerebral symptoms on the asymptomatic ipsilateral side.[39] Putting these data together may support a prognostic role for carotid stenosis ulceration in neurologically asymptomatic patients. Further support for this hypothesis came from observations by Fisher and colleagues,[40] who demonstrated that an asymptomatic carotid plaque in patients with contralateral ischemic neurological events had a higher incidence of ulcers and thrombus than in patients without prior neurological symptoms.

The utility of conventional angiography in accurately detecting carotid plaque ulceration is limited to ~60%.[41] However, the availability of ultra-high resolution digital subtraction angiography may improve these rates.[42,43]

Distal internal carotid artery or middle cerebral artery stenosis (tandem lesions)

Tandem lesions, or distal stenoses, are present in approximately 2% of patients with significant ICA lesions.[43] The most common site for tandem lesions is the carotid siphon, followed by the horizontal middle cerebral artery segment. The two main problems in the management of in-tandem stenosis are:

- to determine if the neurological symptoms, if any, are due to hemodynamic changes or embolic changes
- to decide which lesion causes the symptoms.

Some authors feel that the presence of in-tandem stenosis is a relative contraindication to revascularization.[44] Other authors have reported reversal of intracranial stenosis following carotid surgery.[45]

Several studies have looked at the risk of stroke in individuals with tandem lesions following CEA. Schuler et al found no statistical difference in operative, perioperative, and late strokes in individuals with or without in-tandem lesions following CEA. They also found relief of symptoms to be the same in all groups.[46] However, none of the patients had siphon stenosis >70%. Roederer et al operated on symptomatic patients who had symptomatic stenosis between 20 and 100% and found that concomitant siphon disease was not associated with recurrent symptoms.[47] However, only 9% of these patients had >50% stenosis at the siphon, making this conclusion questionable. Mackey et al showed no difference in short-term and long-term outcome among 597 patients, although the incidence of recurrent transient ischemic attack was 9.7% in the intracranial disease group and 6.5% in the no intracranial disease group ($p = 0.22$).[48] Further analysis of the data, however, showed that only 49 patients had carotid siphon stenosis and, of these, only seven patients had stenosis >80%. Mattos et al found that, among 393 patients, the perioperative and late ipsilateral stroke-free rates were similar in both groups that were with and without siphon stenosis (0.0% vs 0.6%, respectively).[49] Long-term ipsilateral stroke-free rates were also not significantly different in subgroups with siphon stenosis between 20% and 49% and for those with stenosis >50%. At this time, adequate angiographic evaluation of both the carotid siphon and the circle of Willis is recommended prior to revascularization, as the hemodynamic effect of sequential lesions tend to be additive if both lesions are severe enough to reduce flow and tend to be governed by the more severe lesion.[50,51] However, the exact risk of stroke due to in-tandem lesions is still in question.

Collateral circulation

This topic is discussed in detail in Chapter 3. Collateral circulation plays a pivotal role in the pathophysiology of ischemia in patients with chronic occlusion of the ICA.[52] Insufficient collateral flow may predispose to ischemia and infarction in ICA occlusion. Inadequate collateral blood flow may be the result of poor functioning of collateral pathways distal to the ICA occlusion. In ICA occlusion, the circle of Willis, including the anterior and posterior communicating arteries, may be the major collateral pathway that can rapidly compensate for decreased cerebral perfusion pressure. On the other hand, collateral pathways through the ophthalmic artery and leptomeningeal vessels may be recruited when collateral flow through the circle of Willis is inadequate. Thus, poor function of circle of Willis collaterals, which may lead to the recruitment of ophthalmic or leptomeningeal collaterals, may cause hemodynamic impairment.[53] Because the common carotid artery is clamped during endarterectomy, preoperative determination of collateral blood flow is also helpful in determining whether a shunt across the carotid bifurcation during CEA will be necessary.[54]

Concomitant brain arteriovenous malformations and carotid disease

Brain arteriovenous malformations (BAVMs) are characterized by a conglomerate of abnormal vessels lacking a capillary bed. Blood flows through feeding arteries into the BAVMs – the nidus – and from there into draining veins. The nidus functions as an arteriovenous shunt and is characterized by abnormal vessels with thin or irregular muscularis and elastica, hypertrophy of the media, and various amounts of sclerotic tissue. No normal brain tissue is found within the nidus. Epidemiological studies report a detection rate for brain AVMs ranging between 0.89 and 1.34 per 100 000 person-years.[55–58]

Clinically, BAVMs present as intracranial hemorrhage – the most feared presentation, seizures, headaches, or rarely as a progressive neurological deficit.[59] There is controversy regarding treating unruptured BAVMs,[60] but the general consensus is to treat a ruptured BAVM because of the risk of recurrent hemorrhage.[61] Various studies suggest that 38–70% of brain BAVMs present initially with hemorrhages.[55–59] The overall risk of intracranial hemorrhage in patients with known BAVM is 2–4% per year.[62] Ruptured AVMs are at increased risk for rebleeding, particularly during the first year after the initial hemorrhage. Typical rates for hemorrhagic presentation within 12 months of initial clinical presentation are 7–33% in patients with hemorrhagic presentation and 0–3% in patients with non-hemorrhagic presentation.[63,64] Hemorrhage rates progressively converge with time for both patient groups after 1 year.

Clinical and angiographic features associated with the risk for hemorrhagic presentation are male gender, small BAVM size, location in the basal ganglia or posterior fossa, deep venous drainage, single or only few draining veins, high pressure in the feeding arteries as measured during angiography, and intranidal and flow-related feeding artery aneurysms.[65]

AVMs are not well visualized on cranial computed tomography (CCT). MRI is the neuroimaging of choice for detection of BAVMs. Most patients undergoing cerebral angiography will have undergone some form of neuroimaging, but incidental detection of a brain AVM on cerebral angiography is an extremely unlikely event.

There is no published case report of a patient treated with angioplasty or stent-assisted angioplasty of an extracranial cerebral artery harboring AVMs on the brain in the distal territory of the artery. Theoretically, the increased blood flow after successful angioplasty to the BAVM-containing brain will lead to an increased pressure in the feeding arteries and this may predispose to its rupture. In addition, BAVMs have feeding artery or intranidal aneurysms. Both aneurysm types have been associated with an increased risk for BAVM rupture.[66]

A complicating factor is also the requirement for antithrombotic treatment after stent-assisted angioplasty with acetylsalicylic acid and clopidogrel to prevent stent occlusion. It is unknown if this combination increases the risk for BAVM rupture. MRI studies suggest clinically asymptomatic small hemorrhages in patients with BAVM.

Treatment decisions need to be individualized for a given patient. The treatment risk is estimated by the Spetzler–Martin grade. This grading system assigns 1 point to AVMs <3 cm in largest diameter, 2 points to AVMs 3–6 cm in largest diameter, and 3 points for AVMs >6 cm. A further point is added if the AVM is located in functionally critical brain (such as language, motor, sensory, or visual cortex), and another point if the AVM has a deep venous drainage. The current American Heart Association multidisciplinary management guidelines for the treatment of brain AVMs recommend the following approach:[61]

1. Surgical extirpation is strongly suggested as the primary treatment for Spetzler–Martin grade I and II if surgically accessible with low risk.
2. Radiation therapy alone is recommended for Spetzler–Martin grade I or II if the AVM is <3 cm in size and surgery has an increased surgical risk based on location and vascular anatomy.
3. Brain AVMs of Spetzler–Martin grade III can often be treated by a multimodal approach with embolization followed by surgical extirpation. If the lesion has a high surgical risk based on location and vascular anatomy, radiation therapy may be performed after embolization.
4. AVMs of Spetzler–Martin grade IV and V are often not amenable to surgical treatment alone because of the high procedural risk. These AVMs can be approached by a combined multimodal approach of embolization, radiosurgery, and/or surgery.
5. In general, embolization should only be performed if the goal is complete AVM eradication with other treatment modalities. The only exception is palliative embolization in patients with an AVM of Spetzler–Martin grade IV or V with venous outflow obstruction or true steal phenomenon in order to reduce arterial inflow to control edema or to reduce the amount of shunt, respectively.

In the rare case of concurrent BAVM and steno-occlusive cerebrovascular disease, a cerebral angiography needs to be performed to evaluate the presence of high-risk hemorrhagic features of the BAVM. If these are present, it may be preferable to treat the BAVM prior to treatment of the steno-occlusive arterial lesion. For BAVM, definitive treatment is usually achieved by staged embolization and microsurgical resection (Figure 12.3). In BAVMs that are not amenable to surgical resection either because of their deep location or eloquent brain areas and of small size, radiosurgery is the main treatment option and may be preceded by staged endovascular embolization. However, radiation-induced BAVM obliteration is not achieved in a significant number of BAVMs and takes up to 3 years to be completed.[67]

Concomitant intracranial aneurysms and carotid disease

Intracranial aneurysms are responsible for subarachnoid hemorrhage (SAH) – a condition that carries a high risk for death and permanent disability. The incidence of SAH due to ruptured intracranial aneurysms is 6–8 per 100 000 person years and leads to sudden death in 12% of affected patients. The 30-day mortality is as high as 67%.[68] Survivors remain neurologically severely impaired secondary to irreversible brain damage in approximately 50% of cases.[69,70] Despite improvements in the management of SAH patients, mortality and morbidity rates remain overall largely unchanged through the years. Aneurysms increase in frequency with age beyond the third decade.

Cerebral angiography is considered the gold standard for aneurysm detection. Retrospective and prospective studies performed for aneurysm-unrelated conditions and using different imaging modalities report detection rates for incidental, unruptured aneurysms between 1.0% and 7.4% (mean 3.7%)[71-76] and between 2.4 and 41% (mean 6.0%),[77-85] respectively. The large variation in the reported incidence rates is explained by different patient cohorts included in the study, i.e. patients with familial saccular aneurysms or collagen tissue diseases.

For asymptomatic, incidental aneurysms, rupture rates depend largely on aneurysm size. The International Study of Unruptured Intracranial Aneurysms (ISUIA) reported a mean annual rupture rate of 0.05% for aneurysms <10 mm, 1% for aneurysms ≥10 mm but <25 mm, and 6% for ≥25 mm size.[86] In a subsequent paper, the same group found more specific 5-year cumulative rupture rates depending on size and location.[87] Again, rupture rates increased with aneurysm size. Furthermore, aneurysms located in the posterior circulation were more likely to rupture compared with aneurysms in the anterior circulation (Table 12.1). For high-risk aneurysms, the rupture risk exceeds the perioperative risk for endovascular coiling or open neurosurgical clipping.

The main question is how often are incidental aneurysms found in patients with symptomatic or asymptomatic extracranial carotid stenosis. In these patient groups, incidental aneurysms were found between 1% and 9% (mean 3.2%).[85,88-91] The largest prospective series reporting incidental aneurysm detection by angiography in patients with CAS is from the NASCET.[90]

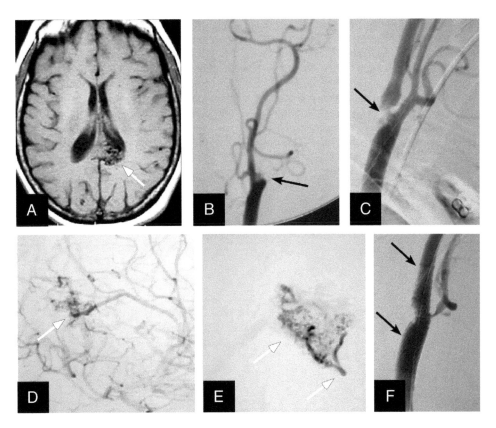

Figure 12.3 A 55-year-old woman with symptomatic carotid stenosis and an incidental brain arteriovenous malformation (AVM). (A) T1-weighted axial MRI brain scan shows an AVM of the left atrial choroid and corpus callosum (white arrow). (B) Right common carotid arteriography in lateral projection shows origin occlusion of the right internal carotid artery (arrow). (C) Left common carotid arteriography in the lateral projection demonstrates high-grade internal carotid stenosis (arrow). (D) Cerebral arteriography in an oblique projection during the arterial phase discloses the presence of a choroidal AVM (white arrow). (E and F) Following treatment of carotid stenosis using stent angioplasty (black arrows), the woman underwent super-selective arteriography and embolization (white arrows), then radiosurgery for the AVM.

Table 12.1 Five-year cumulative aneurysmal rupture rates (percent) according to size and location. Findings of the International Study of Unruptured Intracranial Aneurysms

Vessel location	Patients (*N*)	Aneurysm size (mm)			
		<7	7–12	13–24	≥25
Cavernous carotid artery	210	0	0	3%	6.4%
Anterior cerebral circulation*	1037	0	2.6%	14.5%	40%
Posterior cerebral circulation†	445	2.5%	14.5%	18.4%	50%

*Anterior circulation includes intracranial internal carotid (excluding cavernous portion), anterior cerebral artery, anterior communicating artery, and middle cerebral artery.

†Posterior circulation includes intracranial vertebral artery, basilar artery, posterior cerebral artery, posterior inferior and anterior cerebellar arteries, superior cerebellar artery, and posterior communicating artery.

Modified from The Lancet, 362: Wiebers DO, Whisnant JP, Huston J 3rd et al. Unruptured intracranial aneurysms: natural history, clinical outcome, and risks of surgical and endovascular treatment, 103–10, 2003, with permission from Elsevier.[87]

Among the 2885 patients included, 90 (3.1%) harbored an incidental intracranial aneurysm and in 56 (1.9%) patients the aneurysm was located distal to the symptomatic stenosis. In the vast majority (96%), these aneurysms were <10 mm in maximal diameter, and thus belonged to the low rupture risk group according to the findings of the ISUIA. Not surprisingly, only one patient suffered an SAH 6 days after successful CEA during an average follow-up period of 5 years. These data

suggest that carotid revascularization is safe in patients with small, <10 mm large aneurysms. However, the NASCET results cannot be applied for larger aneurysms. In addition, patients undergoing carotid stenting require antithrombotic treatment with acetylsalicylic acid and clopidogrel, whereas patients after CEA typically receive only acetylsalicylic acid. The combination of two platelet inhibitors may have an effect on the rupture rate of incidental intracranial aneurysms. Furthermore, in disorders

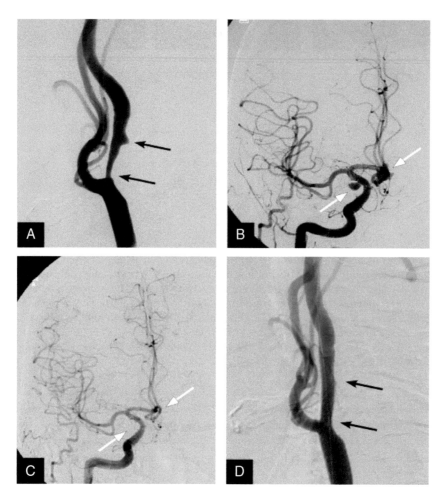

Figure 12.4 A 67-year-old woman with asymptomatic carotid stenosis following cranial radiation therapy for a skull-base brain tumor. Surveillance MRI brain scan demonstrated interval development of two cerebral aneurysms. (A) Right common carotid arteriography in the lateral projection demonstrates high-grade stenosis of the right internal carotid artery origin (black arrows). (B) Cerebral arteriography confirms the presence of right posterior communicating artery and anterior communicating artery aneurysms (white arrows). (C) Cerebral arteriography after surgical clipping confirms exclusion of the two aneurysms (white arrows). (D) After a recovery period, the woman then underwent stent-angioplasty under distal filtration protection for presumed radiation-induced carotid stenosis (black arrows). A similar patient treated for carotid stenosis refused surgical aneurysm treatment and died of aneurysmal subarachnoid hemorrhage several months later.

that are prone to saccular aneurysm formation – such as familial history of cerebral aneurysms, autosomal dominant polycystic kidney disease, extracranial internal carotid artery medial fibrodysplasia, Takayasu's arteritis, or α_1-antitrypsin deficiency – carotid revascularization may not be a safe procedure.

In summary, in patients with hemodynamically significant carotid stenosis and incidental intracranial aneurysm, an individual treatment plan between endovascular surgeon, neurosurgeon, and vascular neurologist, depending on the patient's overall medical condition and preferences, is recommended prior to angioplasty or stent-assisted angioplasty of the carotid stenosis (Figure 12.4). The treatment plan should follow the current recommendations of the American Heart Association for the treatment of intracranial aneurysms.[91,92]

SUMMARY

Carotid and cerebral angiography remains an important tool in the diagnosis of both symptomatic and asymptomatic atherosclerotic disease. Despite the development of non-invasive techniques such as MR angiography and ultrasound, conventional angiography is still considered by many as the gold standard diagnostic technique in the detection of carotid stenosis due to its high sensitivity. In addition, angiography can provide additional information regarding plaque morphology, collateral circulation, and tandem lesions, which may contribute to overall stroke risk and influence choice of revascularization procedure. However, the routine use of conventional angiography in the detection of asymptomatic CAS is not recommended because it is an invasive procedure and may be associated with complications. It should be limited to asymptomatic CAS patients who have inconclusive results from non-invasive diagnostic techniques such as carotid ultrasound and MR angiography, particularly those patients who require carotid revascularization.

REFERENCES

1. O'Leary DH, Polak JF, Kronmal RA et al. Distribution and correlates of sonographically detected carotid artery disease in the Cardiovascular Health Study. The CHS Collaborative Research Group. Stroke 1992; 23: 1752–60.
2. Caplan LR, Gorelick PB, Hier DB. Race, sex and occlusive cerebrovascular disease: A review. Stroke 1986; 17: 648–55.
3. Wityk RJ, Lehman D, Klag M et al. Race and sex differences in the distribution of cerebral atherosclerosis. Stroke 1996; 27: 1974–80.
4. Li H, Wong KS. Racial distribution of intracranial and extracranial atherosclerosis. J Clin Neurosci 2003; 10: 30–4.
5. Moniz D. L'encéphalographie artérielle; son importance dans la localization des tumeurs cerebrales. Rev Neurol 1927; 2: 72–90.
6. Sjöqvist O. Uber intrakranielle aneurysmen der arteria carotis und deren beziehung zur ophthalmoplegischen migraine. Nervenarzt 1936; 9: 233–41.
7. Millikan C, Siekert R, Whisnant J. Cerebral Vascular Diseases. New York: Grune and Stratton, 1955.
8. Fisher C. Clinical syndromes in cerebral arterial occlusion. In: Fields W, ed. Pathogenesis and Treatment of Cerebrovascular Disease. Springfield, IL: Charles C Thomas, 1961.
9. Fisher C, Gore I, Okabe N, White P. Atherosclerosis of the carotid and vertebral arteries; extracranial and intracranial. J Neuropathol Exp Neurol 1965; 24: 455–76.
10. DeBakey ME. Carotid endarterectomy revisited. J Endovasc Surg 1996; 3: 4.
11. Barnett HJ, Taylor DW, Eliasziw M et al. Benefit of carotid endarterectomy in patients with symptomatic moderate or severe stenosis. North American Symptomatic Carotid Endarterectomy Trial Collaborators. N Engl J Med 1998; 339: 1415–25.
12. The European Carotid Surgery Trialists' Collaborative Group. Randomised trial of endarterectomy for recently symptomatic carotid stenosis: final results of the MRC European Carotid Surgery Trial (ECST). Lancet 1998; 351: 1379–87.
13. Endarterectomy for asymptomatic carotid artery stenosis. Executive Committee for the Asymptomatic Carotid Atherosclerosis Study. JAMA 1995; 273: 1421–8.
14. Kerber CW, Cromwell LD, Loehden OL. Catheter dilation of proximal carotid stenosis during distal bifurcation endarterectomy. Am J Neuroradiol 1980; 1(4): 348–9.
15. Hennerici M, Hulsbomer HB, Hefter H, Lammerts D, Rautenberg W. Natural history of asymptomatic extracranial arterial disease. Results of a long-term prospective study. Brain 1987; 110(Pt 3): 777–91.
16. Mackey AE, Abrahamowicz M, Langlois Y et al. Outcome of asymptomatic patients with carotid disease. Asymptomatic Cervical Bruit Study Group. Neurology 1997; 48: 896–903.
17. Alvarez-Linera J, Benito-Leon J, Escribano J, Campollo J, Gesto R. Prospective evaluation of carotid artery stenosis: elliptic centric contrast-enhanced MR angiography and spiral CT angiography compared with digital subtraction angiography. AJNR Am J Neuroradiol 2003; 24: 1012–19.
18. Cosottini M, Pingitore A, Puglioli M et al. Contrast-enhanced three-dimensional magnetic resonance angiography of atherosclerotic internal carotid stenosis as the noninvasive imaging modality in revascularization decision making. Stroke 2003; 34: 660–4.
19. Cosottini M, Calabrese R, Puglioli M et al. Contrast-enhanced three-dimensional MR angiography of neck vessels: does dephasing effect alter diagnostic accuracy? Eur Radiol 2003; 13: 571–81.
20. Nederkoorn PJ, Elgersma OE, van der Graaf Y et al. Carotid artery stenosis: accuracy of contrast-enhanced MR angiography for diagnosis. Radiology 2003; 228: 677–82.
21. Hathout GM, Duh MJ, El-Saden SM. Accuracy of contrast-enhanced MR angiography in predicting angiographic stenosis of the internal carotid artery: linear regression analysis. AJNR Am J Neuroradiol 2003; 24: 1747–56.
22. Nederkoorn PJ, Mali WP, Eikelboom BC et al. Preoperative diagnosis of carotid artery stenosis: accuracy of noninvasive testing. Stroke 2002; 33: 2003–8.
23. Anzalone N, Scomazzoni F, Castellano R et al. Carotid artery stenosis: intraindividual correlations of 3D time-of-flight MR angiography, contrast-enhanced MR angiography, conventional DSA, and rotational angiography for detection and grading. Radiology 2005; 236: 204–13.
24. Patel SG, Collie DA, Wardlaw JM et al. Outcome, observer reliability, and patient preferences if CTA, MRA, or Doppler ultrasound were

used, individually or together, instead of digital subtraction angiography before carotid endarterectomy. J Neurol Neurosurg Psychiatry 2002; 73: 21–8.

25. Johnston DC, Goldstein LB. Clinical carotid endarterectomy decision making: noninvasive vascular imaging versus angiography. Neurology 2001; 56: 1009–15.

26. Wholey MH, Wholey MH. Momentum growing for carotid stent placement. Diagn Imaging 1998; 20: 65–9.

27. Wong JH, Findlay JM, Suarez-Almazor ME. Regional performance of carotid endarterectomy: appropriateness, outcomes, and risk factors for complications. Stroke 1997; 28: 891–8.

28. Biller J, Feinberg WM, Castaldo JE et al. Guidelines for carotid endarterectomy: a statement for healthcare professionals from a special writing group of the stroke council, American Heart Association. Circulation 1998; 97: 501–9.

29. Williams MA, Nicolaides AN. Predicting the normal dimensions of the internal and external carotid arteries from the diameter of the common carotid. Eur J Vasc Surg 1987; 1: 91–6.

30. Rothwell PM, Gibson RJ, Slattery J, Warlow CP. Prognostic value and reproducibility of measurements of carotid stenosis. A comparison of three methods on 1001 angiograms. European Carotid Surgery Trialists' Collaborative Group. Stroke 1994; 25: 2440–4.

31. Vanninen R, Manninen H, Koivisto K et al. Carotid stenosis by digital subtraction angiography: reproducibility of the European Carotid Surgery Trial and the North American Symptomatic Carotid Endarterectomy Trial measurement methods and visual interpretation. AJNR Am J Neuroradiol 1994; 15: 1635–41.

32. Staikov IN, Arnold M, Mattle HP et al. Comparison of the ECST, CC, and NASCET grading methods and ultrasound for assessing carotid stenosis. European Carotid Surgery Trial. North American Symptomatic Carotid Endarterectomy Trial. J Neurol 2000; 247: 681–6.

33. Rothwell PM, Gutnikov SA, Warlow CP. Reanalysis of the final results of the European Carotid Surgery Trial. Stroke 2003; 34: 514–23.

34. Eliasziw M, Streifler JY, Fox AJ et al. Significance of plaque ulceration in symptomatic patients with high-grade carotid stenosis. North American Symptomatic Carotid Endarterectomy Trial. Stroke 1994; 25: 304–8.

35. AbuRahma AF, Covelli MA, Robinson PA, Holt SM. The role of carotid duplex ultrasound in evaluating plaque morphology: potential use in selecting patients for carotid stenting. J Endovasc Surg 1999; 6: 59–65.

36. Iannuzzi A, Wilcosky T, Mercuri M et al. Ultrasonographic correlates of carotid atherosclerosis in transient ischemic attack and stroke. Stroke 1995; 26: 614–19.

37. Kessler C, von Maravic M, Bruckmann H, Kompf D. Ultrasound for the assessment of the embolic risk of carotid plaques. Acta Neurol Scand 1995; 92: 231–4.

38. Rothwell PM, Villagra R, Gibson R, Donders RC, Warlow CP. Evidence of a chronic systemic cause of instability of atherosclerotic plaques. Lancet 2000; 355: 19–24.

39. Nicolaides AN, Kakkos S, Griffin M, Geroulakos G, Ioannidou E. Severity of asymptomatic carotid stenosis and risk of ipsilateral hemispheric ischaemic events: results from the ACSRS study. Eur J Vasc Endovasc Surg 2005; 30: 275–84.

40. Fisher M, Paganini-Hill A, Martin A et al. Carotid plaque pathology: thrombosis, ulceration, and stroke pathogenesis. Stroke 2005; 36: 253–7.

41. Young GR, Humphrey PR, Nixon TE, Smith ET. Variability in measurement of extracranial internal carotid artery stenosis as displayed by both digital subtraction and magnetic resonance angiography: an assessment of three caliper techniques and visual impression of stenosis. Stroke 1996; 27: 467–73.

42. Elgersma OE, Buijs PC, Wust AF et al. Maximum internal carotid arterial stenosis: assessment with rotational angiography versus conventional intraarterial digital subtraction angiography. Radiology 1999; 213: 777–83.

43. Beneficial effect of carotid endarterectomy in symptomatic patients with high-grade carotid stenosis. North American Symptomatic Carotid Endarterectomy Trial Collaborators. N Engl J Med 1991; 325: 445–53.

44. Goldstein LB, McCrory DC, Landsman PB et al. Multicenter review of preoperative risk factors for carotid endarterectomy in patients with ipsilateral symptoms. Stroke 1994; 25: 1116–21.

45. Day AL, Rhoton AL, Quisling RG. Resolving siphon stenosis following endarterectomy. Stroke 1980; 11: 278–81.

46. Schuler JJ, Flanigan DP, Lim LT et al. The effect of carotid siphon stenosis on stroke rate, death, and relief of symptoms following elective carotid endarterectomy. Surgery 1982; 92: 1058–67.

47. Roederer GO, Langlois YE, Chan AR et al. Is siphon disease important in predicting outcome of carotid endarterectomy? Arch Surg 1983; 118: 1177–81.

48. Mackey WC, O'Donnell TF Jr, Callow AD. Carotid endarterectomy in patients with intracranial vascular disease: short-term risk and long-term outcome. J Vasc Surg 1989; 10: 432–8.

49. Mattos MA, van Bemmelen PS, Hodgson KJ et al. The influence of carotid siphon stenosis on short- and long-term outcome after carotid endarterectomy. J Vasc Surg 1993; 17: 902–10, discussion 910–11.

50. Beckmann CF, Levin DC, Kubicka RA, Henschke CI. The effect of sequential arterial stenoses on flow and pressure. Radiology 1981; 140: 655–8.

51. Guppy KH, Charbel FT, Loth F, Ausman JI. Hemodynamics of in-tandem stenosis of the internal carotid artery: when is carotid endarterectomy indicated? Surg Neurol 2000; 54: 145–52, discussion 152–3.

52. Liebeskind DS. Collateral circulation. Stroke 2003; 34: 2279–84.

53. Yamauchi H, Kudoh T, Sugimoto K et al. Pattern of collaterals, type of infarcts, and haemodynamic impairment in carotid artery occlusion. J Neurol Neurosurg Psychiatry 2004; 75: 1697–701.

54. Schwartz RB, Jones KM, LeClercq GT et al. The value of cerebral angiography in predicting cerebral ischemia during carotid endarterectomy. AJR Am J Roentgenol 1992; 159: 1057–61.

55. Stapf C, Mast H, Sciacca RR et al; New York Islands AVM Study Collaborators. The New York Islands AVM Study: design, study progress, and initial results. Stroke 2003; 34: e29–33.

56. ApSimon HT, Reef H, Phadke RV, Popovic EA. A population-based study of brain arteriovenous malformation: long-term treatment outcomes. Stroke 2002; 33: 2794–800.

57. Hillman J. Population-based analysis of arteriovenous malformation treatment. J Neurosurg 2001; 95: 633–7.

58. Al-Shahi R, Bhattacharya JJ, Currie DG et al; Scottish Intracranial Vascular Malformation Study Collaborators. Scottish Intracranial Vascular Malformation Study (SIVMS): evaluation of methods, ICD-10 coding, and potential sources of bias in a prospective, population-based cohort. Stroke 2003; 34: 1156–62.

59. Hofmeister C, Stapf C, Hartmann A et al. Demographic, morphological, and clinical characteristics of 1289 patients with brain arteriovenous malformation. Stroke 2000; 31: 1307–10.

60. Stapf C, Mohr JP, Choi JH, Hartmann A, Mast H. Invasive treatment of unruptured brain arteriovenous malformations is experimental therapy. Curr Opin Neurol 2006; 19: 63–8.

61. Ogilvy CS, Stieg PE, Awad I et al; Special Writing Group of the Stroke Council, American Stroke Association. AHA Scientific Statement: Recommendations for the management of intracranial arteriovenous malformations: a statement for healthcare

professionals from a special writing group of the Stroke Council, American Stroke Association. Stroke 2001; 32: 1458–71.

62. Ondra SL, Troupp H, George ED, Schwab K. The natural history of symptomatic arteriovenous malformations of the brain: a 24-year follow-up assessment. J Neurosurg 1990; 73: 387–91.

63. Mast H, Young WL, Koennecke HC et al. Risk of spontaneous haemorrhage after diagnosis of cerebral arteriovenous malformation. Lancet 1997; 350: 1065–8.

64. Halim AX, Johnston SC, Singh V et al. Longitudinal risk of intracranial hemorrhage in patients with arteriovenous malformation of the brain within a defined population. Stroke 2004; 35: 1697–702.

65. Choi JH, Mohr JP. Brain arteriovenous malformations in adults. Lancet Neurol 2005; 4: 299–308.

66. Stapf C, Mohr JP, Pile-spellmi et al. Concurrent arterial aneurysms in brain arteriovenous malformations with hemorrhagic presentation.J Neurol Neurosurg Psychiatry 2002; 73: 294–8.

67. Maruyama K, Kawahara N, Shin M et al. The risk of hemorrhage after radiosurgery for cerebral arteriovenous malformations. N Engl J Med 2005; 352: 146–53.

68. Huang J, van Gelder JM. The probability of sudden death from rupture of intracranial aneurysms: a meta-analysis. Neurosurgery 2002; 51: 1101–5, discussion 1105–7.

69. Hijdra A, Braakman R, van Gijn J, Vermeulen M, van Crevel H. Aneurysmal subarachnoid hemorrhage. Complications and outcome in a hospital population. Stroke 1987; 18: 1061–7.

70. Roos YB, de Haan RJ, Beenen LF et al. Complications and outcome in patients with aneurysmal subarachnoid haemorrhage: a prospective hospital based cohort study in the Netherlands. J Neurol Neurosurg Psychiatry 2000; 68: 337–41.

71. Jakubowski J, Kendall B. Coincidental aneurysms with tumours of pituitary origin. J Neurol Neurosurg Psychiatry 1978; 41: 972–9.

72. Wakai S, Fukushima T, Furihata T, Sano K. Association of cerebral aneurysm with pituitary adenoma. Surg Neurol 1979; 12: 503–7.

73. Atkinson JL, Sundt TM Jr, Houser OW, Whisnant JP. Angiographic frequency of anterior circulation intracranial aneurysms. J Neurosurg 1989; 70: 551–5.

74. Ujiie H, Sato K, Onda H et al. Clinical analysis of incidentally discovered unruptured aneurysms. Stroke 1993; 24: 1850–6.

75. Sugai Y, Hamamoto Y, Ookubo T, So K. [Angiographical frequency of unruptured incidental intracranial aneurysms]. No Shinkei Geka 1994; 22: 429–32. [in Japanese].

76. Bourekas EC, Newton HB, Figg GM, Slone HW. Prevalence and rupture rate of cerebral aneurysms discovered during intraarterial chemotherapy of brain tumors. AJNR Am J Neuroradiol 2006; 27: 297–9.

77. Wakabayashi T, Fujita S, Ohbora Y et al. Polycystic kidney disease and intracranial aneurysms. Early angiographic diagnosis and early operation for the unruptured aneurysm. J Neurosurg 1983; 58: 488–91.

78. Iwata K, Misu N, Terada K, et al. Screening for unruptured asymptomatic intracranial aneurysms in patients undergoing coronary angiography. J Neurosurg 1991; 75: 52–5.

79. Chapman AB, Rubinstein D, Hughes R et al. Intracranial aneurysms in autosomal dominant polycystic kidney disease. N Engl J Med 1992; 327: 916–20.

80. Nagashima M, Nemoto M, Hadeishi H, Suzuki A, Yasui N. Unruptured aneurysms associated with ischaemic cerebrovascular diseases. Surgical indication. Acta Neurochir (Wien) 1993; 124: 71–8.

81. Nakagawa T, Hashi K. The incidence and treatment of asymptomatic, unruptured cerebral aneurysms. J Neurosurg 1994; 80: 217–23.

82. Ruggieri PM, Poulos N, Masaryk TJ et al. Occult intracranial aneurysms in polycystic kidney disease: screening with MR angiography. Radiology 1994; 191: 33–9.

83. Leblanc R, Melanson D, Tampieri D, Guttmann RD. Familial cerebral aneurysms: a study of 13 families. Neurosurgery 1995; 37: 633–8, discussion 638–9.

84. Ronkainen A, Puranen MI, Hernesniemi JA et al. Intracranial aneurysms: MR angiographic screening in 400 asymptomatic individuals with increased familial risk. Radiology 1995; 195: 35–40.

85. Griffiths PD, Worthy S, Gholkar A. Incidental intracranial vascular pathology in patients investigated for carotid stenosis. Neuroradiology 1996; 38: 25–30.

86. Unruptured intracranial aneurysms – risk of rupture and risks of surgical intervention. International Study of Unruptured Intracranial Aneurysms Investigators. N Engl J Med 1998; 339: 1725–33.

87. Wiebers DO, Whisnant JP, Huston J 3rd et al. Unruptured intracranial aneurysms: natural history, clinical outcome, and risks of surgical and endovascular treatment. Lancet 2003; 362: 103–10.

88. Pappada G, Fiori L, Marina R et al. Incidence of asymptomatic berry aneurysms among patients undergoing carotid endarterectomy. J Neurosurg Sci 1997; 41: 257–62.

89. Yeung BK, Danielpour M, Matsumura JS et al. Incidental asymptomatic cerebral aneurysms in patients with extracranial cerebrovascular disease: is this a case against carotid endarterectomy without arteriography? Cardiovasc Surg 2000; 8: 513–18.

90. Kappelle LJ, Eliasziw M, Fox AJ, Barnett HJ. Small, unruptured intracranial aneurysms and management of symptomatic carotid artery stenosis. North American Symptomatic Carotid Endarterectomy Trial Group. Neurology 2000; 55: 307–9.

91. Bederson JB, Awad IA, Wiebers DO et al. Recommendations for the management of patients with unruptured intracranial aneurysms: a statement for healthcare professionals from the Stroke Council of the American Heart Association. Stroke 2000; 31: 2742–50.

92. Johnston SC, Higashida RT, Barrow DL et al; Committee on Cerebrovasculor Imaging of the American Heart Association Council on Cardiovascular Radiology. Recommendations for the endovascular treatment of intracranial aneurysms: a statement for healthcare professionals from the Committee on Cerebrovascular Imaging of the American Heart Association Council on Cardiovascular Radiology. Stroke 2002; 33: 2536–44.

13

Carotid endarterectomy in patients with asymptomatic carotid artery stenosis

William A Gray and E Sander Connoly

Take-Home Messages

1. Among patients with asymptomatic carotid artery stenosis (CAS) who are at low risk for surgery, carotid endarterectomy (CEA) and 'usual medical care' is superior to 'usual medical care' alone for reduction of ischemic stroke if the perioperative complication rate is <3%.
2. In Asymptomatic Carotid Surgery Trial (ACST), CEA reduced both non-disabling and disabling stroke, as well as ipsilateral and contralateral strokes.
3. The benefit of CEA in patients with asymptomatic carotid artery disease is more pronounced in men than women.
4. The number of low surgical risk patients that need to be treated with CEA to prevent 1 stroke at 5 years can be as low as 16 patients (if perioperative complication rate is 2%) or as high as 500 patients (if perioperative complication rate is 8%).
5. The results of CEA in randomized clinical trials cannot be automatically transferred to routine clinical practice. Institution-specific assessment of the risk of CEA should be a prime consideration in clinical decision-making.
6. Complications after CEA are higher in patients who are 'high surgical risk' compared to those who are 'low surgical risk'.

INTRODUCTION

The management of any asymptomatic condition, such as abdominal aortic aneurysm, carotid artery stenosis (CAS), valvular heart disease, or even coronary artery disease, with surgical or even an endovascular procedure in an attempt to prevent the possibility of a future, potentially catastrophic, event can be a difficult undertaking for both patients and physicians alike. Specific factors considered during the consultation with the patient should include risks of the natural history of the condition, and alternatively the risks of the operation, procedure, or medication. Add to these relatively quantifiable factors certain, less objective, features such as the life expectancy of the patient and the patient's tolerance for 'active' (intervention) vs 'passive' (natural history) risk taking. A further complicating feature is

the assignment of an individual patient's risk from population data. As an example, the per year risk of aneurysm rupture for any given diameter size is reasonably known for a population, but interpolating these data to the individual patient becomes problematic. Many of the evidence-based data may be in populations which are not identical in some, if not many, factors, such as age, medical comorbidities, etc., of the patient the physician is trying to counsel, thus confounding the physician's attempts to give accurate assessments of each side of the equation.

Decision-making as to which patient should undergo carotid revascularization has been discussed in detail in previous chapters. In this Chapter we will examine the surgical option for carotid revascularization of patients with asymptomatic extracranial carotid artery disease.

CAROTID ENDARTERECTOMY

Carotid endarterectomy (CEA) for obstructive atherosclerotic carotid disease was first reported in 1954 by Eastcott et al,[1] who operated on a 66-year-old woman who had 33 episodes of transient cerebral ischemia; following the operation, her symptoms resolved. Another report, published in 1975 by DeBakey,[2] claimed to have actually performed the procedure a year earlier, and reported that the patient had done well for many years after the operation. CEA had gained initial popularity in the 1970s, until a report by Brott and Thalinger[3] in 1984 demonstrated poor outcomes in their survey of results from the Cincinnati and northern Kentucky area, with a 14.3% risk of stroke and death. Based on this report, and others, CEA activity in the USA fell significantly through the 1980s.

Although practiced extensively for 50 years, the evidence that endarterectomy was safe and effective was not definitively demonstrated until 40 years after its advent in the normal surgical risk asymptomatic patient. Several prospective randomized clinical trials conducted in the late 1980s through the 1990s changed perspectives regarding the patient with asymptomatic disease and normal surgical risk.[4–6] Not discussed here are two earlier trials in asymptomatic patients, since either trial design or patient volume limit meaningful conclusions.[7,8]

In a procedure as established as this, there have naturally been several methods developed over the years for its deployment (regional anesthesia, eversion, etc.), all with their respective advocates; however, none has been shown to significantly affect safety outcomes. Accordingly, CEA will be discussed here in a generic fashion, to include all techniques.

EFFECTIVENESS OF CAROTID ENDARTERECTOMY IN ASYMPTOMATIC CAROTID ARTERY STENOSIS: EVIDENCE FROM RANDOMIZED CONTROLLED TRIALS

The Veterans Affairs Study

In the first well-designed trial to assess the role of endarterectomy in the asymptomatic patient, Hobson et al[4] published the results of the Veterans Affairs (VA) trial for asymptomatic carotid stenosis in 1993, representing over 9 years of recruitment and follow-up study. Men with an angiographic $\geq$50% stenosis were randomized to medical therapy or endarterectomy and followed for a mean of 48 months. In this analysis of 444 patients, a significant reduction was observed in the primary combined endpoint of periprocedural stroke and death along with ongoing ipsilateral stroke: 8.0% in the surgical group and 20.6% in the medical group ($p < 0.001$). Whereas the surgical group also appeared to benefit when stroke was analyzed alone (4.7% in the surgical group and 9.4% in the medical group, $p = 0.056$), there were no differences between groups when all stroke and death were compared (surgical, 41.2%; medical, 44.2%; relative risk = 0.92; 95% CI 0.69–1.22). The lack of women in the cohort studied, the lack of a defined medical therapy in the control arm, the relatively low grade of CAS included, and the underpowered nature of this study are obvious drawbacks. Nevertheless, it was the first trial to suggest an advantage of endarterectomy over medical care in patients with asymptomatic CAS.

The Asymptomatic Carotid Atherosclerosis Study

Both confirming and expanding on the VA trial findings in a more heterogeneous population, the multicenter Asymptomatic Carotid Atherosclerosis Study results were published in 1995.[5] This landmark trial randomized 1662 patients with carotid stenosis of >60% and no significant comorbidities to either medical therapy or surgery. Patients undergoing CEA also underwent cerebral angiography to confirm their stenosis. After 2.7 years of follow-up, the trial was stopped when it reached its significance boundary and the results were reported as 5-year outcomes based on Kaplan–Meier estimates. There was a significant advantage in the surgical group compared with the non-surgical cohort, with an absolute reduction in the combined primary endpoint of 30-day perioperative stroke and death and ipsilateral stroke to 5 years, of 5.9% (11% vs 5.1%, $p = 0.004$).

There are reasonable criticisms of this trial from many quarters. The most significant have to do with outcomes related to presurgical diagnostics, and with the medical therapy in the non-surgical cohort:

- Whereas the stroke and death risk in the surgical arm was a low 2.3% at 30 days, it included a 1.2% stroke risk incurred from the preprocedural angiography; accordingly, the surgical procedure appears to be even safer. The complications associated with diagnostic angiography in this trial have been widely used as justification to operate on these patients without angiographic confirmation of stenosis, especially given the 93% concordance of the angiogram with the Doppler noted in ACAS. However, the ACAS angiographic risk is at least twice the current accepted standard.[9] Relying on duplex ultrasound in clinical practice as the sole imaging modality prior to CEA cannot be justified because of the wide variability in accuracy among various laboratories. Wong and colleagues[10] have shown that almost 1 in 5 patients underwent CEA inappropriately, and that the most common cause was overestimation of the degree of stenosis severity by duplex ultrasound.

- Patients randomized to medical therapy in ACAS did not have specific medical therapy other than an antiplatelet regimen of aspirin mandated as part of the trial, nor were lipid levels and/or blood pressure targets either stipulated or reported. Therefore, many observers feel that the full potential benefit of medical therapy was not realized and may have been underestimated.

- Although prior studies had suggested a difference in natural history of stroke based on worsening stenosis severity, no differences were noted in treatment effect among varying levels of stenosis. This trial was not powered to detect such differences and the actual stenoses treated were, in the majority, >70%. If such differences exist, however, the net effect would be to blunt any benefit for the entire population due to the inclusion of lower-grade stenosis.

- Although the results of the study demonstrated effectiveness of endarterectomy in a broad asymptomatic patient population, apparent sex differences were noted. The study was underpowered to detect such differences, but when the 5-year primary endpoint outcomes for men and women in the surgical group are analyzed (absolute and relative risk reductions are 8% and 66% for men, and 1.4% and 17% for women, respectively) the comparison is nevertheless provocative.

- Whereas the trial did use independent neurological assessments prior to and after surgical intervention to assess patient outcomes, results are reported for the 30-day status. This almost certainly led to an underestimation of minor strokes resulting from endarterectomy, since many minor events will be resolved in the first few weeks, as demonstrated in the ARCHeR trial (ACCULINK for Revascularization of Carotids in High Risk Patients).[11]

- Patients with significant comorbidities were excluded from this trial in order to minimize confounding variables, which is appropriate when evaluating a surgical intervention (rather than a treatment strategy). As a result, however, the value of endarterectomy, and medical therapy for that matter, in a population of patents with asymptomatic carotid stenosis at increased risk for surgery was not defined by this study.

In spite of these concerns and shortcomings, ACAS unequivocally changed the management of the asymptomatic patient with carotid stenosis in the USA. Routine angiography was largely abandoned in favor of duplex alone, and patients were offered surgery with asymptomatic stenosis usually >80% in acknowledgment of data suggesting that the natural history had an inflection point at approximately this value where the risk of stroke increased from about 1% per year to about 3–5% per year (Chapter 7). This trial opened the doors in the USA to CEA in asymptomatic patients, and today estimates are that >70% of endarterectomies in the USA are performed on asymptomatic patients.[12]

The Asymptomatic Carotid Surgery Trial

In 2004, the publication of the Asymptomatic Carotid Surgery Trial (ACST) addressed many of the perceived shortcomings of ACAS.[6] This trial was designed to address a similar population of patients studied in ACAS: specifically, patients with asymptomatic stenosis >60% by Doppler were randomized to either immediate or deferred endarterectomy groups. About 90% of patients in the surgical group underwent endarterectomy (50% had surgery within the first month) and approximately 10% of the deferred group had undergone surgery at the time the trial outcome analysis was completed (3.4 years) (Figure 13.1). Medical therapy consisted of antiplatelet, antihypertensive and, increasingly throughout the trial, antilipid medication. Whereas approximately 75% of the patients were on these three therapies at the time of analysis, targets were not established nor values reported, so that the adequacy of medical therapy could not be assessed. Stenosis severity was divided by deciles from 60% to 90% by

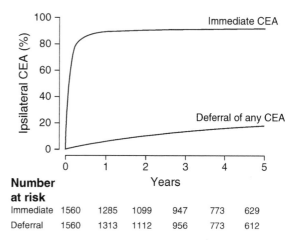

Number at risk						
	0	1	2	3	4	5
Immediate	1560	1285	1099	947	773	629
Deferral	1560	1313	1112	956	773	612

Figure 13.1 Proportion of patients with ipsilateral CEA by time from randomization in ACST, with numbers alive and still under observation at various times. (From Halliday et al.[6])

duplex; routine angiography was not performed. Kaplan–Meier estimates of the 5-year outcomes were presented.

With roughly twice the number of patients as ACAS (3120 vs 1662) and a decade separating the two reports, the outcomes were remarkably similar, with a robust advantage of surgery over medical therapy (Table 13.1). Of note, the difference between the groups would probably have been greater than demonstrated if the assigned therapies had been carried out promptly (surgery) and the assignments followed (medical crossover to surgery had been event-driven rather than patient/physician choice).

Further detail of these results are shown in Figure 13.2. There appears to be, in every subgroup analyzed, a relatively static 3% risk of perioperative stroke and death. Accordingly, the effects of surgical revascularization

become apparent at approximately 2 years, and if the analysis is limited to only ipsilateral non-operative stroke, an even greater differential between the groups is seen, and, regardless of the stroke type analyzed, the benefits of surgery persist.

When the results are further subjected to subgroup analysis, several important clarifications become apparent (Figure 13.3). First, women (about one-third of the cohort in the study) also demonstrated a benefit from surgery, albeit somewhat smaller than men, erasing the concern initially raised by ACAS. The corollary fact is important and inescapable: men have twice the benefit (8.21% vs 4.08%) than women from carotid endarterectomy for asymptomatic CAS. Secondly, patients under the age of 75 benefited from surgery, regardless of their age group; those older died more frequently,

Table 13.1 A comparison between ACST and ACAS. From Halliday et al.[6]

	ACST		ACAS		Total	
	Immediate	Deferral	Immediate	Deferral	Immediate	Deferral
Number of patients	1560	1560	825	834	2385	2394
Follow-up (years)	3.4	3.4	2.7	2.7	3.1	3.1
CEA undertaken	1348	3.4	724	2.7	2072	3.1
Procedural morbidity*						
Death[†]	15	2	3	1	18	3
Non-fatal stroke	25	9	16	2	41	11
Non-procedural stroke						
Fatal (within 5 years)[‡]	12	44	6	9	18	53
Non-fatal	30	76	35	74[‡]	65	150
5-year risk (%) of stroke or procedural morbidity[§]	6.4	11.7	5.1	11.0	6.0	11.5
Other deaths						
Other vascular	144	127	37	50	161	177
Neoplastic	64	47	15	13	79	60
Respiratory	9	11	10	9	19	20
Other/unknown	20	19	12	9	32	28

*Perioperative events in ACST, angiography or perioperative events in ACAS. (One patient in the deferral arm of ACST had a procedural stroke after having another stroke.) Note that absolute numbers suffering procedural morbidity and non-procedural stroke cannot be simply be added to assess net benefit: instead, life table methods must be used, as in Figure 13.2.

[†]Net 5-year risk of procedural death or stroke death in ACST is 21% versus 4.2%, p = 0.006.

[‡]p < 0.0001.

[§]Procedural morbidity or ipsilateral strode in ACAS.

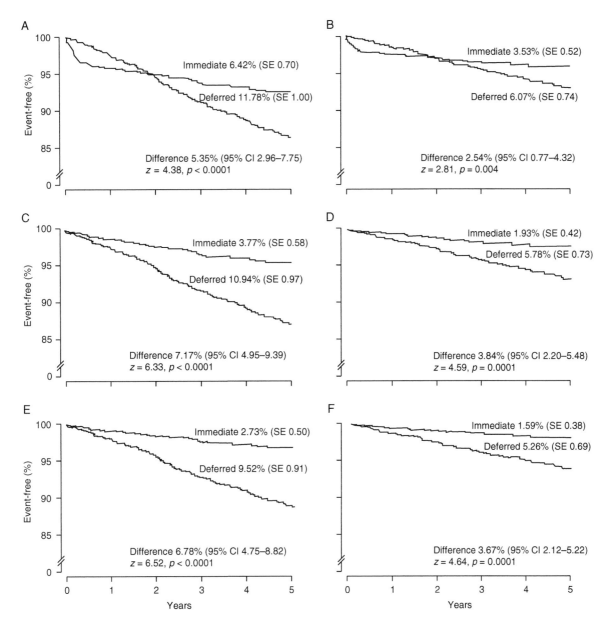

Figure 13.2 Five-year risks of various types of stroke. (A) Any type of stroke or perioperative death. (B) Fatal or disabling stroke or perioperative death. (C) Any type of non-perioperative stroke. (D) Fatal or disabling non-perioperative stroke. (E) Non-perioperative carotid territory ischemic stroke. (F) Fatal or disabling non-perioperative carotid territory ischemic stroke. A and B include perioperative morbidity and C–F do not. A, C, and E involve strokes of any severity; B, D, and F involve only those that were fatal or involved at least moderate long-term disability (requiring some help with daily affairs: modified Rankin score 3, 4, or 5). In E, five of the 30 strokes among those allocated immediate CEA were in patients who had not yet received it, and eight of the 105 strokes among those allocated deferral were in patients who had already undergone a CEA during the trial: z = difference/SE; p values are two-sided. (From Halliday et al.[6])

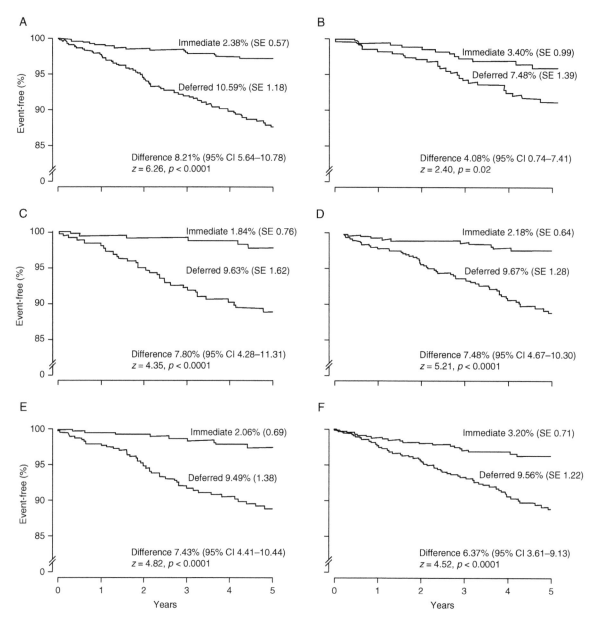

Figure 13.3 (A) Men. (B) Women. (C) Age <65 years. (D) Age 65–74 years. (E) Carotid diameter reduction by ultrasound < 80% (mean 69%). (F) Carotid diameter reduction by ultrasound 80–99%/mean 87%). Five-year risks of non-perioperative carotid territory ischemic stroke in selected subgroups: z = difference/SE; p values are two-sided. (From Halliday et al.[6])

thus limiting any observed benefit. Lastly, Doppler stenosis severity <80% or >80% did not appear to influence the benefit conferred by surgery.

There are several other observations that merit highlighting, as they bear on the role of endarterectomy in these patients, and occasionally cause confusion among providers counseling patients:

- In both groups, half the non-perioperative strokes were disabling or fatal; this contravenes the conventional wisdom regarding strokes in general, that only one-third will be fatal/disabling. It appears that stroke related to carotid disease carries a potentially worse outcome, and therefore its avoidance becomes more pressing.

- In addition to preventing stroke on the treated side, the incidence of contralateral stroke was, interestingly, significantly reduced in the surgical group (11 vs 35, $p = 0.0004$) and was unexplained by any differences in contralateral CEA. Such an observation is not readily explained by the available data; chief among the possibilities is the speculation that maintenance of intracranial collateral support somehow reduces cerebral infarction. More importantly, an accounting of only ipsilateral strokes would have underestimated the benefits of immediate endarterectomy.
- Roughly half the patients had ultrasound plaque analysis that assessed the degree of echolucency, and these results were then assessed in terms of clinical outcomes. No correlation with stroke occurrence could be made relative to plaque composition.
- Much like the VA trial, the all-cause mortality did not differ between the two groups at 5 years. This secondary endpoint has been used to defer surgery in patients with asymptomatic stenosis, but it is not a logical inference. In any directed intervention there are specific preventive goals associated with the therapy: in this case, stroke prevention. This varies significantly from many of the goals of medical therapies (e.g. antihypertensives), which are meant to not only affect the organ system being treated but to also have a salutary effect on broader, secondary outcomes: e.g. stroke, renal failure, myocardial infarction (MI), etc. When performing a surgical or prophylactic procedure such as endarterectomy, neither the operator nor the patient has an expectation of a mortality difference; rather, the explicit benefit sought is that the patient's remaining life will be free of stroke.

The ACST trial follow-up is ongoing, with further results expected at the 10-year follow-up period.

CAN THE RESULTS OF PROSPECTIVE RANDOMIZED CLINICAL TRIALS BE TRANSFERRED TO ROUTINE CLINICAL PRACTICE?

There is concern among clinicians that the low operative risks in ACAS and ACST (<3%) are not consistently matched in routine clinical practice. A perioperative complication rate higher than 3% would significantly reduce the benefit of surgery in asymptomatic patients (Table 13.2). Only surgeons who could document low complication rates were selected in both ACAS and ACST. In ACAS, 40% of initial applicants were rejected and, subsequently, surgeons who had adverse operative outcomes during the trial were barred from

further participation.[13] In ACST, surgeons were required to provide evidence of an operative risk of ≤6% for their last 50 patients having an endarterectomy for asymptomatic stenosis, but none were excluded on the basis of their operative risk during the trial.

Several studies have highlighted the dissociation between surgical outcomes in clinical trials vs that in routine clinical practice. Rothwell and Goldstein[14] compared the operative risks in ACAS with the results of a meta-analysis of the 46 surgical case series that published operative risks for asymptomatic stenosis during ACAS and the 5 years after publication.[15] Operative mortality was 8 times higher than in ACAS (1.11% vs 0.14%; $p = 0.01$), and the risk of stroke and death was ~3 times higher among comparable studies in which outcome was assessed by a neurologist (4.3% vs 1.5%; $p < 0.001$). Even after community-wide performance measurement and feedback, the overall risk for stroke or death after endarterectomy performed for asymptomatic stenosis in 10 US states was 3.8% (including 1% mortality).[16] Therefore, the results of the randomized clinical trials cannot be automatically transferred to routine clinical practice. Institution-specific assessment of the risk of CEA should be a prime consideration in clinical decision-making.

Table 13.2 Projected impact of operative risk of carotid endarterectomy on its 5-year efficacy in patients with asymptomatic carotid artery disease

| Operative risk (%) | ACAS 60–99% | |
	ARR at 5 years	NNT at 5 years
0	8.2%	12
2	6.2%	16
4	4.2%	24
6	2.2%	45
8	0.2%	500
10	n/a	n/s

ARR, absolute risk reduction; NNT, number needed to treat with carotid endarterectomy.
Modified from ACAS.[5]

CAROTID ENDARTERECTOMY IN NEUROLOGICALLY ASYMPTOMATIC BUT HIGH-RISK PATIENTS

Although the VA study,[4] ACAS,[5] and ACST[6] appear to have established the role of CEA in asymptomatic carotid disease, many subsets of patients with carotid lesions have comorbidities that increase their risk of surgery and potentially limit its benefit. Many of these conditions were excluded from the aforementioned trials appropriately in order to limit confounding variables. Thus, it leaves open the question as to the place of surgical therapy in these commonly encountered patients, since there has never been a randomized trial specifically evaluating the benefit in high-risk patients of endarterectomy vs medicine.

However, there are studies comparing CEA to carotid artery stenting in high surgical risk patients. The best prospective adjudicated data available comes from the Stenting and Angioplasty with Protection in Patients at High Risk for Endarterectomy (SAPPHIRE) trial.[17] Whereas there was no medical arm and only 72% of the patients were asymptomatic (>80% stenosis), several important observations can be made. The definition of 'high risk' was quite variable, with age >80 years, recurrent stenosis after prior ipsilateral CEA, previous radical neck surgery, previous neck irradiation, contralateral laryngeal nerve palsy, contralateral carotid occlusion, 'severe pulmonary disease', and clinically significant cardiac disease – congestive heart failure (CHF), positive stress test, and need for coronary artery bypass graft (CABG) surgery – representing the inclusion criteria. The 30-day major adverse event rate (stroke, death, and Q-wave MI) in asymptomatic patients was 9.2%. Almost an identical rate of major adverse events in high-risk patients was reported by Halm and colleagues[12] in an analysis of 2124 patients who underwent CEA in 1997–1998 in six hospitals in New York State (Table 13.3). Thus, while it is hard to ferret out the contribution of every specific risk factor to the high event rate in these patients, it is clear that high-risk patients experience more frequent surgical complications than low-risk patients.

What does 'high surgical risk' really mean?

What is less clear from the SAPPHIRE trial is to what degree the different high-risk criteria drive outcome from surgery and to what degree some of these factors impact natural history in unoperated patients. For instance, a contralateral nerve palsy is unlikely to impact on the future risk of stroke to the same degree as a contralateral carotid occlusion, and the need for open heart surgery to repair two valves and four coronaries is much more likely to be associated with reduced longevity than previous radical neck surgery for a benign process. To get some idea of which high-risk features surgeons consider most important and which tend to

Table 13.3 Rates of major perioperative complications after carotid endarterectomy in patients with asymptomatic carotid artery disease according to the degree of comorbidity

Outcome	Comorbidity category (%)				Trend test p value
	None	Low	Moderate	High	
N	390	680	253	90	
Death	0.26	0.59	0.79	1.11	0.25
Non-fatal stroke	1.03	1.62	1.98	4.44	0.04
Death/stroke*	1.28	2.21	2.77	5.56	0.02
Non-fatal MI†	0.0	0.74	1.58	3.33	0.008

*Combined outcome of death or non-fatal stroke.

†Non-fatal myocardial infarction (MI) in a patient who did not suffer stroke.

Modified from Halm et al.[12]

drive surgeons away from the decision to perform endarterectomy, it is instructive to look at some of the high surgical risk registries most of which are unadjudicated. These features can be divided to medical comorbidities and anatomic high surgical risk features.

Medical comorbidities

Increased surgical risk has been reported with CHF (perioperative stroke and death = 8.6–25%);[10,18] angina (range of perioperative stroke, death, and MI = 9.9–12%),[10,19] and renal insufficiency (range of perioperative stroke, death, and MI = 8.2–43%).[10,20,21] Although the severity of these disease states is not clearly delineated, the fact that patients are at higher risk for operative complications combined with the decreased longevity expected with these diseases generally weights the decision away from surgery. When surgery is still being considered, such as when transcranial Dopplers show decreased autoregulatory capacity or when the asymptomatic stenosis is rapidly progressive, consideration is often given to awake endarterectomy, as increased complications in these patients are often cardiac in nature.

In addition to these conditions, patients in need of open heart surgery for either symptomatic coronary disease or valvular pathology, who also exhibit high-grade asymptomatic stenosis, are at increased risk for surgical complications, regardless of whether they undergo cardiac surgery prior to CEA, after CEA, or synchronously with it.[22] Carotid artery stenting may become a reasonable alternative for these patients (see Chapter 14).

Finally, there are the issues of extreme old age (>75 years). With regard to age, there are data on both sides of this issue; however, most of the data point to a high rate of perioperative stroke and death (range of 7–9.9%).[10,18,19,23] The most important consideration with advanced age is whether or not the patient is going to live long enough to benefit from the operative intervention. If there is any doubt, most clinicians favor medical management. (see Risk stratification section)

Anatomic high surgical risk features

Anatomic high surgical risk features include contralateral occlusion, recurrent stenosis after prior ipsilateral CEA, previous radical neck surgery, previous neck irradiation, contralateral laryngeal nerve palsy, and carotid bifurcation above C2.

With regard to contralateral carotid occlusion, there are data on both sides of the issue. Whereas the North American Symptomatic Carotid Endarterectomy Trial (NASCET) showed a marked increased risk of complications in this cohort (14% perioperative stroke and death),[24] ACAS showed no increased risk; however, CEA was not beneficial in this patient cohort. Similarly, patients with restenosis after prior ipsilateral CEA are also at high risk for perioperative complications (range of perioperative stroke and death 7.6–10.9%).[25,26]

With respect to the other anatomic high-risk features (previous radical neck surgery, previous neck irradiation, contralateral laryngeal nerve palsy, and carotid bifurcation above C2), it is unlikely to be associated with an increased risk of death and stroke but more likely to be associated with a higher rate of local complications, most notably nerve palsies. Given the non-inferiority data in SAPPHIRE, these patients are generally referred for stenting.

SUMMARY

The VA Cooperative Study Trial, ACAS, and ACST serve as the basis for recommending and performing endarterectomy in patients with asymptomatic carotid stenosis. Each trial either established, reinforced, or expanded the benefit of surgery in the population studied. Whereas reasonable argument could be made that optimal medical therapy has never been fairly compared to surgery, it is also important to note three facts referable to medical therapy. First, there are no data demonstrating the effectiveness of medical therapy in preventing carotid stenosis-related stroke. The only available data for the absolute effect of medical therapy on all-cause stroke prevention are in broad populations and not in those with established carotid disease. A favorable effect of medical therapy on stroke prevention in patients with carotid stenosis would most likely be secondary to reduction of stroke from non-carotid etiologies and thus be equally distributed between both groups. Secondly, the effect of medical therapy in patients with established stenosis would have to be fairly significant in order to blunt the benefits of CEA, particularly in certain subgroups such as men under 75 years of age. Therefore, based on the data available, it appears reasonable that for asymptomatic carotid stenosis of >60% (preferably >70–80%) in patients under 75 years, revascularization should be considered if the projected complication rate is <3%. Proper Risk Stratification (as discussed in the Risk Stratification section) would help steer this therapy to those patients who may gain the most in terms of stroke prevention. Whereas, the role of CEA in patients with comorbidities remains an open question, there are increasing data to suggest that stenting may be better for some of these patients and medical management for others.

REFERENCES

1. Eastcott HH, Pickering GW, Robb CG. Reconstruction of the internal carotid artery in a patient with intermittent attacks of hemiplagia. Lancet 1954; 267: 994–6.

2. DeBakey ME. Successful carotid endarterectomy for cerebrovascular insufficiency. Nineteen-year follow-up. JAMA 1975; 233(10): 1083–5.

3. Brott T, Thalinger K. The practice of carotid endarterectomy in a large metropolitan area. Stroke 1984; 15(6): 950–5.

4. Hobson RW, Weiss DG, Fields WS et al. Efficacy of carotid endarterectomy for asymptomatic carotid stenosis. N Engl J Med 1993; 328: 221–7.

5. Executive Committee for the Asymptomatic Carotid Atherosclerosis Study. Endarterectomy for asymptomatic carotid stenosis. JAMA 1995; 273: 1421–8.

6. Halliday A, Mansfield A, Marro J et al. MRC Asymptomatic Carotid Surgery Trial (ACST) Collaborative Group. Prevention of disabling and fatal strokes by successful carotid endarterectomy in patients without recent neurological symptoms: randomised controlled trial. Lancet 2004; 363: 1491–502.

7. Mayo Asymptomatic Carotid Endarterectomy Study Group. Results of a randomized controlled trial of carotid endarterectomy for asymptomatic carotid stenosis. Mayo Clin Proc 1992; 67: 513–18.

8. The CASANOVA Study Group. Carotid surgery versus medical therapy in asymptomatic carotid stenosis. Stroke 1991; 22: 1229–35.

9. Wholey MH, Wholey MH. Momentum growing for carotid stent placement. Diagn Imaging 1998; 20: 65–9.

10. Wong JH, Findlay JM, Suarez-Almazor ME. Regional performance of carotid endarterectomy: appropriateness, outcomes, and risk factors for complications. Stroke 1997; 28: 891–8.

11. Gray WA, Hopking LN, Yadav S et al. For the Acculink for Revascularization of Carotids in High Risk Patients Trial (ARCHeR) Investigators. (In press 2006).

12. Halm EA, Chassin MR, Tuhrim S, Hollier LH et al. Revisiting the appropriateness of carotid endarterectomy. Stroke 2003; 34: 1464–72.

13. Moore WS, Vescera CL, Robertson JT et al. Selection process for surgeons in the Asymptomatic Carotid Atherosclerosis Study. Stroke 1991; 22: 1353–7.

14. Rothwell PM, Goldstein LB. Carotid endarterectomy for asymptomatic carotid stenosis: asymptomatic carotid surgery trial. Stroke 2004; 35: 2425–7.

15. Bond R, Rerkasem K, Rothwell PM. High morbidity due to endarterectomy for asymptomatic carotid stenosis. Cerebrovasc Dis 2003; 16(Suppl): 65.

16. Kresowik TF, Bratzler DW, Kresowik RA et al. Multistate improvement in process and outcomes of carotid endarterectomy. J Vasc Surg 2004; 39: 372–80.

17. Yadav JS, Wholey MH, Kuntz RE et al. Stenting and Angioplasty with Protection in Patients at High Risk for Endarterectomy Investigators. Protected carotid-artery stenting versus endarterectomy in high-risk patients. N Engl J Med 2004; 351(15): 1493–501.

18. Goldstein LB, Samsa GP, Matchar DB et al. Multicenter review of preoperative risk factors for endarterectomy for asymptomatic carotid artery stenosis. Stroke 1998; 29: 750–3.

19. McCrory DC, Goldstein LB, Samsa GP et al. Predicting complications of carotid endarterectomy. Stroke 1993; 24: 1285–91.

20. Rigdon, EE, Monajjem N, Rhodes RS. Is carotid endarterectomy justified in patients with severe chronic renal insufficiency? Ann Vasc Surg 1997; 11: 115–19.

21. Hamdan AD, Pomposelli FB, Gibbons GW et al. Renal insufficiency and altered postoperative risk in carotid endarterectomy. J Vasc Surg 1999; 29: 1006–11.

22. Naylor AR, Cuffe RL, Rothwell PM, Bell PRF. A systematic review of outcomes following staged and synchronous carotid endarterectomy and coronary artery bypass. Eur J Vasc Endovasc Surg 2003; 25: 380–9.

23. Rothwell PM, Slattery J, Warlow CP. Clinical and angiographic predictors of stroke and death from carotid endarterectomy: systematic review. BMJ 1997; 315: 1571–7.

24. Gasecki AP, Eliasziw M, Ferguson GG, Hachinski V, Barnett HJ. Long-term prognosis and effect of endarterectomy in patients with symptomatic severe carotid stenosis and contralateral carotid stenosis or occlusion: results from NASCET. North American Symptomatic Carotid Endarterectomy Trial (NASCET) Group. J Neurosurg 1995; 83: 778–82.

25. Meyer FB, Piepgras DG, Sundt TM Jr, et al. Recurrent carotid stenosis. Sundt's Occlusive Cerebrovascular Disease, 2nd edn. Philadelphia: WB Saunders, 1994: 310–21.

26. Das MB, Hertzer NR, Ratliff NB et al. Recurrent carotid stenosis: a five-year series of 65 reoperations. Ann Surg 1985; 202: 28–35.

14

Carotid artery stenting in patients with asymptomatic carotid artery stenosis

William A Gray and Issam D Moussa

Take-Home Messages

1. When a decision is made to proceed with carotid revascularization in a patient with asymptomatic carotid stenosis, institution-specific risk assessment for appropriateness of carotid endarterectomy (CEA) and carotid artery stenting (CAS) should be performed and the patient triaged accordingly.
2. CAS with embolic protection has been shown to be at least as effective as CEA in preventing stroke in high surgical risk patients with symptomatic or asymptomatic carotid artery disease.
3. Minimizing complications and improving outcome of CAS in asymptomatic patients is heavily dependent on proper patient selection and operator experience.
4. Advanced age, complex aortic arch and carotid artery anatomy, and prolonged procedure time are risk factors for CAS-related periprocedural complications.
5. Among high surgical risk patients with asymptomatic carotid disease, the net benefit of CAS is greatest among those <80 years of age.
6. Although standardizing the technical aspects of a CAS procedure has the advantage of increasing operator proficiency in that particular technique, the overriding goal should be to tailor the CAS technique to the patient's anatomy.
7. The standard of care, in terms of carotid revascularization strategy, in low surgical risk patients with asymptomatic carotid artery disease will be determined by the results of the ongoing prospective randomized trials of CAS vs CEA.
8. Currently, Medicare reimburses CAS in asymptomatic patients only if performed in the context of investigational device exemption (IDE) or post marketing surveillance (PMS) registries (high surgical risk patients) or prospective randomized clinical trials (low surgical risk patients).

INTRODUCTION

Although carotid percutaneous intervention using angioplasty alone was first pioneered in the late 1970s and early 1980s by Mathias and colleagues,[1,2] the field was launched with the advent of stents[3–5] which provided a more secure initial result, and probably more robust long-term patency rates. Subsequent publications of single-center experiences[6] demonstrated enough of a safety and efficacy 'signal' with off-the-shelf equipment, which by today's standards are considered primitive, to continue exploring this alternative.

In direct contradistinction to the pathway taken to validation for carotid endarterectomy (CEA), carotid artery stenting (CAS) with embolic protection has taken an entirely opposite tack. Rather than proving safety and efficacy of the technology in the broad swath of patients with carotid stenosis and low frequency of comorbidities such as the Veterans Affairs (VA) cooperative study,[7] Asymptomatic Carotid Atherosclerosis Study (ACAS),[8] and Asymptomatic Carotid Surgery Trial (ACST)[9] investigations, the primary cohort of patients studied with CAS were those with significant comorbidities. This strategy was driven largely by two fundamental factors: the availability of a safe and effective surgical alternative in low-risk patients, and the lack of endovascular skills in the at-large surgical community at the time CAS was introduced in this country (1990s), which resulted in a rejection and opposition to the new technology from the physicians who had been managing this disease domain for several decades.

The introduction of dedicated equipment, nickel–titanium (nitinol) stents and embolic protection systems, led to the launch of multiple registry studies and a multicenter randomized trial in high surgical risk patients.[10–16] Ultimately, these trials led to the Food and Drug Administration (FDA) approval of the ACCULINK stent and ACCUNET filter (Guidant Corporation, Menlo Park, CA) in August 2004 and the Xact stent and the Emboshield filter (Abbott Vascular, Redwood City, CA) in 2005 for use in high surgical risk patients with severe stenosis who are either symptomatic or asymptomatic.

Although there are several single- and multicenter reports of outcomes following CAS, both before and after the advent of embolic protection devices (EPDs),[17–20] this chapter focuses on the pivotal multicenter trials with neurologically audited results. The individual pivotal trials performed for device approval are generally underpowered for subset analysis, each typically having 300–500 patients with ~70–75% of them asymptomatic. Where there are data available from these trials it will be presented, but the focus will primarily be on the larger data sets available from the FDA-mandated post-market approval surveillance registries which had ~90% asymptomatic patients,[21,22] along with the Carotid Revascularization Endarterectomy versus Stenting Trial (CREST) lead-in phase registry,[23] both of which have neurologically audited outcomes reporting and robust-enough numbers to allow some subset analysis and conclusions.

EFFICACY OF CAROTID ARTERY STENTING IN STROKE PREVENTION

Before specifically addressing procedural outcomes in asymptomatic patients, it is critically important to establish the stroke preventive role of CAS, at least relative to the CEA standard, and there are now data available beyond 2 years that demonstrate the efficacy of CAS in this regard. The SAPPHIRE trial,[16] which randomized 334 symptomatic and asymptomatic patients at high risk for surgical intervention to either surgery or stenting, demonstrated that, at 1 year, stenting outcomes for the composite endpoint were better than the surgical control (Figure 14.1). When the incidence of stroke alone is analyzed in the two groups, the results are remarkably overlapping, as shown in Figure 14.2, demonstrating efficacy in stroke prevention at least on par with CEA up to 2 years.[24]

Confirming these results in another trial is the ARCHeR (ACCULINK for Revascularization of Carotids in High-Risk Patients) analysis, which reported 30-day periprocedural stroke, death, and myocardial infarction (MI) and ipsilateral stroke to 3 years.[10] Again, the efficacy of CAS in stroke prevention is demonstrated by the lack of late events (Figure 14.3). The rate of event-free survival was 90.4% (95%CI 88–92.8%) at 1 year and 88.4% at both 2 and 3 years.

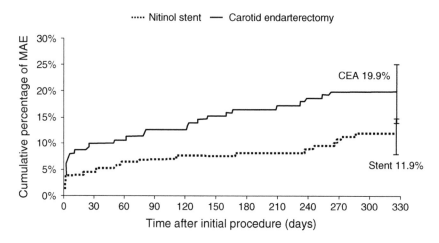

Figure 14.1 Cumulative percentage of major adverse events (MAE) – death, stroke, myocardial infarction – at 360 days in the CAS (11.9%) vs CEA (19.9%), $p = 0.048$ arms of the SAPPHIRE trial in symptomatic and asymptomatic patients. (Adapted from Yadav et al.[16])

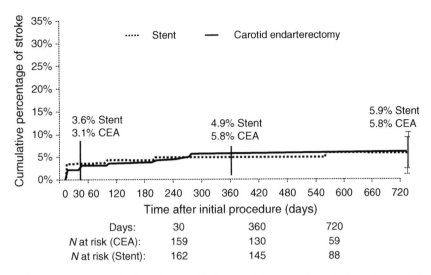

Figure 14.2 Cumulative percentage of all strokes to 30 days and ipsilateral stroke from 31–720 days in all randomized symptomatic and asymptomatic patients in the SAPPHIRE trial. (Adapted from Yadav.[24])

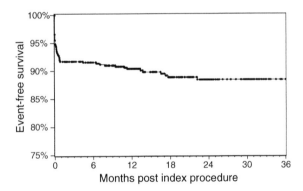

Figure 14.3 Freedom from any stroke, death, or myocardial infarction up to 30 days or ipsilateral stroke beyond 30 days in the ARCHeR trials. (Adapted from Gray.[10])

In a related ARCHeR analysis, the annual incidence of stroke following CAS was approximately 0.9% in a high surgical risk cohort with significant comorbidities by definition.

These two trials, with the longest-term outcome available from the controlled multicenter study of CAS, established the value of stents in extracranial carotid disease in preventing stroke and being at least as useful as carotid surgery in that regard. Given that there are, as yet, no direct data from randomized trials comparing carotid stenting to either CEA or medical therapy specifically in asymptomatic patients, this analysis will

center around the periprocedural (30-day) comparisons between the two revascularization strategies, both direct and historical.

CAROTID ARTERY STENTING WITH EMBOLIC PROTECTION IN ASYMPTOMATIC CAROTID ARTERY DISEASE: CLINICAL OUTCOME DATA

High surgical risk patients

Pivotal device trials

The pivotal device approval trials in high surgical risk patients are listed in Table 14.1. Out of these trials, detailed data on outcome of asymptomatic patients is available for the ARCHeR and SAPPHIRE trials. The SAPPHIRE trial randomized patients between CEA and stenting with the Precise stent and Angioguard filter (Johnson & Johnson/Cordis); the trial cohort included 72% of patients who were asymptomatic.[16] In this non-inferiority trial, a prespecified analysis in the asymptomatic subset demonstrated no difference between CAS and CEA in both the 30-day periprocedural and 1-year outcomes (Figure 14.4), with trends favoring stenting in each case. Specifically, carotid stenting in asymptomatic patients resulted in 6.0% 30-day MAE (major adverse events) rate vs 9.2% in the CEA cohort.

Table 14.1 Carotid artery stenting with embolic protection devices (EPDs) in high surgical risk patients with carotid artery stenosis

Study	Sample size	Stent	EPD	Manufacturer	Status
CAS Registries					
ARCHeR 1–3[10]	581	ACCULINK	ACCUNET	Guidant	Completed
BEACH[11]	747	Wallstent	FilterWire EX/EZ	Boston Scientific	Completed
CABernET[12]	488	NexStent	FilterWire EX/EZ	Boston Scientific	Completed
CREATE[13]	419	Protégé	Spider	eV3	Completed
MAVErIC II[14]	399	Exponent	PercuSurge	Medtronic	Completed
SECuRITY[15]	398	Xact	Emboshield	Abbott	Completed
Randomized trials (CAS vs CEA)					
SAPPHIRE[16]	334	Precise	Angioguard	CORDIS Endovascular	Completed

ARCHeR: ACCULINK for Revascularization of Carotids in High-Risk Patients (Guidant Corporation, Menlo Park, CA).
BEACH: Boston Scientific EPI-A Carotid Stenting Trial for High Risk Surgical Patients (Boston Scientific, Boston, MA).
CABernET: Carotid artery revascularization using the Boston Scientific FilterWire EX/EZ and the EndoTex NexStent trial (Boston Scientific, Boston, MA; EndoTex, Cupertino, CA).
CREATE: The Carotid Revascularization with ev3 Arterial Technology Evolution (ev3 Inc., Plymouth, MN).
MAVErIC: Evaluation of the Medtronic AVE Self-Expanding Carotid Stent System in the Treatment of Carotid Stenosis (Medtronic Vascular, Santa Rosa, CA).
SECuRITY: Registry Study to Evaluate the Neuroshield Bare Wire Cerebral Protection System and XAct Stent in Patients at High Risk for Carotid Endarterectomy (Abbott Vascular, Redwood City, CA).
SAPPHIRE: Stenting and Angioplasty with Protection in Patients at High Risk for Endarterectomy (CORDIS, NJ)

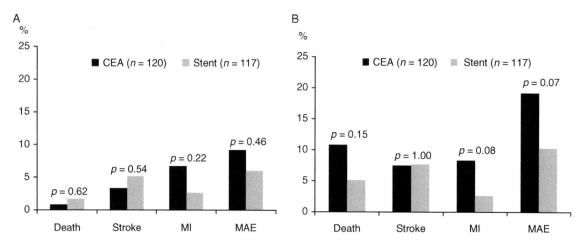

Figure 14.4 Frequency of major adverse events (MAE) – death, stroke, myocardial infarction (MI) – in randomized asymptomatic patients in the SAPPHIRE trial (intention-to-treat analysis): (A) at 30 days; (B) at 360 days.

These results were further supported by data generated from the ARCHeR studies.[10] The inclusion and exclusion criteria from the ARCHeR studies, which are generally representative of these investigations and define the high surgical risk patients treated in the CAS trials, are listed in Table 14.2. These generally follow the categories of patients listed previously with documented poor outcomes in surgical registries. Of the 581 high surgical risk patients treated with the ACCULINK stent and ACCUNET embolic filter system in this non-randomized registry, 76% were asymptomatic. While the overall rate of periprocedural adverse events

Table 14.2 Key eligibility criteria from the ARCHeR trials

Key inclusion criteria

General criteria:

    Age ≥ 18 years old

    Symptomatic with a stenosis ≥50%, or

    Asymptomatic with a stenosis ≥80% by

    angiography

Major criteria for high risk

need one or more for entry:

    Ejection fraction <30% or NYHA class ≥III

    Dialysis-dependent renal failure

    Restenosis after previous CEA

    FEV_1 <30% (predicted)

    Surgically inaccessible lesion

    Prior radiation to neck

    Prior radical neck surgery

    Spinal immobility

    Tracheostomy stoma

    Contralateral laryngeal nerve paralysis

or need two or more of the following for entry:

    Need open heart surgery within 30 days

    Two or more diseased coronary arteries

    Contralateral ICA occlusion

    Unstable angina

    MI within 30 days and need carotid

    revascularization

Key exclusion criteria

Patient has an evolving stroke

Patient has a history of major ipsilateral stroke

Patient has a neurological deficit not due to stroke

    that would confound the neurological assessment

Patient has had a recent (<7 days) stroke

Patient had hemorrhagic transformation of an ischemic

    stroke within the past 60 days

Knowledge of cardiac sources of emboli

Adapted from Gray.[10]

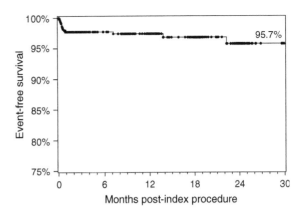

Figure 14.5 Freedom from periprocedural death and major stroke and ipsilateral major stroke at 2.5 years in the ARCHeR trials. (Adapted from Gray.[10])

The results of these pivotal trials suggest rates of adverse outcomes in high surgical risk patients which approach those from the normal-risk CEA landmark trials, but are underpowered to draw significant conclusions. Subsequent studies that enrolled a broader patient population with respect to surgical risk provide some of the additional numbers to aid in further comparisons with the CEA historical controls.

Post-marketing surveillance registries

The primary intent of the FDA-mandated post-marketing surveillance (PMS) registries was to both assess the transfer of stent technology into the clinical, non-trial, setting and to survey for any unanticipated device-related events. On both counts, data from the Carotid RX ACCULINK®/RX ACCUNET™Post-Approval Trial to Uncover Unanticipated or Rare Events (CAPTURE, Guidant Corporation)[21] and Carotid Artery Stenting With Emboli Protection Surveillance (CASES, Johnson & Johnson/Cordis)[22] demonstrate no device-related issues and successful outcomes across operator experience. These registries also represent the largest neurologically audited outcomes databases available in stenting or surgical carotid intervention and allow subset analyses with a reasonably robust statistical power. The only drawback to using data from these two registries is that they include, in part, learning curves of multiple operators.

CAPTURE has reported outcomes on 2500 high-surgical risk patients treated using the Guidant filter and stent system at 137 centers across the USA; 90.7% of patients treated were asymptomatic.[21] The 30-day MAE rate (death, stroke, MI) for asymptomatic patients ($n = 2268$) was 4.9% and for asymptomatic patients <80 years old ($n = 1741$) was 4.2% (Figure 14.6A). Moreover, if

(death, stroke, and MI) was 8.3% (95% CI 6.2–10.8%), asymptomatic patients experienced less events (6.8%; 95% CI 4.6–9.5%). Further, at 2.5 years, 95.7% of asymptomatic patients were free from periprocedural death/major stroke and major ipsilateral stroke (Figure 14.5). It is important to note that in the CEA trials previously detailed, the 30-day endpoints did not include MI. If the results from ARCHeR exclude MI, the 30-day periprocedural rate drops to 5.4% (95% CI 3.5–8.0%).

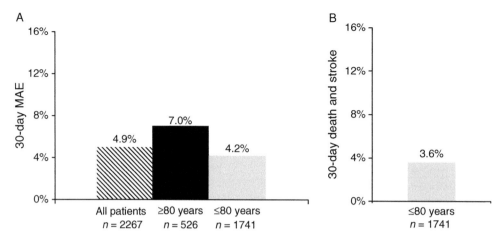

Figure 14.6 (A) Frequency of 30 day major adverse events (MAE) – death, stroke, myocardial infarction – in asymptomatic patients according to age in the CAPTURE registry. (B) Frequency of 30 day death and stroke in asymptomatic patients <80 years old in the CAPTURE registry. (Adapted from Gray.[21])

only the 30-day rate of stroke and death is considered the event rate fell to 3.6% in asymptomatic patients <80 years old (Figure 14.6B). Lastly, CASES-PMS enrolled 974 asymptomatic high surgical risk patients who were treated with Cordis/Johnson and Johnson stent and filter system.[22] The 30-day risk of stroke and death in the entire asymptomatic group was 4.2% (the breakout for patients <80 years old is unavailable).

Low surgical risk patients

Data regarding the role of CAS in low surgical risk patients with asymptomatic carotid artery stenosis are limited. The CREST lead-in registry has reported data on investigators coming online in the CREST becoming familiar with the equipment before embarking on randomization.[23] The 30-day rate of stroke and death in the 960 asymptomatic patients was 4.0%, and, if limited to only patients <80 years old, is 3.3% (Figure 14.7A). The 30-day rate of death and major stroke in patients <80 years old was 1.4% (Figure 14.7B).

There are three prospective clinical randomized trials of CAS vs CEA in low surgical risk patients that are ongoing (ACT 1, CREST) or in the planning phase (Transatlantic Asymptomatic Carotid Intervention Trial; TACIT) (Table 14.3). The Asymptomatic Carotid Stenosis Stenting versus Endarterectomy Trial (ACT 1, Abbott Vascular) is in the enrollment phase and it will randomize up to 1658 patients to CAS with the Abbott system or CEA in a 3:1 scheme. The asymptomatic arm of the CREST will randomize up to 1400 patients between CEA and CAS. Based on current rates of enrollment, these trials may have data available on 1-year follow-up by 2009 or 2010.

THE CAROTID ARTERY STENTING PROCEDURE IN ASYMPTOMATIC PATIENTS

Needless to say, the technical aspects of carotid artery stenting do not differ according to symptom status. However, since the net benefit of carotid revascularization in asymptomatic patients is lower than that in symptomatic patients, tolerance for complications should be significantly lower. The current guidelines call for a ≤3% perioperative rate of stroke and death after CEA for low surgical risk asymptomatic patients.[25] This goal can certainly be achieved with CAS, but only through proper patient selection, adequate preprocedure patient preparation, careful procedural planning and execution, and fastidious postprocedural management.

Patient selection

The decision regarding which asymptomatic patients should be considered for carotid revascularization is discussed in the Risk Stratification section of this book (Chapters 7–11). Once a decision has been made to proceed with carotid revascularization, institution-specific risk assessment for appropriateness of CEA and CAS should be performed and the patient triaged accordingly (Figure 14.8). Currently, CAS is accessible to asymptomatic high surgical risk patients under the PMS registries, and to asymptomatic low surgical risk patients in the context of prospective randomized trials. To optimize patient selection for CAS, it is crucial to consider the clinical and anatomic features that may increase the risk of complications. As a rule of thumb,

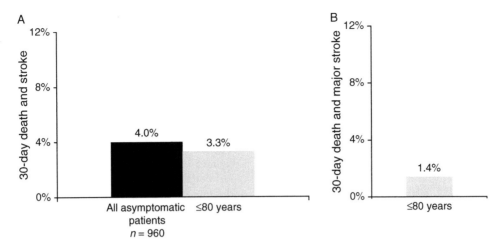

Figure 14.7 (A) Frequency of 30-day death and stroke in asymptomatic patients according to age in the CREST lead-in registry. (B) Frequency of 30-day death and major stroke in asymptomatic patients <80 years old in the CREST lead-in registry. (Adapted from Roubin.[23])

Table 14.3 Prospective randomized controlled trials of carotid artery stenting with distal protection in low surgical risk asymptomatic patients in the USA

Study	Sample size	Stent`	EPD	Status
ACT 1	1658	Xact	Emboshield	Enrolling
CREST	1400	ACCULINK	ACCUNET	Enrolling
TACIT	2400	TBD	TBD	Planned

ACT 1: Asymptomatic Carotid Stenosis Stenting versus Endarterectomy Trial.
CREST: Carotid Revascularization Endarterectomy versus Stenting Trial.
TACIT: Transatlantic Asymptomatic Carotid Intervention Trial.

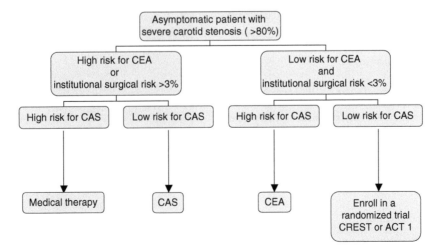

Figure 14.8 An algorithm to triage patients with asymptomatic carotid artery disease who need carotid revascularization to carotid endarterectomy (CEA) vs carotid artery stenting (CAS).

the higher the number of high-risk features, the higher the likelihood of CAS-related complications.

Clinical high-risk features

Age >80 years old
Most of the data indicate that the rate of complications after CAS is higher in patients >80 years old compared with patients <80 years old.[26] The higher complication rate in these patients is most likely a consequence of higher prevalence of complex anatomic features as well as impaired cerebrovascular reserve. However, age alone should not exclude patients from undergoing CAS if it is otherwise indicated. On the other hand, advanced age combined with other clinical or anatomic risk factors should preclude these patients from intervention.

Chronic renal insufficiency
Chronic renal insufficiency (CRI) is a known risk factor for occurrence of a first-time stroke in patients with asymptomatic carotid occlusive disease who are treated conservatively.[27] CRI is also associated with higher peri-procedural complications after CEA[28] and CAS.[13,29] Although the presence of CRI alone should not preclude performance of CAS, the presence of additional high-risk features should increase the threshold of intervention, particularly in asymptomatic patients.

Several precautionary measures can be taken to reduce contrast-related morbidity in these patients:

- preprocedure carotid magnetic resonance angiography (MRA) to define the cerebrovascular anatomy and the potential working views, thereby reducing intraprocedural iodinated contrast volume
- preprocedure intravenous hydration and renal protective pharmacotherapy (acetylcysteine, sodium bicarbonate)
- use of gadolinium and saline with iodinated contrast to reduce the total volume of the latter.

Anatomic high-risk features

As there are well-defined anatomic features that increase the risk of complications after CEA, there are also anatomic features that increase the risk of CAS. The three most important anatomic high-risk features are:

- type III aortic arch, particularly in the presence of moderate to severe atherosclerosis
- severe common or internal carotid artery (ICA) tortuosity
- severe lesion calcifications.

A type III aortic arch may lead to prolonged catheter manipulation and difficulty in accessing the common carotid artery (CCA), with potentially higher risk of aortic arch plaque embolization (Figure 14.9). Excessive vessel tortuosity proximal or distal to the carotid stenosis increases the difficulty of EPD delivery and potentially deployment, and it increases the likelihood of vascular spasm. Occasionally, extreme tortuosity may even preclude a patient from undergoing intervention (Figure 14.10). Finally, severe calcification, particularly in combination with tortuosity, can cause difficulties in device delivery, lesion dilation, and stent expansion (Figure 14.11).

Although operator experience, appropriate device selection, and technique modification can increase technical success, the potential for complications remains higher than that in simpler anatomy.

Preprocedure patient preparation

Fundamental to optimal patient preparation prior to CAS is an adequate antiplatelet regimen and proper hydration. Although no comparative clinical trials exist as to the optimal preprocedure antiplatelet regimen, there is consensus that these patients should receive a similar regimen to that of patients undergoing coronary stenting. The standard antiplatelet regimen comprises aspirin 325 mg/day and clopidogrel 75 mg/day for at least 1 week prior to the procedure. In patients who do not receive this regimen, some clinicians advocate a loading dose of aspirin (650 mg) and clopidogrel (600 mg) at least 6 hours before the procedure. Currently, there is no role for elective use of glycoprotein IIb/IIIa receptor antagonists.

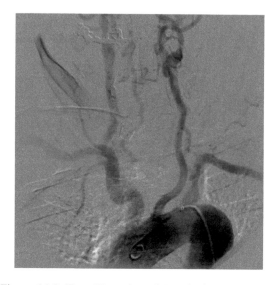

Figure 14.9 Type III aortic arch in a high surgical risk patient with asymptomatic severe left internal carotid artery stenosis.

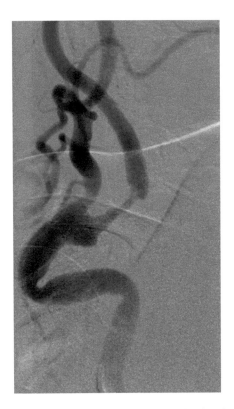

Figure 14.10 Severe tortuosity of the right distal common carotid artery in a high surgical risk patient with asymptomatic right internal carotid artery stenosis.

All patients should be adequately hydrated to reduce the incidence and severity of intraprocedural hypotension.

Traditionally, all antihypertensive medications are withheld on the day of the procedure. This is done to avoid excessive hypotension after CAS, particularly in patients with known severe coronary artery disease or critical aortic stenosis. In the absence of these conditions, however, the decision to withhold antihypertensive medications, other than β-blockers, should be done on a case by case basis. In patients with poorly controlled hypertension or those who are on multiple drugs, withholding antihypertensive medications can lead to difficulty in controlling blood pressure post procedure. Uncontrolled hypertension, along with pre-existing severe carotid stenosis, particularly if bilateral, increases the risk of hyperperfusion syndrome after CEA as well as after CAS.[30,31]

Procedure planning and execution

A comprehensive discussion of the technical aspects of the CAS procedure is beyond the scope of this chapter. In this section we will briefly touch upon key elements of procedural planning and execution.

Diagnostic angiography

In the absence of preprocedure anatomic imaging – MRA or computed tomographic angiography (CTA) – aortic arch angiography is essential for proper procedural planning. Aortic arch angiography provides information

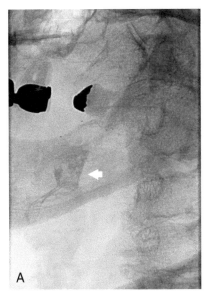
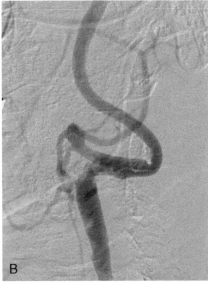

Figure 14.11 Severely calcified left carotid bulb stenosis (A, white arrow) with 90° bend distal to the stenosis (B).

regarding arch type, extent of atherosclerotic disease, arch anomalies, and presence or absence of ostial CCA disease. This information help the operator choose the most appropriate diagnostic cerebral angiography catheter and plan and anticipate the level of difficulty in accessing the CCA. In type I arch (Figure 14.12), a simple curve diagnostic catheter is adequate (JB1, Bernstein, vertebral, etc.), whereas in type II (Figure 14.13) or type III arches (Figure 14.14), a double-curved catheter may be needed (Vitek, Simmons, etc.). A double-curved catheter

may also be needed in patients where an arm access is necessary (Figure 14.15).

Carotid and intracerebral angiography should define lesion severity, the degree of tortuosity and calcification of the CCA/ICA, presence or absence of tandem extra- or intracranial atherosclerotic disease (Figure 14.16), the extent and source of collateral circulation, particularly if a balloon-occlusive EPD is to be used (Figure 14.17), and the presence or absence of large intracranial aneurysms or arteriovenous malformations (Chapter 12).

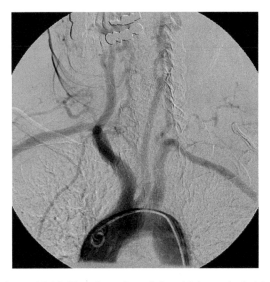

Figure 14.12 Type I aortic arch in a high surgical risk patient with asymptomatic left internal carotid artery stenosis.

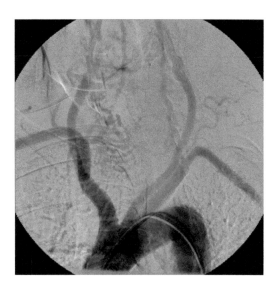

Figure 14.13 Type II aortic arch in a high surgical risk patient with asymptomatic left internal carotid artery stenosis.

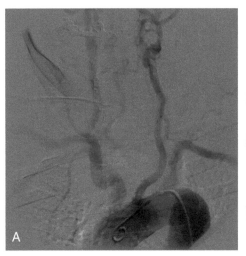
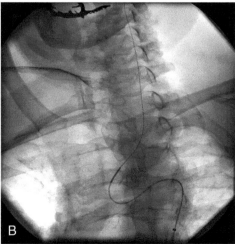

Figure 14.14 (A) Type III aortic arch in a high surgical risk patient with asymptomatic left internal carotid artery stenosis. (B) The use of the Vitek catheter to engage the left common carotid artery.

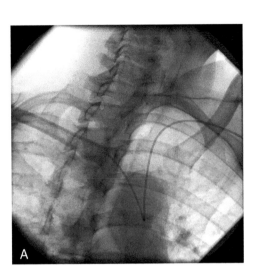
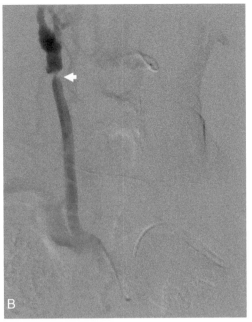

Figure 14.15 Severe right distal common carotid artery stenosis (CEA restenosis) in a high surgical risk patient with infrarenal aortic occlusion. (A) Use of the Simmons 1 catheter to engage the innonimate artery from the left brachial artery. (B) Note the severe right distal common carotid artery stenosis (white arrow).

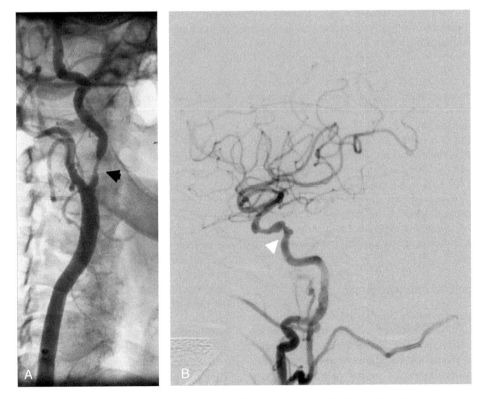

Figure 14.16 (A) Right internal carotid artery stenosis (black arrow) in a high surgical risk asymptomatic patient. (B) Intracranial tandem carotid siphon stenosis (white arrow).

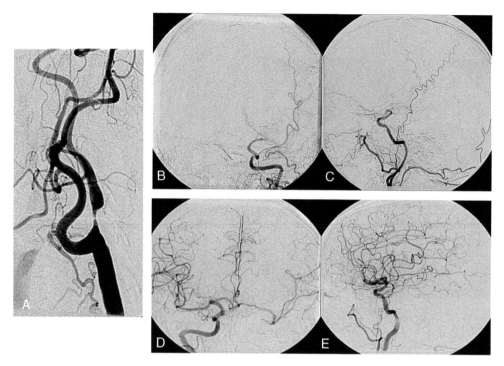

Figure 14.17 (A) Severe left internal carotid artery stenosis (LICA) in a high surgical risk asymptomatic patient. (B, C) Anteroposterior and lateral views of the left intracranial carotid circulation. Note lack of antegrade flow in the LICA proximal to its bifurcation. (D, E) Anteroposterior and lateral views of the right intracranial carotid circulation. Note that the left intracranial circulation is supplied by the right anterior cerebral artery through the anterior communicating artery.

Needless to say, complications of carotid angiography should be kept to a minimum; the death and stroke rate of carotid angiography in ACAS[8] (1.2%) is an unacceptable standard in today's practice. In a review of 634 patients undergoing carotid and vertebrobasilar arteriography, Wholey and Wholey reported a stroke and morbidity rate of 0.34%.[32] Neurological events associated with carotid angiography are often due to excessive and prolonged manipulation of the diagnostic catheter in the aortic arch. Operator experience and proper choice of diagnostic catheters are paramount in reducing these complications.[33]

Common carotid artery access

Although many operators develop a preference for one access technique over another and tend to use it in the majority of cases, it is advisable that the access technique be tailored to the patient-specific anatomy. Four factors need to be considered prior to choosing an access technique:

- aortic arch type
- the degree of tortuosity of the origin of the CCA

- lesion location (distal CCA vs ICA)
- external carotid artery (ECA) patency.

Based on these variables, the operator can then choose an access technique using a sheath-based or a guiding catheter-based platform.

The standard technique utilizing a sheath-based platform was popularized by Roubin and colleagues.[34] In this technique, a double-curved 5 Fr catheter (VTK, Cook Inc., Bloomington, IN) and an 0.038 inch angled-tip hydrophilic-coated wire are used to cannulate the external carotid artery (ECA). The hydrophilic-coated wire is then exchanged for a soft-tipped, stiff, 0.035 inch guidewire (e.g. Supracore, Guidant Inc., Indianapolis, ID) and the Vitek catheter is removed. A 6 Fr 90 cm sheath (Shuttle, Cook Inc.) is then introduced over the wire and positioned in the distal portion of the CCA, a few centimeters below the bifurcation. In cases where the stenosis is located in the distal segment of the CCA, the above technique is modified by placing the tip of the 5 Fr catheter and stiff guidewire (Amplatz Super Stiff J-wire, MediTech, Natick, MA) assembly below the lesion in the CCA and the 6 Fr sheath is advanced over this assembly.

Alternatively, the sheath-based technique can be performed using the 'telescoping method'. With this technique, the 90 cm sheath is introduced and positioned at the level of the proximal descending aorta and the dilator retrieved. A long 125 cm 5 Fr diagnostic cerebral catheter is then introduced through the sheath and advanced over a 0.035 inch or 0.038 inch angled-tip hydrophilic guidewire (depending on the shape of the diagnostic catheter) to the ECA. The sheath is then advanced over the assembly of the diagnostic catheter and the guidewire to the distal CCA. One disadvantage

of this approach is the mismatch between the size of the diagnostic catheter (5 Fr) and the size of the sheath (6 Fr). This may cause the tip of the sheath to scrape the arterial wall at the origin of the CCA. Using a 6 Fr cerebral catheter instead can provide a smoother transition.

On the other hand, a guiding catheter-based platform (8 Fr, 90 cm) is preferable in patients with complex aortic arch anatomy and tortuous origin of the CCA because it is available in various tip shapes and provides better trackability and torque control (Figure 14.18). CCA access using guide catheters is typically done

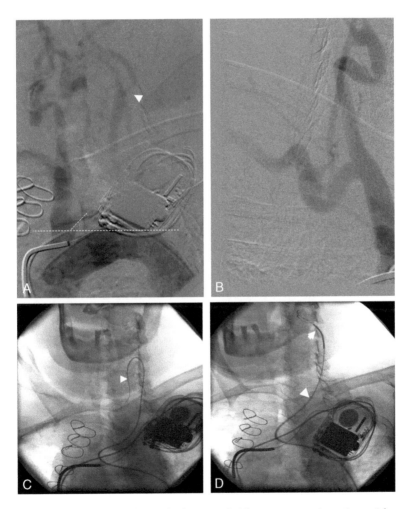

Figure 14.18 (A) Type II bovine aortic arch in a high surgical risk asymptomatic patient with severe left internal carotid artery (LICA) stenosis (white arrow). (B) Note the acute angle take-off of the left common carotid artery. (C) The sheath-based approach using a Vitek catheter over a 0.038 inch hydrophilic guidewire (white arrow) failed in securing access to the left common carotid artery. (D) A guiding catheter-based approach (8 Fr 90 cm hockey stick) using the telescoping method over a 6.5 Fr JB1 hydrophilic catheter and a 0.038 inch hydrophilic guidewire (white arrow) secured access to the left common carotid artery (white arrowhead). (E) Baseline left carotid angiography demonstrating a severe LICA stenosis. (F) Final left carotid angiography after implantation of a self-expandable stent with distal protection.

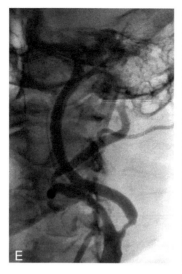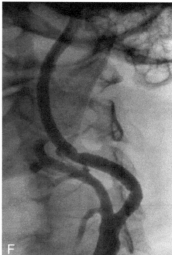

Figure 14.18 (*Continued*).

using the 'telescoping technique' described above. However, in situations where this technique is not successful, such as in extreme type III arch, the 'remote access technique' can be helpful. This can be achieved by engaging the ostium of the left CCA or the innominate artery directly with the guiding catheter and using a high-support 0.014 inch coronary guidewire 'buddy wire' to stabilize the guiding catheter (Figure 14.19).

Embolic protection devices

There is universal consensus that EPDs are beneficial in reducing cerebral embolic complications with CAS. There are three categories of EPDs: distal occlusion balloons,[14] distal filter devices (Figure 14.20),[10–13,15–16] and flow-reversal devices.[35] Although there are clear differences among these devices in design, profile, deployment method, and technical performance (Table 14.4), once an EPD is deployed there is no proof of differences in clinical outcome. Currently, the only EPDs approved for clinical use in the United States are the ACCUNET filter (Guidant Corporation, Menlo Park, CA), the Emboshield filter (Abbott Vascular, Redwood City, CA), and the Spider filter (ev3 Inc., Plymouth, MN). The choice of one category of EPDs vs the other depends on the particular anatomy. The Advantages and disadvantages of the various EPD categories are listed in Table 14.5. The anatomic features that need to be considered when choosing an EPD include:

- angle of origin of the ICA
- degree of ICA tortuosity distal to the lesion, particularly at the exit point
- adequacy of the landing zone
- adequacy of collateral circulation when distal balloon occlusion or flow-reversal is considered.

Techniques for facilitating EPD delivery are described elsewhere.

Self-expanding carotid stents

There is consensus that self-expandable stents are preferable to balloon expandable stents due to the propensity of the latter for compression. Stent length should be adequate to cover the entire lesion and extend to the distal portion of the CCA (in the majority of cases where the lesion is located at or in proximity of the bifurcation). The nominal diameter of the self-expandable stent should be at least 1–2 mm larger than the distal reference of the lesion (ICA), but also large enough to provide good apposition to the common carotid artery. A wide variety of self-expandable open cell (Figure 14.21) and closed cell (Figure 14.22) carotid stents are available, each with its unique attributes (Table 14.6). Although tailoring stent choice (in terms of conformability, lesion coverage and radial strength) to the specific anatomy makes intuitive sense, there is no proof that one stent is superior to others in terms of clinical outcome. Currently, only the ACCULINK (Guidant Corporation, Menlo Park, CA) and the Xact (Abbott Vascular, Redwood City, CA) stents are approved for clinical use in the USA.

Operator experience

Along with proper patient selection, operator experience is critical to the success of CAS, but is also the most difficult element to define. Defining the relationship

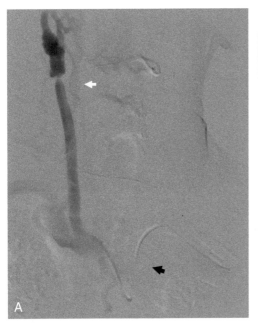
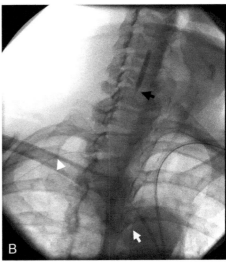

Figure 14.19 (A) Severe right distal common carotid artery stenosis (CEA restenosis) (white arrow) in a high surgical risk patient with infrarenal aortic occlusion. Note the use of a Simmons 1 catheter to engage the innonimate artery from the left brachial artery (black arrow). (B) Use of the 'remote access technique' utilizing an 8 Fr 90 cm EBU 3.5 guiding catheter (white arrow) engaged in the innonimate artery. Note the 'buddy wire' in the right subclavian artery (white arrowhead) and the filter wire and predilatation balloon across the lesion (black arrow).

between operator experience and the clinical outcome of patients undergoing CAS is a difficult task. Operator experience is typically measured based on the number of procedures performed and the outcome of these procedures. However, this process is confounded by lack of adjustment for patient's characteristics. Several reports have indicated that operator experience, as measured by the number of CAS procedures performed, correlateas with clinical outcome.[36,37] The lack of effect of operator experience on patient outcome in the CAPTURE registry is most likely due to patient selection bias. An alternative measure that incorporates operator experience and patient-related factors is the duration of the CAS procedure as reflected by filter deployment time. This measure has been shown to be an independent predictor of periprocedural complications with a filter deployment time >20 minutes doubling the risk of stroke and death.[13]

Intraprocedural complications and management

Intraprocedural complications that are specific to CAS can be divided into three categories:

- hemodynamic depressive response (hypotension and bradycardia)
- cerebral embolism
- complications at the carotid stent site, such as slow flow, spasm, and perforation.

We will limit our discussion to the first two categories of complications.

Hypotension and bradycardia

Most experts agree that hypotension and bradycardia during CAS are related to carotid bulb distention during balloon inflation and stent deployment. Distention of the carotid bulb leads to stimulation of the baroreceptors, which in turn causes reflex inhibition of adrenergic output to the peripheral vasculature and increased cardiac parasympathetic stimulation.[38] Hypotension and bradycardia with CAS are more commonly observed in patients with de-novo carotid bulb lesions as opposed to those with post-CEA restenosis,[39,40] and in patients with severely calcified lesions,[40] particularly when an oversized balloon is used for stent expansion.[41] Anecdotal experiences also suggest that stent oversizing

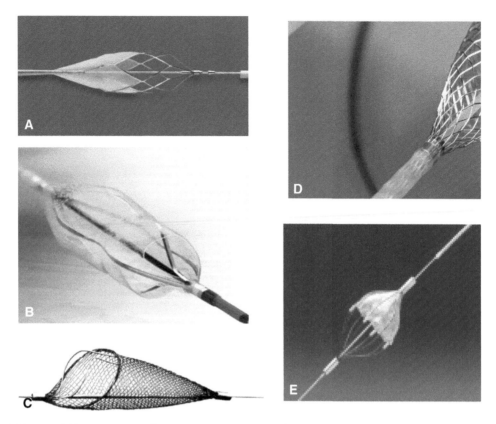

Figure 14.20 Distal filter protection devices: (A) AccuNet (Guidant Corporation, Menlo Park, CA); (B) Emboshield (Abbott Vascular, Redwood City, CA); (C) Spider (ev3 Inc., Plymouth, MN); (D) Filterwire EZ (Boston Scientific, Boston, MA); (E) ANGIOGUARD (Cordis, Warren, NJ).

may contribute to a prolonged hemodynamic depressive response. It has been suggested that the presence of diabetes mellitus reduces the chances of hypotension and bradycardia with CAS,[40] presumably because of an impaired ability to develop reflex bradycardia.[42]

Transient episodes of hypotension and bradycardia during CAS should not be labeled as a 'complication' because it is an expected hemodynamic alteration that occurs in 19–68% of CAS procedures[13,39,41,43,44] and can be readily managed with intravenous fluids, atropine, and vasopressors in most patients.[13] On the other hand, if these hemodynamic alterations become persistent and do not immediately respond to volume expansion, atropine and/or an intravenous bolus of a vasopressor they can be associated with adverse clinical outcome.[40]

To reduce the chances of hypotension and bradycardia with CAS, some operators advocate routine pretreatment with a bolus of intravenous atropine (0.6–1.0 mg) prior to predilatation. Other operators, however, argue that the routine use of atropine may lead to potential complications, such as confusion, urinary retention,

and arrhythmias, and that there is no proof that routine prophylactic pharmacological treatment is associated with improved outcome. A more balanced approach would be to emphasize the role of preprocedure volume expansion and use of atropine only for those patients who manifest hemodynamic depressive response after initial predilatation[44] or for those patients with pre-existing critical aortic stenosis who may not tolerate a prolonged hemodynamic depressive response.

Cerebral embolism

The incidence of cerebral embolism during CAS has diminished with the use of EPDs,[45] and if it occurs it is often clinically silent.[46] In a minority of patients, however, cerebral embolism can lead to a transient or permanent neurological deficit. Studies with brain MRI diffusion-weighted imaging have demonstrated that cerebral embolism during CAS is often ipsilateral to the treated vessel, but it can also affect the contralateral hemisphere and the posterior circulation.[47] The frequency

Table 14.4 Embolic protection devices

Study	Manufacturer	Protection mechanism	Pore size (μm)	Crossing profile	Diameter (mm)
Distal occlusion balloons					
GuardWire® Temporary Occlusion and Aspiration System	Medtronic	Latex balloon	NA	2.7 Fr	3.0–6.0
Distal filter devices					
RX ACCUNET	Guidant/Abbott	Polyurethane filter	125	3.5–3.7 Fr	4.5–7.5
ANGIOGUARD XP	Cordis Endovascular	Polyurethane filter	100	3.2–3.9 Fr	4.0–8.0
Filter EZ™	Boston Scientific	Polyurethane filter	110	3.2 Fr	3.5–5.5
Emboshield	Abbott	Polyurethane filter	140	3.7–3.9 Fr	3.0–6.0
Interceptor® PLUS	Medtronic	Nitinol mesh filter	100	2.7 Fr	5.5–6.5
Rubicon	Rubicon Medical	Polyurethane filter	110	2.1–2.7 Fr	4.0–6.0
SpideRX™	eV3	Nitinol filter	100–150	2.9 Fr	3.0–7.0
Flow-reversal devices					
Mo.Ma	Invatec	Flow reversal	NA	NA	NA
Parodi Anti-Emboli System	ArteriA	Flow reversal	NA	NA	NA

Approved by the FDA for clinical use in the USA with carotid artery stenting: RX ACCUNET, Emboshield, SpideRX™.
Not approved by the FDA for clinical use in the USA with carotid artery stenting: GuardWire® Temporary Occlusion and Aspiration System, ANGIOGUARD XP, Filter EZ™ Interceptor® plus, Rubicon, Mo.Ma, Parodi Anti-Emboli System.

Table 14.5 Advantages and disadvantages of different categories of embolic protection devices

Study	Advantages	Disadvantages
Distal occlusion balloons	• Complete protection of distal ICA • Low crossing profile and high flexibility • One size fits all	• Interruption of antegrade blood flow through the ICA Potential dissection/spasm in distal ICA Potential embolization through a patent ECA • No angiographic visualization during the procedure
Distal filter devices	• Preservation of antegrade flow • Angiographic visualization preserved	• Larger crossing profile and lower flexibility compared with occlusion balloons No protection during filter introduction • Possible filter occlusion with debri
Flow-reversal devices	• Complete protection prior to lesion crossing • Ability to use any wire for lesion crossing • Ability to treat highly tortuous ICAs	• Complete interruption of antegrade blood flow • Potential dissection in CCA/ECA • More complex to use than filters • Large introducer size

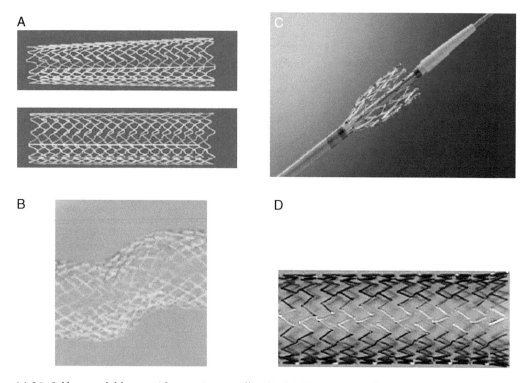

Figure 14.21 Self-expandable carotid stents (open cell): (A) ACCULINK (Guidant Corporation, Menlo Park, CA); (B) Exponent (Medtronic Vascular, Santa Rosa, CA); (C) Precise (Cordis, Warren, NJ); (D) Protégé (ev3 Inc., Plymouth, MN).

of clinical ischemic neurological events in asymptomatic patients undergoing protected CAS has been reviewed earlier in the chapter. The majority of these events manifest during the procedure. In the CREATE registry, about 70% of strokes manifested during the procedure, 13% during the first 24 hours, and 17% between 1 and 30 days postprocedure.[13]

Management of patients who suffer from an intraprocedural stroke due to cerebral embolism depends on the severity of the neurological deficit. Patients with a minor deficit should be treated medically. In patients with a major neurological deficit, an attempt at neuro rescue should be considered if local expertise is available.[48] The use of glycoprotein IIb/IIIa receptor antagonists and thrombolytic therapy is associated with an unacceptable rate of intracranial hemorrhage.[49]

Postprocedure complications and management

The majority of CAS-related complications occur during the procedure. However, serious cerebrovascular complications can still occur afterwards such as hyperperfusion syndrome and intracranial bleeding,

delayed ischemic stroke, and rarely subacute stent thrombosis.[50]

Hyperperfusion syndrome

Along with major ischemic stroke, hyperperfusion syndrome is the most feared complication after CAS because it can result in cerebral hemorrhage. Cerebral hyperperfusion syndrome (CHS) after carotid revascularization, CEA, or CAS, is characterized by ipsilateral headache, hypertension, seizures, and focal neurological deficit and manifests on brain imaging as generalized or focal hemispheric brain edema.[51] This condition can be self-limited,[52] but if not treated properly it can result in intracerebral or subarachnoid hemorrhage and death. Occasionally, cerebral hemorrhage can be the first presenting sign of CHS.[53,54]

The incidence of CHS after CAS ranges from 1.2% to 5%[31,55] and it results in cerebral hemorrhage in about 1% of patients.[13,31] Risk factors for CHS and intracranial hemorrhage after CAS are bilateral severe carotid artery stenosis, which is commonly associated with diminished cerebrovascular reserve, and postprocedure hypertension.[31] Concomitant administration of

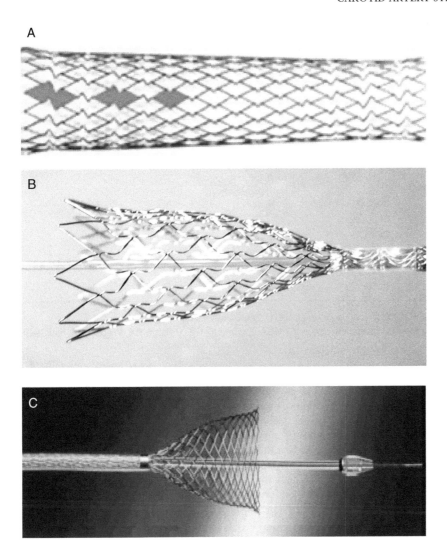

Figure 14.22 Self-expandable carotid stents (closed cell): (A) Xact (Abbott Vascular, Redwood City, CA); (B) NexStent (Boston Scientific, Boston, MA/EndoTex, Cupertino, CA); (C) Carotid Wallstent (Boston Scientific, Boston, MA).

warfarin in addition to the dual antiplatelet therapy may increase the risk of intracranial hemorrhage.[13] Preventive treatment strategies should focus on proper hypertension management prior to CAS and control of postprocedure blood pressure to limit the excessive rise in cerebral perfusion, particularly in high-risk patients.

Delayed ischemic stroke

Cerebral embolism during CAS is not the only cause of stroke associated with the procedure. About 30% of CAS-related strokes occur 1–30 days postprocedure[13] and these strokes tend to occur more commonly in symptomatic rather than asymptomatic patients.[56] The mechanism of delayed postprocedural stroke is unclear, but some clinicians propose a role for platelet embolization from the stented segment. Other causes include stent thrombosis or an alternative source of cerebral embolization.

SUMMARY

Carotid artery stenting with embolic protection in asymptomatic patients has demonstrated safety and

Table 14.6. Self-expandable carotid stents

Study	Manufacturer	Material	Lesion coverage	Radial force	Comformability
Open cell design					
RX ACCULINK	Guidant	Nitinol	+	+±	++
Exponent RX	Medtronic	Nitinol	+±	+±	++
Protégé RX	eV3	Nitinol	+	++	++
Closed cell design					
NexStent	Boston Scientific/ EndoTex	Nitinol	++	++	+
Precise RX	CORDIS	Nitinol	+±	++	++
Xact	Endovascular Abbott	Nitinol	+++	++	+
Carotid Wallstent Monorail	Boston Scientific	Cobalt-alloy	+++	+	+

Approved by the FDA for clinical use in the USA: RX ACCULINK, Xact.

Not approved by the FDA for clinical use in the USA: Exponent® RX, Protégé RX, Precise RX, NexStent, Wallstent.

long-term efficacy in multiple neurologically controlled settings, including randomized trials, lead-in registries, and PMS registries in over 4750 high-to-moderate surgical risk patients. Specifically, in the cohort of patients <80 years old, stroke and death rates approach normal-risk historical controls. Nevertheless at the time of this writing, Medicare reimbursement covers only patients with symptomatic stenosis and high surgical risk. For standard surgical risk patients, the ongoing prospective randomized clinical trials comparing CAS with CEA will define the standard of care.

Most importantly, asymptomatic patients with carotid artery disease need to undergo a rigorous risk stratification process: first, to establish the need for carotid revascularization; and secondly, to choose the optimal revascularization strategy (CAS vs CEA). Proper patient selection based on demographic, clinical, and angiographic features, meticulous procedure planning and execution, and fastidious postprocedural management are essential steps to insure a low complication rate with CAS.

REFERENCES

1. Mathias K. A new catheter system for percutaneous transluminal angioplasty (PTA) of carotid artery stenoses. Fortschr Med 1977; 95(15): 1007–11.
2. Bockenheimer SA, Mathias K. Percutaneous transluminal angioplasty in arteriosclerotic internal carotid artery stenosis. AJNR Am J Neuroradiol 1983; 4(3): 791–2.
3. Diethrich EB, Gordon MH, Lopez-Galarza LA, Rodriguez-Lopez JA, Casses F. Intraluminal Palmaz stent implantation for treatment of recurrent carotid artery occlusive disease: a plan for the future. J Interv Cardiol 1995; 8(3): 213–18.
4. Roubin GS, Yadav S, Iyer SS, Vitek J. Carotid stent-supported angioplasty: a neurovascular intervention to prevent stroke. Am J Cardiol 1996; 78(3A): 8–12.
5. Theron JG, Payelle GG, Coskun O, Huet HF, Guimaraens L. Carotid artery stenosis: treatment with protected balloon angioplasty and stent placement. Radiology 1996; 201(3):627–36.
6. Yadav JS, Roubin GS, Iyer S et al. Elective stenting of the extracranial carotid arteries. Circulation 1997; 95(2): 376–81.
7. Hobson RW, Weiss DG, Fields WS et al. Efficacy of carotid endarterectomy for asymptomatic carotid stenosis. N Engl J Med 1993; 328: 221–7.
8. Executive Committee for the Asymptomatic Carotid Atherosclerosis Study. Endarterectomy for asymptomatic carotid stenosis. JAMA 1995; 273: 1421–8.
9. Halliday A, Mansfield A, Marro J et al; MRC Asymptomatic Carotid Surgery Trial (ACST) Collaborative Group. Prevention of disabling and fatal strokes by successful carotid endarterectomy in patients without recent neurological symptoms: randomised controlled trial. Lancet 2004; 363: 1491–502.
10. Gray WA. Hopkins NL, Yadav S et al for the ARCHeR Trial Collaborators. Protected carotid stenting in high-surgical-risk patients: The ARCHeR results. J Vasc Surg 2006; 44: 258–69.
11. White C. BEACH investigators. Presented at the 2005 International Stroke Conference, New Orelans, LA.
12. Hopkins LN. CABernET investigators. Carotid artery revascularization using the Boston Scientific FilterWire EX/EZ and the Endo Tex NexStent: 30-day pivotal group results. Presented at Transcatheter Cardiovascular Therapeutics Conference 2004 Washington, DC.
13. Safian RD, Bresnahan JF, Jaff MR et al. CREATE Pivotal Trial Investigators. Protected carotid stenting in high-risk patients with severe carotid artery stenosis. J Am Coll Cardiol 2006; 47: 2384–9.

14. Ramee SR. MAVErIC Investigators. MAVErIC II: a prospective registry of carotid stenting with the Exponent stent and distal protection with the GuideWire in high risk patients: 30-day results. Presented at Transcatheter Cardiovascular Therapeutics Conference 2004 Washington, DC.

15. Whitlow P; SECuRITY Investigators. SECuRITY: multicenter evaluation of carotid stenting with a distal protection filter. Presented at Transcatheter Cardiovascular Therapeutics Conference 2003 Washington, DC.

16. Yadav JS, Wholey MH, Kuntz RE et al; Stenting and Angioplasty with Protection in Patients at High Risk for Endarterectomy Investigators. Protected carotid-artery stenting versus endarterectomy in high-risk patients. N Engl J Med 2004; 351(15): 1493–501.

17. Roubin GS, New G, Iyer SS et al. Immediate and late clinical outcomes of carotid artery stenting in patients with symptomatic and asymptomatic carotid artery stenosis: a 5-year prospective analysis. Circulation 2001; 103(4): 532–7.

18. Wholey MH, Al-Mubarek N, Wholey MH. Updated review of the global carotid artery stent registry. Catheter Cardiovasc Interv 2003; 60(2): 259–66.

19. Reimers B, Schluter M, Castriota F et al. Routine use of cerebral protection during carotid artery stenting: results of a multicenter registry of 753 patients. Am J Med 2004; 116(4): 217–22.

20. CaRESS Steering Committee. Carotid Revascularization Using Endarterectomy or Stenting Systems (CaRESS) phase I clinical trial: 1-year results. J Vasc Surg 2005; 42: 213–19.

21. Gray WA for the CAPTURE Investigators. Carotid RX ACCULINK® /RX ACCUNET™ Post-Approval Trial to Uncover Unanticipated or Rare Events. Presented at the American College of Cardiology Scientific Sessions 2006 Atlanta, GA.

22. Gray WA. CASES Steering Committee. Carotid Artery Stenting With Emboli Protection Surveillance (CASES Registry). Personal Communication.

23. Roubin GS. CREST lead-in Phase Registry Investigators. Presented at the American College of Cardiology Scientific Sessions 2006 Atlanta, GA.

24. Yadav JS. Two year follow-up of the SAPPHIRE trial. Presented at Transcatheter Cardiovascular Therapeutics Conference 2005 Washington, DC.

25. Goldstein LB, Adams R, Alberts MJ et al; American Heart Association; American Stroke Association Stroke Council. Primary prevention of ischemic stroke. A guideline from the American Heart Association/American Stroke Association Stroke Council: cosponsored by the Atherosclerotic Peripheral Vascular Disease Interdisciplinary Working Group; Cardiovascular Nursing Council; Clinical Cardiology Council; Nutrition, Physical Activity, and Metabolism Council; and the Quality of Care and Outcomes Research Interdisciplinary Working Group. Stroke 2006; 113(24): e873–923.

26. Hobson RW II, Howard VJ, Roubin GS et al. Carotid artery stenting is associated with increased complications in octogenarians: 30-day stroke and death rates in the CREST lead-in phase. J Vasc Surg 2004; 30: 1106–11.

27. Nicolaides AN, Kakkos S, Griffin M, Geroulakos G, Ioannidou E. Severity of asymptomatic carotid stenosis and risk of ipsilateral hemispheric ischaemic events: results from the ACSRS study. Eur J Vasc Endovasc Surg 2005; 30: 275–84.

28. Hamdan AD, Pomposelli FB Jr, Gibbons GW, Campbell DR, LoGerfo FW. Renal insufficiency and altered postoperative risk in carotid endarterectomy. J Vasc Surg 1999; 29: 1006–11.

29. Saw J, Gurm HS, Fathi RB et al. Effect of chronic kidney disease on outcomes after carotid artery stenting. Am J Cardiol 2004; 94: 1093–6.

30. Wong JH, Findlay JM, Suarez-Almazor ME. Hemodynamic instability after carotid endarterectomy: risk factors and associations with operative complications. Neurosurgery 1997; 41: 35–41.

31. Abou-Chebl A, Yadav JS, Reginelli JP et al. Intracranial hemorrhage and hyperperfusion syndrome following carotid artery stenting: risk factors, prevention, and treatment. J Am Coll Cardiol 2004; 43(9): 1596–601.

32. Wholey MH, Wholey MH. Momentum growing for carotid stent placement. Diagn Imaging 1998; 20: 65–9.

33. Krings T, Willmes K, Becker R et al. Silent microemboli related to diagnostic cerebral angiography: a matter of operator's experience and patient's disease. Neuroradiology 2006; 48(6): e387–93.

34. Vitek JJ, Roubin GS, Al-Mubarek N, New G, Iyer SS. Carotid artery stenting: technical considerations. AJNR Am J Neuroradiol 2000; 21: 1736–43.

35. Reimers B, Sievert H, Schuler GC et al. Proximal endovascular flow blockage for cerebral protection during carotid artery stenting: results from a prospective multicenter registry. J Endovasc Ther 2005; 12(2): 156–65.

36. Ahmadi R, Willfort A, Lang W et al. Carotid artery stenting: effect of learning curve and intermediate-term morphological outcome. J Endovasc Ther 2001; 8(6): 539–46.

37. Al-Mubarak N, Roubin GS, Hobson RW. Credentialing of stent operators for the Carotid Revascularization Endarterectomy vs. Stenting Trial (CREST). Stroke 2000; 31: 292.

38. Timmers HJ, Wieling W, Karemaker JM, Lenders JWM. Denervation of carotid baro- and chemoreceptors in humans. J Physiol 2003; 553: 3–11.

39. Qureshi AI, Luft AR, Sharma M et al. Frequency and determinants of postprocedural hemodynamic instability after carotid angioplasty and stenting. Stroke 1999; 30: 2086–93.

40. Gupta R, Abou-Chebl A, Bajzer CT, Schumacher C, Yadav JS. Rate, predictors, and consequences of hemodynamic depression after carotid artery stenting. J Am Coll Cardiol 2006; 47: 1538–43.

41. Dangas G, Laird JR Jr, Satler LF et al. Postprocedural hypotension after carotid artery stent placement: predictors and short- and long-term clinical outcomes. Radiology 2000; 215: 677–83.

42. Lloyd-Mostyn RH, Watkins PJ. Defective innervation of heart in diabetic autonomic neuropathy. Br Med J 1975; 3: 15–17.

43. Mendelsohn FO, Weissman NJ, Lederman RJ et al. Acute hemodynamic changes during carotid artery stenting. Am J Cardiol 1998; 82: 1077–81.

44. Leisch F, Kerschner K, Hofmann R et al. Carotid sinus reactions during carotid artery stenting: predictors, incidence and influence on clinical outcome. Catheter Cardiovasc Interv 2003; 58: 516–23.

45. Boltuch J, Sabeti S, Amighi J et al. Procedure-related complications and early neurological adverse events of unprotected and protected carotid stenting: temporal trends in a consecutive patient series. J Endovasc Ther 2005; 12(5): 538–47.

46. Cosottini M, Michelassi MC, Puglioli M et al. Silent cerebral ischemia detected with diffusion-weighted imaging in patients treated with protected and unprotected carotid artery stenting. Stroke 2005; 36: 2389–93.

47. Pinero P, Gonzalez A, Mayol A et al. Silent ischemia after neuroprotected percutaneous carotid stenting: a diffusion-weighted MRI study. AJNR Am J Neuroradiol 2006; 27(6): 1338–45.

48. Green DW, Sanchez LA, Parodi JC et al. Acute thromboembolic events during carotid artery angioplasty and stenting: etiology and a technique of neurorescue. J Endovasc Ther 2005; 12(3): 360–5.

49. Wholey MH, Wholey MH, Tan WA et al. Management of neurological complications of carotid artery stenting. J Endovasc Ther 2001; 8: 341–53.

50. Buhk JH, Wellmer A, Knauth M. Late in-stent thrombosis following carotid angioplasty and stenting. Neurology 2006; 66: 1594–6.

51. van Mook WN, Rennenberg RJ, Schurink GW et al. Cerebral hyperperfusion syndrome. Lancet Neurol 2005; 4(12): 877–88.

52. Pilz G, Klos M, Bernhardt P et al. Reversible cerebral hyperperfusion syndrome after stenting of the carotid artery – two case reports. Clin Res Cardiol 2006; 95(3): 186–91.

53. McCabe DJH, Brown MM, Clifton A. Fatal cerebral reperfusion hemorrhage after carotid stenting. Stroke 1999; 30: 2483–6.

54. Al-Mubarak N, Roubin GS, Vitek JJ et al. Subarachnoidal hemorrhage following carotid stenting with the distal-balloon protection. Catheter Cardiovasc Interv 2001; 54(4): 521–3.

55. Meyers PM, Higashida RT, Phatouros CC et al. Cerebral hyperperfusion syndrome after percutaneous transluminal stenting of the craniocervical arteries. Neurosurgery 2000; 47(2): 335–43.

56. Hauth EA, Drescher R, Jansen C et al. Complications and follow-up after unprotected carotid artery stenting. Cardiovasc Intervent Radiol 2006; 29(4): 511–18.

15

Asymptomatic carotid atherosclerotic stenosis: guidelines and future directions

Shyam Prabhakaran and Ralph L Sacco

CURRENT GUIDELINES

Based on the Asymptomatic Carotid Atherosclerosis Study (ACAS) and the Asymptomatic Carotid Surgery Trial (ACST), current American Stroke Association evidence-based recommendations support carotid endarterectomy (CEA) in selected patients with 60–99% asymptomatic carotid stenosis if performed by a surgeon with a <3% surgical complication rate. Patient selection criteria regarding comorbid conditions, life expectancy, patient preference, and demographics, including gender, are crucial.[1] It is also recommended that other treatable causes of stroke are thoroughly investigated and intensive medical therapy instituted for coexisting medical conditions. These recommendations for endarterectomy are given class IA grade based on the weight of evidence from two randomized trials.

Despite these recommendations, considerable debate remains regarding:

1. Risk stratification and appropriate patient selection, given the narrow risk–benefit margin and lower absolute stroke risk among asymptomatic vs symptomatic patients.
2. Choice of revascularization procedure.
3. Role of generalized screening.

In this chapter, we will discuss some of these controversies, examine the gaps in the current state of knowledge regarding the management of asymptomatic carotid stenosis, and discuss future directions.

Risk stratification

Presence of atherosclerotic carotid stenosis is a well-established risk factor for transient ischemic attack (TIA) and ischemic stroke.[2–4] Compared to patients with symptomatic carotid stenosis, the absolute risk of first stroke with asymptomatic carotid artery disease is considerably lower.[3,5] In observational studies, the annual risk of ipsilateral stroke among those with asymptomatic stenosis >50% ranged from 1.0 to 3.4%, increasing with advancing degree of stenosis.[6–13] Therefore, as only some patients with asymptomatic carotid stenosis develop stroke or TIA, predicting which patients will develop ischemic symptoms remains a challenge.

Among asymptomatic individuals, the risk of stroke increases modestly with advancing degree of stenosis [6–13] and may depend on the rate of progression of stenosis, the adequacy of collateral vessels, the morphological characteristics of the plaque, and other stroke risk factors.[11,14–16] For example, heterogeneous, echolucent, and ulcerated plaques may better predict stroke risk[16,17] and serve as markers of vulnerable or unstable carotid plaques. In addition, cerebral vasoreactivity to carbon dioxide challenge and transcranial Doppler detection of embolic signals have been shown to be useful markers of elevated risk.[18,19] In the Asymptomatic Carotid Stenosis and Risk of Stroke (ACSRS) study, degree of stenosis was linearly related to ipsilateral hemispheric ischemic events, along with a history of contralateral TIA, elevated serum creatinine, and plaque morphological type on ultrasound.[20,21]

Given this complexity and the heterogeneity of risk, the evaluation of patients with asymptomatic carotid stenosis requires not only an appreciation of the associated stroke risk but also knowledge of subclinical, clinical, and intraplaque features that help stratify risk. Risk stratification based on some of these features may be particularly important among patients with 60–79% stenosis, in whom the appropriate management is more uncertain. Therefore, stroke risk is not a simple algorithm determined solely by degree of stenosis.

Practical considerations

Other considerations in the risk–benefit calculation for CEA deserve mention. First, nearly 40% of ipsilateral strokes in patients with asymptomatic carotid stenosis may be attributable to small-artery disease or cardio-embolism.[13] Therefore, it is imperative that a thorough evaluation be conducted to assess and treat other potential risk factors for ischemic stroke. Secondly, since most of these prospective studies and clinical trials occurred in an era before the widespread use of statins that may halt or regress carotid atherosclerosis in some patients,[22–29] some have argued that the previously calculated outcome rates may not accurately reflect the actual risk for asymptomatic carotid stenosis in the setting of multimodal intensive medical therapies.[30] However, at the last clinical follow-up of ACST in 2002–03, more than 90% of the survivors were on antiplatelet therapy, 81% were on anti-hypertensive agents, and 70% were on lipid-lowering treatment with similar stroke risks as in ACAS done a decade earlier.[31] These data suggest that use of standard medical therapies has increased over time, with similar absolute and relative risk reductions (RRRs), but does not address the issue of whether increased intensity of medical therapy (with specific treatment goals for dyslipidemia, diabetes, and hypertension) might lower absolute stroke risks.

Risk reduction strategies

Two general strategies have emerged in the management of asymptomatic carotid stenosis >60%:

- medical therapy aimed at halting plaque progression and reducing stroke risk
- revascularization therapy by endarterectomy or angioplasty and stenting to remove or reduce carotid stenosis.

Medical

The medical approach is critical for all patients with carotid plaque (even those managed by surgery or endovascular modalities) and employs aggressive risk factor modification and management of associated vascular risk factors such as hypertension, diabetes mellitus, dyslipidemia, and cigarette smoking.[1] The overall vascular risk reduction in patients with prior cardiovascular or cerebrovascular ischemic events achieved by medical measures can be as high as 75% if multimodal therapies are employed.[32] Moreover, several studies have also demonstrated that plaque progression can be retarded using 'statin' therapy.[22,23,27] Therefore, medical

therapy remains a keystone in the management of individuals with asymptomatic carotid stenosis.

Surgical

The second approach employs carotid revascularization, including surgical and endovascular approaches. Several large studies have evaluated the efficacy of CEA in asymptomatic carotid stenosis.[31,33–36] Although the primary analysis of both ACAS and ACST favored CEA, various subgroups are worth evaluating in the application of the evidence into practice.

In ACAS, the benefit was most notable among men (RRR = 66% in men vs 17% in women), explained partly by a 1.7% complication rate in men compared with 3.6% in women. In contrast to ACAS, the surgical benefits in ACST extended to both men and women. However, no benefit was seen in patients >75 years old. Pooled data from ACAS and ACST suggest that surgical benefit is greater in men than in women (pooled interaction $p = 0.01$; men, odds ratio [OR] = 0.49, 95% CI 0.36–0.60, women, OR = 0.96, 95% CI 0.63–1.45).[37] Another subgroup with discrepant results is the group with contralateral carotid occlusion, which showed benefit from immediate surgery in ACST but not in ACAS. These data suggest that specific subgroups might have greater benefits from CEA than others, which requires careful preoperative assessment and selection.

Other considerations include the ability to reduce perioperative risk. First, the surgical benefit is highly dependent on surgical risk, and any benefit is eliminated when surgical complication rates exceed 2.7–3.1%, as reported in the randomized trials. These rates, while attainable in most academic centers, have not been observed in community-based practice, where the overall risk of stroke or death following CEA for asymptomatic stenosis was estimated at 3.8%.[38] In making a recommendation for surgery, some have suggested that referring physicians and patients have access to audited surveys of operators' records and that furthermore, neurologists or trained examiners of the nervous system should be required to evaluate the preoperative risk and postoperative complications of all patients who have CEA.[30]

Whereas CEA would not be expected to alter overall mortality, other competing vascular causes of morbidity and mortality among patients with asymptomatic carotid stenosis need to be considered in the overall prognosis. In fact, when one considers all stroke or death as primary outcomes, the benefit of CEA is diminished.[31,36] Because the stroke risk reduction following CEA begins to accrue after 2 years among asymptomatic patients, long-term benefits of endarterectomy also may be considered. However, long-term natural history studies are lacking. A small study found that the 10-year and 15-year stroke risks of asymptomatic carotid stenosis >50% were lower than expected (approximately 1% per year), whereas risk of myocardial infarction or vascular death was considerably higher.[7] With annual risk of stroke with medical treatment remaining consistently low at 10 and 15 years, the authors concluded that benefit from CEA in such patients may not increase substantially with longer follow-up. However since only 35 patients in this study had ≥70% stenosis, further study with larger cohorts may be needed to better answer this question.

Endovascular

In the last decade, endovascular techniques have been developed to offer non-invasive alternatives to surgical CEA. Advocates of carotid angioplasty and stenting cite the less-invasive approach, reduced cranial nerve and wound complications, utility in high-risk patients unsuitable for general anesthesia and surgery, and ability to access lesions more cephalad along the carotid artery. In addition, it may be preferable in those with prior neck surgery or radiation due to the difficulty of CEA in these scenarios. However, unlike CEA, the long-term outcomes from carotid angioplasty and stenting have not been well studied.[39,40] Critics also emphasized that, initially, carotid angioplasty and stenting had high rates of procedure-related strokes.[41] However, these have been allayed substantially with the introduction of new devices and increased technical expertise. With the advent of distal protection devices that have further reduced the risks of embolic stroke during the procedure, more recent studies have suggested that the short-term stroke risk with carotid angioplasty and stenting may be lower than CEA, especially in high-risk individuals. In the Stenting and Angioplasty with Protection in Patients at High Risk for Endarterectomy (SAPPHIRE) study,[42] patients with asymptomatic carotid stenosis >80% constituted over 70% of trial patients. In this group, the 1-year cumulative incidence of death or ipsilateral stroke was lower among stented patients (9.9% vs 21.5% $p = 0.02$) compared with patients who underwent endarterectomy. However, no interaction was found between asymptomatic stenosis and receipt of a carotid artery stent ($p = 0.55$). Procedural complications were not different between groups (5.4% and 6%), although higher than the ACAS and ACST, which is partly explained by the high-risk population. Ongoing studies comparing carotid angioplasty and stenting with CEA in lower-risk individuals (similar to those enrolled in

ACAS and ACST) are necessary before any further conclusions can be made regarding the safety, efficacy, and long-term durability of carotid stenting and angioplasty in asymptomatic carotid stenosis.[39,43–45] While prospective, randomized clinical trials comparing CEA to carotid stenting in low-surgical risk symptomatic patients have recently been completed (Stent-protected percutaneous angioplasty of the carotid vs. Endartectormy trial (SPACE), periprocedured rate of death or stroke was 6.3% vs. 6.8% in patients treated with CEA and carotid stenting, respectively), prospective, randomized clinical trials in low-surgical risk asymptomatic patients are still under way or in the planning phase.

- the Asymptomatic Carotid Stenosis, Stenting versus Endarterectomy Trial (ACT 1)
- the Carotid Revascularization Endarterectomy versus Stenting Trial (CREST) for both asymptomatic and symptomatic patients
- the Transatlantic Asymptomatic Carotid Intervention Trial (TACIT)
- the ACST-2.

Practical considerations

The intermediate-risk patient with 60–79% asymptomatic carotid stenosis presents a management challenge (Figure 15.1). In this group, a search for high-risk features (i.e. heterogeneous plaque morphology, impaired vasoreactivity, emboli detection) is paramount. If no high-risk features are found, many clinicians do not consider revascularization for this intermediate group, offering maximal medical therapy and serial surveillance for progression of stenosis by ultrasonography.[11,14] By contrast, in patients with ≥80% stenosis, carotid revascularization in addition to maximal medical therapy is strongly recommended, but the above factors still deserve consideration.

The decision between endovascular and surgical revascularization is complex and involves assessing the patient's age, medical comorbidities, anatomic considerations of the carotid lesion, surgical and endovascular technical expertise, and patient preferences. In patients who are deemed high risk for CEA or have difficult anatomy that makes CEA more challenging, angioplasty and stenting may be the only plausible options. Given the clinical equipoise between surgery and endovascular approaches at the moment, we recommend enrollment in ongoing clinical trials comparing angioplasty and stenting versus CEA in low risk patients for patients with ≥80% stenosis who are low risk for CEA. If such a patient is not eligible or is unwilling to enroll in a study, CEA is a reasonable option.

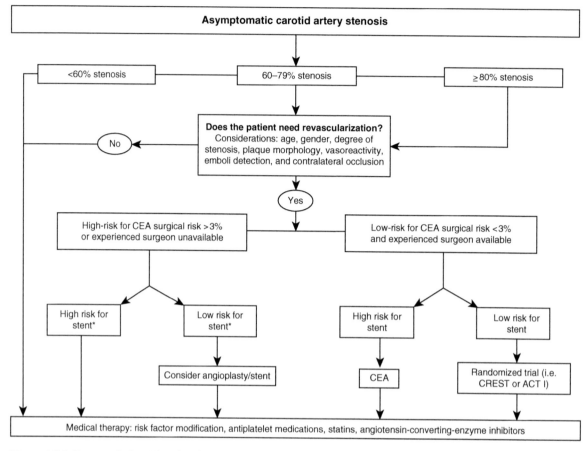

Figure 15.1 Proposed algorithm for the management of asymptomatic carotid stenosis (based on anatomic considerations). Abbreviations: CEA, carotid endarterectomy; CREST, Carotid Revascularization Endarterectomy versus Stenting Trial; ACT I, Asymptomatic Carotid Stenosis, Stenting versus Endarterectomy Trial.

The role of screening

Given the prevalence of occult carotid artery disease, the known ischemic stroke risk, and the potential benefits of medical and surgical intervention, the role of early detection via non-invasive screening has been raised.[46] Based on several population-based studies,[47–49] approximately 5–10% of patients >65 years old (as high as 50% in one study)[50] have asymptomatic carotid artery stenosis >50% and 1% have >80% stenosis. With an aging population and the widespread use of non-invasive screening for carotid stenosis, the detection of asymptomatic disease will only increase.

Previous studies suggested that, given the low overall prevalence of carotid artery stenosis >50%, screening the general population would not be cost-effective.[51,52] However, selective screening among patients with risk factors for carotid artery stenosis where the prevalence of the disease is >20% might be cost-effective.[53] Using a community health screening program, one study reported

that ultrasound screening for carotid stenosis >50% might be useful in the select group of patients with multiple stroke risk factors.[54] Other studies have also suggested that screening for asymptomatic stenosis may be more fruitful in high-risk groups such as individuals with peripheral or coronary arterial disease or hyperlipidemia, current smokers, and hypertensives.[55–57] However, there is still a great deal of uncertainty regarding whom to screen for asymptomatic carotid stenosis and whether it is cost-effective from a public health perspective. For now, it cannot be recommended in unselected patients.

Practical considerations

While screening for carotid stenosis is not feasible at a population level, prudent and cost-effective use of non-invasive imaging, such as ultrasonography or magnetic resonance imaging, in select individuals at high risk for vascular disease is reasonable. For example, in patients with significant coronary or peripheral artery disease awaiting coronary or peripheral arterial revascularization, screening is more likely to detect asymptomatic carotid artery stenosis and may alter subsequent management.[58] Currently, we favor the use of ultrasonographic screening in such high-risk patients.

FUTURE DIRECTIONS

The cascade of events leading to carotid plaque formation and rupture involves endothelial damage, lipid deposition, inflammation, and coagulation and platelet activation. In recent years, exciting research in this area has yielded some interesting results and introduced the concept of the 'unstable' carotid plaque, which through in-situ hemorrhage, thrombosis, and inflammation, may result in plaque rupture with secondary embolization and/or perfusion failure.[59] This complex pathobiology may yield keys to understanding stroke mechanisms and provide novel targets for medical therapies.

The links between inflammation, carotid atherosclerosis, and plaque rupture may be critical to elucidating these mechanisms. Histological and immunological investigations into the underlying pathophysiology of the unstable carotid plaque have observed that echolucent and irregular plaques are associated with plaque rupture.[60–62] Increased white blood cell count is highly predictive of carotid atherosclerosis in asymptomatic individuals.[63] Other clinicians have observed that inflammatory markers, such as C-reactive protein (CRP), metalloproteinases, and cytokines, are elevated in patients with complex or unstable carotid plaques.[64–66] In addition, a strong positive association was observed between CRP and intraplaque inflammatory cell infiltrate, implying that plaque instability and rupture may be mediated by an inflammatory cascade.[67] Hence, an inflammatory pathway may be important in the conversion from an asymptomatic to a symptomatic carotid plaque, and these and other novel markers may help clinicians identify patients at highest risk.

Besides biomarkers, emerging imaging technologies, including high-resolution magnetic resonance imaging (MRI) of carotid plaque and molecular imaging, may help in risk stratification by identification of vulnerable plaques.[68] In a recent prospective study using MRI, presence of thin or ruptured fibrous cap, intraplaque hemorrhage, lipid–necrotic core ratio, and maximum plaque wall thickness were predictors of ipsilateral cerebrovascular events.[69] Another study found that indium-labeled platelet scintigraphy may be useful in identifying plaque thrombosis.[70]

Another recent advance has been in the measurement of potential carotid plaque precursors. Carotid intima–media thickness (IMT), which has been associated with

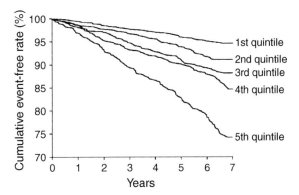

Figure 15.2 Unadjusted cumulative event-free rates for the combined endpoint of myocardial infarction or stroke, according to quintile of combined intima–media thickness. (adapted from O'Leary et al.[74]

systemic atherosclerosis, may be a subclinical predictor of stroke and myocardial infarction (Figure 15.2).[71–74] A recent study has also found that carotid IMT is a risk factor for stroke and cardiovascular events, independent of carotid plaque.[75] Thus, carotid IMT may be an intermediate and earlier stage in the causal pathway of plaque formation[76] and amenable to earlier initiation of treatments such as lipid-lowering therapies.[23–26,28,29]

SUMMARY

Atherosclerotic carotid stenosis elevates the risk of ischemic stroke among asymptomatic individuals. However, since the risk is dependent on many other factors, including demographics and medical comorbidities, intrinsic plaque characteristics, and cerebral vascular reserve, the optimal management of patients with asymptomatic carotid stenosis requires individualized care that integrates these considerations in calculating risks and benefits of treatments. A comprehensive evaluation in these patients and assessment of global vascular risk may allow clinicians to better select patients for medical, interventional, and combined strategies. The improving endovascular technology and the results of ongoing clinical trials will probably guide the choice between CEA and CAS in the future. The scientific advances in the development of subclinical biomarkers and imaging correlates of plaque instability may also be of great utility in identifying high-risk persons, allowing for more precise risk stratification, selecting persons for earlier treatments, encouraging the development of novel medications, and ultimately preventing the potentially devastating consequences of ischemic stroke.

REFERENCES

1. Goldstein LB, Adams R, Alberts MJ et al. Primary prevention of ischemic stroke. A guideline from the American Heart Association/American Stroke Association Stroke Council: cosponsored by the Atherosclerotic Peripheral Vascular Disease Interdisciplinary Working Group; Cardiovascular Nursing Council; Clinical Cardiology Council; Nutrition, Physical Activity, and Metabolism Council; and the Quality of Care and Outcomes Research Interdisciplinary Working Group. Stroke 2006; 113(24): e873–923.

2. Bock RW, Gray-Weale AC, Mock PA et al. The natural history of asymptomatic carotid artery disease. J Vasc Surg 1993; 17: 160–9, discussion 170–1.

3. Bogousslavsky J, Despland PA, Regli F. Prognosis of high-risk patients with nonoperated symptomatic extracranial carotid tight stenosis. Stroke 1988; 19: 108–11.

4. Satiani B, Porter RM Jr, Biggers KM, Das BM. Natural history of nonoperated, significant carotid stenosis. Ann Vasc Surg 1988; 2: 271–8.

5. Bogousslavsky J, Despland PA, Regli F. Asymptomatic tight stenosis of the internal carotid artery: long-term prognosis. Neurology 1986; 36: 861–3.

6. Norris JW, Zhu CZ, Bornstein NM, Chambers BR. Vascular risks of asymptomatic carotid stenosis. Stroke 1991; 22: 1485–90.

7. Nadareishvili ZG, Rothwell PM, Beletsky V, Pagniello A, Norris JW. Long-term risk of stroke and other vascular events in patients with asymptomatic carotid artery stenosis. Arch Neurol 2002; 59: 1162–6.

8. Meissner I, Wiebers DO, Whisnant JP, O'Fallon WM. The natural history of asymptomatic carotid artery occlusive lesions. JAMA 1987; 258: 2704–7.

9. Mackey AE, Abrahamowicz M, Langlois Y et al. Outcome of asymptomatic patients with carotid disease. Asymptomatic Cervical Bruit Study Group. Neurology 1997; 48: 896–903.

10. Hennerici M, Hulsbomer HB, Hefter H, Lammerts D, Rautenberg W. Natural history of asymptomatic extracranial arterial disease. Results of a long-term prospective study. Brain 1987; 110 (Pt 3): 777–91.

11. Chambers BR, Norris JW. Outcome in patients with asymptomatic neck bruits. N Engl J Med 1986; 315: 860–5.

12. Autret A, Pourcelot L, Saudeau D et al. Stroke risk in patients with carotid stenosis. Lancet 1987; 1: 888–90.

13. Inzitari D, Eliasziw M, Gates P et al. The causes and risk of stroke in patients with asymptomatic internal-carotid-artery stenosis. North American Symptomatic Carotid Endarterectomy Trial Collaborators. N Engl J Med 2000; 342: 1693–700.

14. Muluk SC, Muluk VS, Sugimoto H et al. Progression of asymptomatic carotid stenosis: a natural history study in 1004 patients. J Vasc Surg 1999; 29: 208–14, discussion 214–6.

15. Powers WJ. Cerebral hemodynamics in ischemic cerebrovascular disease. Ann Neurol 1991; 29: 231–40.

16. Polak JF, Shemanski L, O'Leary DH et al. Hypoechoic plaque at US of the carotid artery: an independent risk factor for incident stroke in adults aged 65 years or older. Cardiovascular Health Study. Radiology 1998; 208: 649–54.

17. Johnson JM, Ansel AL, Morgan S, DeCesare D. Ultrasonographic screening for evaluation and follow-up of carotid artery ulceration. A new basis for assessing risk. Am J Surg 1982; 144: 614–18.

18. Molloy J, Markus HS. Asymptomatic embolization predicts stroke and TIA risk in patients with carotid artery stenosis. Stroke 1999; 30: 1440–3.

19. Silvestrini M, Vernieri F, Pasqualetti P et al. Impaired cerebral vasoreactivity and risk of stroke in patients with asymptomatic carotid artery stenosis. JAMA 2000; 283: 2122–7.

20. Nicolaides AN, Kakkos SK, Griffin M et al. Severity of asymptomatic carotid stenosis and risk of ipsilateral hemispheric ischaemic events: results from the ACSRS study. Eur J Vasc Endovasc Surg 2005; 30: 275–84.

21. Nicolaides AN, Kakkos SK, Griffin M et al. Effect of image normalization on carotid plaque classification and the risk of ipsilateral hemispheric ischemic events: results from the Asymptomatic Carotid Stenosis and Risk of Stroke Study. Vascular 2005; 13: 211–21.

22. Corti R, Fuster V, Fayad ZA, Worthley SG et al. Effects of aggressive versus conventional lipid-lowering therapy on simvastatin on human atherosclerotic lesions: a prospective, randomized, double-blind trial with high-resolution magnetic resonance imaging. J Am Coll Cardiol 2005; 46: 106–12.

23. Corti R, Fuster V, Fayad ZA et al. Lipid lowering by simvastatin induces regression of human atherosclerotic lesions: two years' follow-up by high-resolution noninvasive magnetic resonance imaging. Circulation 2002; 106: 2884–7.

24. Crouse JR 3rd, Byington RP, Bond MG et al. Pravastatin, Lipids, and Atherosclerosis in the Carotid Arteries (PLAC-II). Am J Cardiol 1995; 75: 455–9.

25. Furberg CD, Adams HP Jr, Applegate WB et al. Effect of lovastatin on early carotid atherosclerosis and cardiovascular events. Asymptomatic Carotid Artery Progression Study (ACAPS) research group. Circulation 1994; 90: 1679–87.

26. Hodis HN, Mack WJ, LaBree L et al. Reduction in carotid arterial wall thickness using lovastatin and dietary therapy: a randomized controlled clinical trial. Ann Intern Med 1996; 124: 548–56.

27. Lima JA, Desai MY, Steen H et al. Statin-induced cholesterol lowering and plaque regression after 6 months of magnetic resonance imaging-monitored therapy. Circulation 2004; 110: 2336–41.

28. Salonen R, Nyyssonen K, Porkkala E et al. Kuopio Atherosclerosis Prevention Study (KAPS). A population-based primary preventive trial of the effect of LDL lowering on atherosclerotic progression in carotid and femoral arteries. Circulation 1995; 92: 1758–64.

29. Taylor AJ, Sullenberger LE, Lee HJ, Lee JK, Grace KA. Arterial Biology for the Investigation of the Treatment Effects of Reducing Cholesterol (ARBITER) 2: a double-blind, placebo-controlled study of extended-release niacin on atherosclerosis progression in secondary prevention patients treated with statins. Circulation 2004; 110: 3512–17.

30. Barnett HJ. Carotid endarterectomy. Lancet 2004; 363: 1486–7.

31. Halliday A, Mansfield A, Marro J et al. Prevention of disabling and fatal strokes by successful carotid endarterectomy in patients without recent neurological symptoms: randomised controlled trial. Lancet 2004; 363: 1491–502.

32. Yusuf S. Two decades of progress in preventing vascular disease. Lancet 2002; 360: 2–3.

33. Carotid surgery versus medical therapy in asymptomatic carotid stenosis. The CASANOVA Study Group. Stroke 1991; 22: 1229–35.

34. Results of a randomized controlled trial of carotid endarterectomy for asymptomatic carotid stenosis. Mayo Asymptomatic Carotid Endarterectomy Study Group. Mayo Clin Proc 1992; 67: 513–18.

35. Hobson RW 2nd, Weiss DG, Fields WS et al. Efficacy of carotid endarterectomy for asymptomatic carotid stenosis. The Veterans Affairs Cooperative Study Group. N Engl J Med 1993; 328: 221–7.

36. Endarterectomy for asymptomatic carotid artery stenosis. Executive Committee for the Asymptomatic Carotid Atherosclerosis Study. JAMA 1995; 273: 1421–8.

37. Lovett JK, Gallagher PJ, Hands LJ, Walton J, Rothwell PM. Histological correlates of carotid plaque surface morphology on lumen contrast imaging. Circulation 2004; 110: 2190–7.

38. Bunch CT, Kresowik TF. Can randomized trial outcomes for carotid endarterectomy be achieved in community-wide practice? Semin Vasc Surg 2004; 17: 209–13.

39. Bettmann MA, Katzen BT, Whisnant J et al. Carotid stenting and angioplasty: A statement for healthcare professionals from the Councils on Cardiovascular Radiology, Stroke, Cardio-Thoracic and Vascular Surgery, Epidemiology and Prevention, and Clinical Cardiology, American Heart Association. Stroke 1998; 29: 336–8.

40. Brott TG, Brown RD Jr, Meyer FB et al. Carotid revascularization for prevention of stroke: carotid endarterectomy and carotid artery stenting. Mayo Clin Proc 2004; 79: 1197–208.

41. Grotta J. Elective stenting of extracranial carotid arteries. Circulation 1997; 95: 303–5.

42. Yadav JS, Wholey MH, Kuntz RE et al. Protected carotid-artery stenting versus endarterectomy in high-risk patients. N Engl J Med 2004; 351: 1493–501.

43. Roubin GS, Hobson RW 2nd, White R et al. CREST and CARESS to evaluate carotid stenting: time to get to work! J Endovasc Ther 2001; 8: 107–10.

44. Hobson RW 2nd. CREST (Carotid Revascularization Endarterectomy versus Stent Trial): background, design, and current status. Semin Vasc Surg 2000; 13: 139–43.

45. Gray WA. Endovascular treatment of extra-cranial carotid artery bifurcation disease. Minerva Cardioangiol 2005; 53: 69–77.

46. Brott T, Toole JF. Medical compared with surgical treatment of asymptomatic carotid artery stenosis. Ann Intern Med 1995; 123: 720–22.

47. O'Leary DH, Polak JF, Kronmal RA et al. Distribution and correlates of sonographically detected carotid artery disease in the Cardiovascular Health Study. The CHS Collaborative Research Group. Stroke 1992; 23: 1752–60.

48. Hillen T, Nieczaj R, Munzberg H et al. Carotid atherosclerosis, vascular risk profile and mortality in a population-based sample of functionally healthy elderly subjects: the Berlin Ageing Study. J Intern Med 2000; 247: 679–88.

49. Fine-Edelstein JS, Wolf PA, O'Leary DH et al. Precursors of extracranial carotid atherosclerosis in the Framingham Study. Neurology 1994; 44: 1046–50.

50. Pujia A, Rubba P, Spencer MP. Prevalence of extracranial carotid artery disease detectable by echo-Doppler in an elderly population. Stroke 1992; 23: 818–22.

51. Obuchowski NA, Modic MT, Magdinec M, Masaryk TJ. Assessment of the efficacy of noninvasive screening for patients with asymptomatic neck bruits. Stroke 1997; 28: 1330–9.

52. Feussner JR, Matchar DB. When and how to study the carotid arteries. Ann Intern Med 1988; 109: 805–18.

53. Derdeyn CP, Powers WJ. Cost-effectiveness of screening for asymptomatic carotid atherosclerotic disease. Stroke 1996; 27: 1944–50.

54. Qureshi AI, Janardhan V, Bennett SE et al. Who should be screened for asymptomatic carotid artery stenosis? Experience from the Western New York Stroke Screening Program. J Neuroimaging 2001; 11: 105–11.

55. Rockman CB, Jacobowitz GR, Gagne PJ et al. Focused screening for occult carotid artery disease: patients with known heart disease are at high risk. J Vasc Surg 2004; 39: 44–51.

56. Kurvers HA, van der Graaf Y, Blankensteijn JD, Visseren FL, Eikelboom BC. Screening for asymptomatic internal carotid artery stenosis and aneurysm of the abdominal aorta: comparing the yield between patients with manifest atherosclerosis and patients with risk factors for atherosclerosis only. J Vasc Surg 2003; 37: 1226–33.

57. Jacobowitz GR, Rockman CB, Gagne PJ et al. A model for predicting occult carotid artery stenosis: screening is justified in a selected population. J Vasc Surg 2003; 38: 705–9.

58. Durand DJ, Perler BA, Roseborough GS et al. Mandatory versus selective preoperative carotid screening: a retrospective analysis. Ann Thorac Surg 2004; 78: 159–66, discussion 159–66.

59. Fuster V, Moreno PR, Fayad ZA, Corti R, Badimon JJ. Atherothrombosis and high-risk plaque: part I: evolving concepts. J Am Coll Cardiol 2005; 46: 937–54.

60. Croft RJ, Ellam LD, Harrison MJ. Accuracy of carotid angiography in the assessment of atheroma of the internal carotid artery. Lancet 1980; 1: 997–1000.

61. Endo S, Hirashima Y, Kurimoto M et al. Acute pathologic features with angiographic correlates of the nearly or completely occluded lesions of the cervical internal carotid artery. Surg Neurol 1996; 46: 222–8.

62. Estol C, Claasen D, Hirsch W, Wechsler L, Moossy J. Correlative angiographic and pathologic findings in the diagnosis of ulcerated plaques in the carotid artery. Arch Neurol 1991; 48: 692–4.

63. Elkind MS, Cheng J, Boden-Albala B, Paik MC, Sacco RL. Elevated white blood cell count and carotid plaque thickness: the Northern Manhattan Stroke Study. Stroke. 2001; 32: 842–9.

64. Lombardo A, Biasucci LM, Lanza GA et al. Inflammation as a possible link between coronary and carotid plaque instability. Circulation 2004; 109: 3158–63.

65. Sapienza P, di Marzo L, Borrelli V et al. Metalloproteinases and their inhibitors are markers of plaque instability. Surgery 2005; 137: 355–63.

66. Businaro R, Digregorio M, Rigano R et al. Morphological analysis of cell subpopulations within carotid atherosclerotic plaques. Ital J Anat Embryol 2005; 110: 9–15.

67. Alvarez Garcia B, Ruiz C, Chacon P, Sabin JA, Matas M. High-sensitivity C-reactive protein in high-grade carotid stenosis: risk marker for unstable carotid plaque. J Vasc Surg 2003; 38: 1018–24.

68. Nighoghossian N, Derex L, Douek P. The vulnerable carotid artery plaque: current imaging methods and new perspectives. Stroke 2005; 36: 2764–72.

69. Takaya N, Yuan C, Chu B et al. Association between carotid plaque characteristics and subsequent ischemic cerebrovascular events: a prospective assessment with MRI – initial results. Stroke 2006; 37: 818–23.

70. Manca G, Parenti G, Bellina R et al. [111]In platelet scintigraphy for the noninvasive detection of carotid plaque thrombosis. Stroke 2001; 32: 719–27.

71. Bots ML, Hoes AW, Koudstaal PJ, Hofman A, Grobbee DE. Common carotid intima-media thickness and risk of stroke and myocardial infarction: the Rotterdam Study. Circulation 1997; 96: 1432–7.

72. Chambless LE, Folsom AR, Clegg LX et al. Carotid wall thickness is predictive of incident clinical stroke: the Atherosclerosis Risk In Communities (ARIC) study. Am J Epidemiol 2000; 151: 478–87.

73. Ebrahim S, Papacosta O, Whincup P et al. Carotid plaque, intima media thickness, cardiovascular risk factors, and prevalent cardiovascular disease in men and women: the British Regional Heart Study. Stroke 1999; 30: 841–50.

74. O'Leary DH, Polak JF, Kronmal RA et al. Carotid-artery intima and media thickness as a risk factor for myocardial infarction and stroke in older adults. Cardiovascular Health Study Collaborative Research Group. N Engl J Med 1999; 340: 14–22.

75. Rosvall M, Janzon L, Berglund G, Engstrom G, Hedblad B. Incidence of stroke is related to carotid IMT even in the absence of plaque. Atherosclerosis 2005; 179: 325–31.

76. Zureik M, Ducimetiere P, Touboul PJ et al. Common carotid intima-media thickness predicts occurrence of carotid atherosclerotic plaques: longitudinal results from the Aging Vascular Study (EVA) study. Arterioscler Thromb Vasc Biol 2000; 20: 1622–9.

Index

T - #0971 - 101024 - C244 - 246/189/11 [13] - CB - 9781841846132 - Gloss Lamination